GW00568974

The
Information
Sourcebook of
HERBAL
MEDICINE

The Information Sourcebook of

HERBAL MEDICINE

A Detailed Bibliography of
Herbalism and Herbal Pharmacology

A Glossary of Herbal, Medical,
Pharmacological and Pharmacy Terms

A Unique Guide to Computer Databases
for the Herbalist

Medline Citations for Commonly Used
Medicinal Herbs

Edited by David Hoffmann, M.N.I.M.H.

✳ The Crossing Press, Freedom, CA 95019

Copyright © 1994 by David Hoffmann
Cover design by Sheryl Karas
Printed in the U.S.A.

Library of Congress Cataloging-in-Publication Data

The information sourcebook of herbal medicine / edited by David
   Hoffmann.
       p. cm.
   Includes bibliographical references.
   ISBN 0-89594-671-8. —ISBN 0-89594-670-X (pbk.)
    1. Herbs—Therapeutic use.   2. Herbs—Therapeutic use—
Bibliography. 3. Herbs—Therapeutic use—Information services.
I. Hoffmann, David. 1951-
RM666.H33I54 1994
615' .321—dc20   93-44206
                                                CIP

Contents

Foreword

Foreword

It is important to recognize what this book is and what it isn't. It makes no attempt to cover all aspects of the enormous and diverse field of human endeavor called herbalism. The focus is upon the information relevant to the practice of western herbal medicine, known as Phytotherapy in Europe. Because of lack of space there is no coverage of the vast range of information covering the cultivation of herbs, botanical field guides or non-therapeutic uses. There is also no detailed listing of sources in non-western phytotherapy such as Ayurveda, Traditional Chinese Medicine or Unani. It is to be hoped that a similar work will be forthcoming that addresses this need. The book is structured in such a way that it can either be read in sequence as a guide to information sources and retrieval for anyone interested in herbal medicine, or it can be dipped into as needed for specific references.

Chapter 1 is an overview of the world of herbalism, exploring its diversity and the role it plays in the modern world. The rapidly unfolding sociopolitical context that modern herbalists find themselves in is why they need to be cognizant of the range of sources described in the book.

Chapter 2 explores the way access to information is handled in orthodox medicine, but more importantly how access to information is changing the nature of health care. From this context it is clear that medical herbalism is not on the fringe but is a component of the drive to humanize medicine and empower both doctor and patient through the perspectives of holistic healing.

Chapter 3 is a road map of the sources of phytotherapeutic information. Details of the types of relevant information are given covering the resources of libraries, both general and specialized, the Dewey Decimal System, The Library of Congress Classification System, newspaper and periodical indexes. The information available through public relations departments of the herb industry and sources of information from federal agencies are then explained, followed by a description of the services of antiquarian book dealers and how to find out-of-print books. Commercial computer software with herbal information is also listed. A comprehensive bibliography of books relating to western phytotherapy then follows. In addition to books on western herbalism, sections cover ethnobotany, pharmacognosy, pharmacology, toxicology, pharmacopoeias and pharmacy. A listing of peer review journals that cover phytotherapy is given as well as published abstracts, bibliographies and indexes. The growing body of professional phytotherapy journals, newsletters and organizations from around the English-speaking world are also described.

Chapter 4, The On-line Herbalist, is an exploration of the potential offered the herbalist by the computer databases now accessible over telephone lines. Information on the medicinal properties of plants used in traditional medicine is very complex, and the literature is scattered and diverse. It covers data on the plants concerned, the chemical constituents or compounds they contain, pharmacological and ethnobotanical or ethnopharmacological information. There is a description of the available services, both the electronic bulletin boards and commercial on-line services. There follows a detailed description of how to conduct an on-line search of Medline and a unique guide to Medical Subject Headings (MeSH terms) that relate to herbal medicine. An example is used concerning herbs and aspects of immunity.

Chapter 5 is a cornucopia of information that the herbalist might find useful. The derivation of the Latin names of herbs is explained with selected examples of the binomial meanings. Charts listing herbs by their Latin binomial and then their common English names are given for easy cross-reference. Commonly used herbal and medical prefixes and suffixes are defined, followed by a glossary of medical, botanical, herbal and pharmaceutical terms. The last section of the book is lists of citations from the Medline database of published papers on the therapeutic use of a number of important herbs. These are selections from the vast amount available, focusing on clinical relevance.

Chapter 1

Information and the Herbalist

W hy a book on information for herbalists? There was a time not very long ago when all that was needed was a copy of Kloss's *Back to Eden*, Lust's *Herb Book* or Mrs. Grieve's *A Modern Herbal*. How times have changed! Most herbalists today keep extensive book collections, and it would need a well-endowed library to keep up to date with the plethora of potential new additions each year. The discovery of herbalism by the publishing industry is a microcosm of a phenomenon that Dr. Paul Lee has called the Herbal Renaissance. This wonderful description points to the rediscovery of green medicine as part of the rediscovery of the green world by millions of people worldwide as they face the consequences of industrial civilization. The revival of the practice of herbal medicine is a worldwide phenomenon. This renaissance is multifactorial in origin, but representative issues include:

- an experience that the therapy has medical value and complements (rather than replaces) the strengths of "allopathic" medicine.

- growing concerns amongst the general public about drug side effects.

- reaction to the common experience of modern health-care practices as impersonal and demeaning.

Thus a complex of socioeconomic factors is in play in addition to the purely medical. Medical Herbalism, or Phytotherapy as it is known in Europe, is a medical modality that uses therapeutically active plants to treat illness. It is by far the most ancient form of medicine known to humanity, used in all cultures and in all historical periods. Using plants as the basis for Materia Medica does not define how they are used therapeutically, or in what philosophical context the practitioner practices. Thus herbs are a component of Chinese medicine and Ayurvedic medicine and the basis of pharmacology. It has a breadth of use as wide as any form of medicine, as medicinal plants may be used in any condition that is medically treatable. This is not to claim that Herbalism is a panacea for the ills of humanity, but an affirmation that the natural world provides tools for the healing work. An important component of the "herb renaissance" is the way it fits perfectly into the context of holistic medicine, an unfolding perspective on health that is a change both in attitude and approach. What is health when seen in the context of holistic medicine? The World Health Organization has the clearest definition:

> Health is more than simply the absence of illness. It is the active state of physical, emotional, mental and social well-being.

This approach to medicine starts from the assumption that health is a positive and active state, that it is an inherent characteristic of whole and integrated human beings. Some characteristics of holistic medicine are:[1]

- From a holistic standpoint, a person is not a patient with a disease syndrome but a whole being. This wholeness necessitates therapists appreciating the mental, emotional, spiritual, social and environmental aspects of their patients' lives, as well as the physical.

- A holistic practitioner, of whatever specific therapy, has a deep respect for the individual's inherent capacity for self-healing. This enables a relationship of active partnership in the healing process, rather than expert and passive recipient.

- Relating to the whole person is not new. From Hippocrates onwards there has been the caring support of the patient that every doctor, every herbalist, every nurse, is guided towards by their teachers. Naming and emphasizing holistic medicine is an attempt to correct the tendency in modern medicine to equate health care with only the treatment of a "disease entity."

- Holism does not predefine any medical technique or theory. It is a context in which individuals are considered, their physical health as well as mental and emotional state, relationships and life in the world. A medical doctor can be holistic, as can a medical herbalist. A framework becomes apparent that can embrace a range of therapeutic modalities, whether labeled "orthodox" or "alternative."

- Holistic medicine emphasizes the uniqueness of individuals, and the importance of tailoring treatment to meet their broad needs is fundamental.

- The need to understand and treat people in the context of their family, their community and their culture is recognized.

- Holistic medicine emphasizes the promotion of health and the prevention of disease. Therapeutic modalities are employed that mobilize people's innate capacity for healing.

- The role of individuals in their own healing process is emphasized, with much responsibility being handed back to them. While not denying the occasional necessity for swift and authoritative medical or surgical intervention, the emphasis is on helping people understand and help themselves, focusing on education and self-care rather than just treatment and the resulting dependency.

- A unique and important characteristic of any holistic approach is viewing illness as an opportunity for self-discovery, not simply a misfortune. This leads to many important implications for the caring professions, perhaps best exemplified by the hospice movement.

- There is an appreciation of the quality of life in each of its stages and a commitment to improving it, as well as the knowledge of the illnesses that are common to it.

- The therapeutic importance of the setting within which health care takes place is fundamental to holistic practice. Part of the problem with medical care is the alienation and dehumanizing that tends to accompany institutions and laboratories. When the healing process is separated too far from the humanity of the people involved, there is nothing other than chemistry and surgery. The hearts of doctor and patient must meet as well as their skill and symptoms.

- There is a recognition of the social and economic conditions that perpetuate ill health. A commitment to change these factors is a part of holistic medicine. Herbal medicine fits well into this emerging holistic paradigm. It is a therapy that might be seen as ecological healing because of its basis in the shared ecological and evolutionary heritage humanity has with the plant world.

Complementary, Alternative or Orthodox

It is a mistake to talk of Medical Herbalism as a form of alternative medicine. Is it an alternative to Acupuncture, Osteopathy or Psychiatry? Of course not, they complement each other, creating a complex of relationships where the whole is much more than the sum of the parts. All medical modalities are complementary within the perspective of the patient's needs.

There are many therapeutic modalities available other than the form of medicine that has become dominant today. For want of a better term I shall call this "orthodox medicine." It may seem like an overabundance of therapies, but they should be viewed in the same way as the various specialties within orthodox medicine. The emphasis is upon complementary support. These therapies embrace a wide range of techniques, philosophies and terminologies. Some are profoundly holistic medical systems such as TCM, Unani and Ayurveda, while others are focused on specific techniques or conditions, but they all share the dubious honor of being beyond the pale of the orthodox medical establishment. Everyone involved in health care provision will benefit in such a mutually supportive environment, as such cooperative endeavors bear many kinds of fruit. Health service administrators will appreciate the economic savings gleaned from a lessening of dependence upon costly medical technology. A proportion of procedures and treatments that currently utilize expensive drugs or surgery could be undertaken by more appropriate techniques from another healing modality. For example, most run-of-the mill gallbladder removals could be avoided by using Phytotherapy, and some expensive orthopedic techniques could be replaced with skilled osteopathy.

The International Context

Herbalism is a common bond between the peoples and cultures of the world. This shared experience of alleviating suffering through plant medicines bridges cultural divides, religious differences and racial conflicts. The unique knowledge of the herbalist is an invaluable resource that cannot be regained once lost. However, the efforts of ethnopharmacologists to find healing plants so that patentable drugs may be developed misses the central insight of humanity's use of herbs. There is a relationship between a culture and its plant environment, within which the herbalist plays a pivotal role. Herbalism is more than knowledge about healing plants, it is the experience and wisdom that comes from the relationship between humanity and plants. The World Health Organization (WHO) appreciates this and is promoting what it calls traditional medicine. The 30th World Health Assembly, in 1977, adopted a resolution urging interested governments to give:

> "Adequate importance to the utilization of their traditional systems of medicine, with appropriate regulations as suited for their national health systems."[2]

They recognize that all traditions have value, and that any world view as seen from the belief system of any one particular tradition is limited. Thus from the cloisters of a western medical school, the view of reality is as limited and limiting as that from a shaman's hut in West Africa. All perspectives have value in any worldwide approach to health for all. One aspect of this program is the attempt to integrate traditional methods of healing with "western" medicine. They propose some prerequisites for integration, including:

- Provision of valid factual data to overcome the current lack of information. This may then be used to help convince decision-makers, professional health personnel and the population at large of the value of integration.

- Legal recognition of the therapies and therapists to ensure sociopolitical acceptability and access to resources.

- The early establishment of dialogue amongst practitioners of differing systems. This should eliminate prejudice and hopefully develop more acceptable attitudes.

A well-integrated holistic health service would offer the benefits of all approaches to health care, not simply one system or another. There are important possibilities of mutual support between different therapeutic modalities. This may take the form of compensating for any weaknesses inherent within a particular therapy: for example, homeopathic remedies will not put a fractured arm into a splint. From a more positive perspective, cooperation can lead to synergistic support, with the whole of any treatment program being more than the sum of its parts. A geodesic relationship develops where extraordinary potential and strength can flow from cooperation between the therapies. Differences can lead to a celebration of the richness of therapeutic diversity and no longer be a cause for acrimonious debate and conflict.

Practitioners and academics often have firmly held opinions concerning one approach or another, but patients are always more important than their doctors' belief system. Practitioners must identify the limits of both their therapy and themselves. This, however, raises questions about educational standards that cannot be meaningfully explored here. Suffice it to say that an M.D. who attends a short training in acupuncture is no more an Acupuncturist than a D.C. who does a workshop on herbs becomes a Medical Herbalist.

There is a great need for herbalists to be well informed and aware of the diversity of their field of interest. I am grouping a range of activities under the term "Herbalist," but of course the members of these various groups may not agree! There are different forms of Phytotherapy, embracing both the Folk healers and those using a developed medical system, approaches based within the western biomedical model, as well as Oriental approaches, such as

Traditional Chinese Medicine and Ayurveda. Pharmacognosists, phyto-pharmacologists and ethnobotanists also fit the description, as are those involved in the various aspects of the herb industry. There are the many people involved in growing and collecting medicinal plants as well as those in the manufacturing and retail components of the herb industry. Most importantly there is the general public who use and consume herbs.

Herbalism is an inclusive field of human endeavor, embracing all of humanity's relationship with the plant kingdom. It comprises such a diverse range of topics herbalists need to clarify which areas draw them. Some are drawn to working with the plants directly as growers, wild-crafters or medicine makers; while others are drawn to working with people, using the herbs therapeutically. Of course some people can embrace the whole field, but when it comes to searching the published literature such differentiations can be very helpful.

Herbal information appropriate to the various interests exists, but is often unknown to those in different groups. There is thus the need to expand the existing sources of information and build access bridges between these enclaves of interest. For example, for health care professionals who want to add phytotherapy as an adjunct to their existing skills; for people working within the herb industry, both manufacturing and retail; for the general public; and the most challenging is the regulatory and academic "establishment" which has needs it isn't even aware of yet! This raises complex issues about mutual comprehension. Language often blocks communication and shared endeavor in medicine. Apparent vocabulary and jargon disparities may mask fundamental agreements of ideas and approach. On the other hand, lack of clarity obscures important differences in both guiding principles and technique. There is an all too common dogmatic attachment to words and specific formulations of belief, opinion and theory. Open-mindedness and tolerance should be characteristics common to all involved in health care, whether as practitioners, researchers, or patients. Medical modalities that have their foundations outside the biomedical model should not be ignored or discounted simply because they exemplify a different belief system. They should be respected as an enrichment of possibilities and not a challenge to the status quo.

Recent events have profoundly affected Herbalism in the U.S., with the furor surrounding proposed changes in F.D.A. regulations having an unexpected "side effect"—the focusing of attention on Herbalism. This has revealed an identity crisis in the diverse arena that is embraced by the term Herbalism. This is crisis in its Chinese sense, where the word "wei-ji" is constructed from the two characters for "danger" and "opportunity."

All sides in the unfortunately polarized debate triggered by the F.D.A. would benefit from recognizing that the driving forces for each are not the arcana of labeling law, but that the labeling issues are a focus for well-meant concerns resulting from very different world views. There is a profound philosophical debate in play, with the dominant belief system insisting that it alone is a repository of truth. This intellectual construct and world view has the force of law behind it. Practicing medicine without a license is illegal, but if the decision about what constitutes a license is in the hands of intellectual vested interests then the law can become a tool of oppression and not protection. This all comes into focus on relatively minor issues, such as the labeling regulations, as the substantive issues are not being addressed or not even recognized.

The F.D.A. is acting under guidelines intended to protect the public, and people in the natural health field need to acknowledge this. This problem is with the mechanics, not the intention. The herb industry has a major responsibility in this. It is a commercial venture, simply supplying the needs of the herbal movement in general. Just as the pharmaceutical industry is not medicine and a pharmacist is not an M.D., so the herbal product manufacturers are not practitioners or necessarily skilled or knowledgeable in herbal medicine.

There is an unfortunate tendency for people drawn to herbalism to get their information from the advertising literature produced by the herb industry. Such information is generally reliable but selective, and the public is not well enough informed to know the wider picture. A fundamental prerequisite for good communication in this debate is information and an understanding of the perspectives and issues of the various positions. This cannot happen without finding the information in the first place. This book is a contribution to that process.

Where Are the Forgotten Herbs?

Many eclectic remedies are ignored by people who know of them—and others never find out! American medicinal plants are used extensively in Europe, reflecting the respect given internationally to the U.S. herbal tradition. They include a number of herbs that have been slipped into the category of heirloom plants in this country. Of the 232 monographs in the British Herbal Pharmacopoeia, 73 are plants indigenous to North America. These are not the European plants that have become naturalized and used throughout North America, but species such as Balmony (*Chelone glabra*) and Fringe-Tree Bark (*Chionanthus virginicus*). It is exported to Britain in what must be reasonably large quantities. However, there are no reliable statistics on the export of medicinal herbs other than the few monitored by the U.S.D.A. in its annual review of the spice and essential oil trade.[3,4]

In much of the debate over the Rio Bio-diversity treaty, as well as general issues around deforestation, medicine has become an important player. The loss of potentially important medical plants has been posited as a reason for stopping the destruction. Just consider the furor around the taxol and the yew in the Pacific Northwest. It is ironic then that with such issues being acknowledged as valid concerns, there is still little attention given to North American herbal medicine. The case of the purple coneflower, *Echinacea spp.*, is illuminating. A plant with a long history of use in North America, it was becoming forgotten and ignored in the 50s and 60s. However, its value in medicine was recognized in Europe since its introduction at the end of the last century. Extensive German pharmacological and clinical studies clearly demonstrate its value to medicine.[5,6] It is now the top-selling medicinal plant in the U.S. following its reintroduction to the marketplace in the 70s. Marketing strategies utilizing the German research have proved a great success.

The point is that it took Europeans to recognize the value of this American plant. A common plant in the Midwest, it had been ignored by the U.S. pharmaceutical industry. As environmentalists demand protection for endangered rain forests, using concerns about lost medicinals as one rationale, why are the medicinals of North America ignored? This cultural amnesia concerning the cornucopia of medicinal plants can only be sublimated into awareness and use through information, hence this book.

Herbalism and the Economics of the Health Care Crisis

The majority of pharmaceutical products are manufactured from raw materials generated by the petrochemical industry. It has proved impossible to get reliable statistics about how much oil is used by the multinational drug companies. The reference library of the Pharmaceutical Manufacturers Association was unable to supply such figures from their databases. However, it is self-evident that the modern pharmaceutical industry is founded upon a non-renewable resource. Such petrochemical dependence raises immediate concerns when depletion of oil reserves is considered. One study, which the author described as optimistic, estimates exhaustion of planet-wide petroleum reserves by 2060 at current rates of consumption.[7] Domestic petroleum reserves will be exhausted by 2020 if consumption rates remain the same and imports of oil carry on at 80% of needs.[8]

Before stocks are exhausted it can be assumed that market forces and governmental action will act in such a way that some form of rationing will be imposed. This will initially take the form of sharply rising prices: just consider the economic package proposed by Perot in the 1992 election campaign. Without developing the economics of this in detail, it is evident that this will lead to *de facto* economic rationing of pharmaceuticals. The poor and elderly are already experiencing this. Given time, the "middle class" will also be unable to afford petrochemical-based medications.

Judicious utilization of herbal medicine will help ameliorate the trauma caused by the health care crisis. Medicinal plants will not replace the materia medica of modern medicine, but will augment it in those areas where herbal medicine has its strengths. From my years in clinical practice I feel the main therapeutic strengths of phytotherapy are in treating chronic illness, in approaches to preventive medicine and in replacing or reducing the demand for some over-the-counter drugs such as the non-steroidal anti-inflammatories. With the woeful dearth of clinical studies it becomes a judgment call at this stage to say what the strengths are. On one hand the medical establishment would cite the lack of studies as evidence that there are no strengths. A short-sighted attitude that is the epitome of bad science! On the other hand there is the overreaction of people rejecting modern medicine who would claim that "natural means" can cure anything. A shortsighted and potentially dangerous attitude. Thus consumer demand for products made from the increasingly scarce petroleum can be reduced. This will benefit the consumer by reducing costs and has the deeper benefit of reducing the ecological impact of the petrochemical industry. Of course this may also affect the profits of the pharmaceutical industry. Conspiracy theorists may see this as a factor in the intensity of the F.D.A.'s response to herbal products.

For this process of disengagement from the embrace of the pharmaceutical industry to occur there must be readily available information to enable the consumer to make knowledgeable decisions. Yet another reason for this book.

Self-Medication

Demonstrating that herbs are safe and trustworthy medicines is not a straightforward matter. Firstly what form of "proof" is needed? For some there need only be the subjective experience of personal benefit gained from herbal medicine, or it may be a similarly subjective observation of another's experience. For the medical establishment and those who perceive the world from that perspective, such experiences are invalid. There must be objective, quantifiable and reproducible data. Evidence becomes a dispassionate mathematical process rather than a messy human one. Striving for "objectivity" has obscured the reality of people, with all our diversity and idiosyncrasies. So problems arise for the herbalist in a world where the arbiters of medical veracity consider the Cartesian paradigm to be the truth, the whole truth and nothing but the truth.

There are many valid forms of knowledge in addition to those that flow from the "scientific method," and herbalists celebrate this diversity of "ways of knowing." However, there is a need for clarity about what basis is being used in any particular case.

Medical Herbalism is a modern therapy based upon thousands of years of usage and recorded observation. Is there a need to verify such ancient knowledge through animal experimentation? Such moral compromises may be acceptable for the clinical biochemist but are anathema to the herbalist. There is a universally shared ethic of respect and reverence for life amongst herbalists. An extensive historical tradition about the remedies and a daily experience with patients is often all the evidence they require. Using laboratory animals to demonstrate something already well known by practitioners is anathema to the herbalist's work of affirming life, a distortion of the search for knowledge and the desire for health. Most of the research is identifying "active constituents." The problems with this limited approach are numerous, but the main issue is the difference between whole plants in practice and their chemical constituents. The identification of specific chemicals of plant origin that affect human physiology tells us little about the value of the whole plant they were derived from. Little research is done on whole plant activity because of extreme technical difficulties in dealing with such complex biological systems. Biomedical techniques focus on analytical reduction to single or controllable relationships. Herbal medicine is rarely so simple. It is a simple matter to use a plant for an illness, but when looked at in a scientific way, problems immediately arise. The rarity of whole plant studies on people reflects the lack of a way to get valid scientific data in the face of such complexity. This is an insight into the limitations of the scientific method rather than an indictment of Medical Herbalism.

Doubts about the validity of the testing procedures focusing upon "active constituents" for carcinogenic activity have been voiced by the man who initiated the whole field of research, Dr. Bruce Ames.[9] In a recent review Ames discusses reasons why animal cancer tests cannot be used to predict absolute human risks. Such tests, however, may be used to indicate that some chemicals might be of greater concern than others.

Herbals usually list what chemical constituents have been found in an herb. This is an example of the pseudo-science that plagues Herbalism when it tries to become scientifically respectable. There are thousands of different molecules present in each cell of every plant, with each fulfilling a role within the greater whole. Constituent lists are shorthand for both the herbalist and pharmacologist to identify possible actions and uses of the plant. When this information is taken out of context of the whole it becomes meaningless. The rest of the chemical complex within the herb is equivalent to the complex within what we eat. The nutritional matrix of plant biochemistry profoundly modifies the activity of specific chemicals. Assimilation of an "active ingredient," its metabolism, transportation by the blood, availability at its site of activity and many other factors are affected and modified by the whole biochemical complex in the plant.

Both the herbal self-medicator and those legally responsible for their protection have the responsibility to inform themselves about the various issues involved. Whether it be dosage levels or the difference between whole plant effects versus extracted constituent effects, the key is information—hence this book.

1. Gordon, James S., "The Paradigm of Holistic Medicine" in *Health and the Whole Person*, edited by A.C. Hastings, J. Fadiman and J.S. Gordon, Boulder, Westview Press, 1980.
2. WHO Technical Report: 622 (1978) *The promotion and development of traditional medicine.*
3. *U.S. Spice Trade & U.S. Essential Trade*, U.S.D.A. Circular series, FTEA 1-92.
4. U.S. Essential Trade, U.S.D.A. Circular series, FTEA 2-92.
5. Foster, S., *Echinacea, Nature's Immune Enhancer*, Healing Arts Press, Rochester, 1991.
6. Hobbs, C., *The Echinacea Handbook*, Portland, Eclectic Medical Publications, 1989.
7. Ashworth, W., *The Encyclopedia of Environmental Studies*, Facts on File, New York, 1991.
8. Kerr, R.A., Oil and Gas Estimates Plummet, *Science* 241, 1989.
9. Ames, B.N.; Magaw, R.; Gold, L.S., Ranking possible carcinogenic hazards, *Science* (1987 Apr 17) 236 (4799): 271-80.

Chapter 2

Medicine, Information and Healing

Upon this gifted age, in its dark hour, Rains from the sky a meteoric shower Of facts . . . they lie unquestioned, uncombined. Wisdom enough to leech us from our ill Is daily spun, but there exists no loom To weave it into a fabric.
— Edna St. Vincent Millay

A significant part of the history of Western allopathic medicine is the story of the relentless acquisition and control of "medical" information and techniques by a few small, exclusive, all-male guilds. Access to medical care, like religious care, was through a hierarchy of ever more specialized Great Professionals. Membership in the guilds was closely controlled and ultimately depended on an apprenticeship with a master. Organized medicine has not deviated much from this form in the 500 years or so of its supremacy. However, as we now move away from this model of health care *delivery* and towards a new configuration, health *maintenance*, we must develop general access to information. (In this context, "information" is the collected experience of our ancestors and peers, physicians, herbalists, and others.)

To sustain a relationship wherein the healer and client *collaborate* to elicit the body's inner healing mechanisms, we must improve the way we work and share help with one another. There can be no hidden knowledge, no unspoken facts. Mutual respect is enabled by loosening the titles, the labels, by which we identify ourselves. Individuals involved in healing may be called doctor, physician, practitioner, health care worker, nurse, care-giver, etc. Clients have been patients, consumers, supplicants, the ill or the sick. These labels create expectations of both behavior and outcome. They often create barriers, and worse, confuse and distract us from the most important aspect of the healing adventure, the healing. My use of these labels in the following is loose; for me, many are interchangeable. If I mean to refer to a specific professional group, I will specify them formally, e.g., "M.D."

Information Storage and Memories of Healing

For most of the history of health care and medicine, the information used by a practitioner to help his or her client was whatever they remembered of the accumulated memories of all the practitioners who came before. This is called "memory-based" information (yes, even when it's written down and then studied and remembered when the need arises). Practitioners expected their intuition to search their experience and "remember" what might be needed as they examined their patient. The searching of old texts and manuscripts was sometimes done, but in the past as now, the old books were frequently unavailable, slow to search, cumbersome, and not well indexed for problem solving across disciplines. A few great physicians of the past developed some independence from the limitations of their personal memory, and expected to consult texts before proceeding with a project. They also contributed to the literature of health with lengthy, detailed observations of patients in their care. But overall, the information transfer from the human mind to a plan of medical care or cure is often slow, often inadequate to the task, and often misunderstood.

Allopathic medicine, the dominant form in the United States, discovered "evidence-based medicine" and medical information systems approximately 30 years ago. One of the early pioneers to decry the impossibility of remembering all the accumulated wisdom of all physicians, as well as all the particular aspects of any particular patient, was Lawrence Weed, M.D., of the University of Vermont. His seminal book, *Medical Records, Medical Information, and Patient Care,* was published in 1969. He states that physicians should perfect their skills in taking a history, doing a physical examination, reviewing laboratory results, and developing a relationship with the patient and the patient's family. Information storage and processing should be delegated to libraries and computers. Some of his developments, the Problem-Oriented Medical Record and the SOAP format for record keeping, have been widely implemented. These cognitive devices help to organize data about individual patients according to the problems they have, and then enable the search for information, from a client problem-centered point of view. Another integral part of the shift from the "all-knowing" physician is the increasing presence of medical literature, not only in book and magazine form, but in the expansion of the National Library of Medicine and computerized access systems. Within the last 10 years or so, these access systems have become simple enough for even the non-computer literate user. The National Library of Medicine (NLM) can be reached over the telephone through their own in-house access system called Grateful Med, or through CompuServe via PaperChase. Full-text articles are as close as your local Information Store. This shift in the availability of medical and health information has been reflected in the legal concept of "local standards of care" being expanded to encompass the entire country. There is no "local standard" anymore; all physicians and health care workers (theoretically) have access to the same worldwide memory. It has been suggested in the medico-legal literature that NOT to interrogate the medical literature will soon be regarded as *substandard* practice.

Decision-Making Support

Recognition and use of the worldwide information ocean has steadily increased over the last two decades, as the percentage of students entering professional schools with computer skills has increased. As these practitioners enter the world of healing they maintain their connections to the national (and international) electronic information resources connecting them to libraries around the world. As the information base grows, it has formed the necessary precondition for the next level, that of "informatics," of problem-solving/artificial intelligence-like programs that assist in the sorting and resolution of a particular set of symptoms or diagnostic choices. Use of these "information systems" ranges from casual, as a memory jogger for remembering unusual diseases or atypical presentations, to rigorous, with availability of predictive power, and sensitivity statistics for a particular set of symptoms, signs, or laboratory results. For example, Mac-On-Call and Quick Medical Reference are two of several software programs available for the home or office personal computer that assist in remembering or choosing a diagnosis or treatment options.

Pharmaceutical information for the allopathic and osteopathic practitioners changes very rapidly with the introduction of every new drug, or discovery of a new adverse or side effect. Drug information learned in medical school is generally outdated within five years. New antibiotics, pain killers, chemotherapeutics, and psychotropics appear every week. Dozens of new drugs are making their way through the regulatory process, and many more are expected as gene therapy and the new biologics are developed and tested. Very few drugs are ever removed from the marketplace, so the total list gets longer and longer. Ongoing seminars and articles continually inform practitioners of new, better, faster, longer acting, shorter acting, more powerful, expensive prescription pharmaceuticals. The ethics of relying on the producers of drugs for information about their products have recently been addressed by national medical groups, but, nevertheless, surveys have shown that the majority of physicians do acquire much of their knowledge of new drugs from the drug company advertisements, or the representatives that visit every doctor's office regularly.

The *Physician's Desk Reference* (PDR), a very large book produced in-house by the pharmaceutical industry, has also been available in portable electronic form for some years now. The *Non-Prescription PDR* is much smaller, not reflecting the huge diversity of OTC drugs presented to the public. OTC is the acronym for "over the counter," and refers to substances available to people without a doctor's prescription (aspirin, cold and allergy preparations, vitamins, etc.) but still regulated by the Federal Drug Administration. In general usage, OTC would *not* include herb or plant substances as they are not sold in drugstores. Information about non-prescription drugs is frequently ignored by health care workers, despite the large numbers of adverse reactions and effects that occur because of both proper and improper use. A flexible software drug database, AskRx, is now also available to individual practitioners, and allows searching by side effects, by indicated uses, and by interactions, and is more useful for solving complex clinical problems. Portable electronic information tools will assist all kinds of practitioners in the future. Problem-solving will focus on choices, rather than finding the one "best" solution.

Collaboration: New Doctor-Patient Relationships

There is no question that the nature of information access is changing; perhaps the health and medical "guilds" (AMA et al) are only just now learning how to take advantage of the new opportunities offered by global communication and the availability of electronic and specialty libraries. Besides the obvious advantages of comprehensive information, this worldwide communications network promises to radically alter the relationship between the practitioner and his or her client.

As health care workers we must now recognize that we exist in a democratically semi-accessible sea of information. While the information is at least "theoretically" available to all, there is no such claim made about the availability of the medicines themselves, or access to health care generally. It is this "bottleneck" at the gatekeeper level, the doctor level, that has provided much of the impetus to consumer-driven self-help movements, and to collaboration with non-traditional and alternative practitioners. This information "highway" is available to anyone with a need, i.e. both ourselves, our colleagues and our clients. No longer can we, as individual practitioners, rest assured that we are the sole proprietors of the best approach to any particular problem. Nor can we assume that our memory will always serve us with the most appropriate response. As we get older and more experienced we learn that there are many ways to resolve a particular problem, and many ways to serve a client. Decisions are made based on combinations of factors:

- The wishes of the client, and his or her problem or intention.
- Personal-biological factors of the client as determined by the doctor.
- In the context of *as many choices as possible*. Multiple choices are required to optimize the fit between client desires and outcome. And, if you don't like any of your choices, you haven't thought of them all yet.

This process shifts health care from regarding the doctor as repository and source of health itself, to seeing the healing process begin when a physician is recruited by the client to assist him or her in a search for the "best" path to a particular health or medical goal. This recognizes that there is not a single "best" path, but that a course of action must be determined with a particular client, with the assistance of that client himself. The patient requests that the practitioner assist him to become a partner in a problem-solving quest. This collaborative model of health care relationship may reflect similar shifts occurring in some government, industry, and educational organizations. More reliance on teamwork, less on authoritarian power structures occurs. More power, and shared responsibility, to the client emerges. This restructuring has occurred before in our social evolutionary history. When human social groups become less like agriculturally based, authoritarian nuclear family structures and look more like tribal, hunter-gatherer affiliations, the role of the authority figure declines. Some sociologists describe this shift occurring in the United States as land/home ownership declines and both men and women spend much of their time out "gathering" a living. This results in a redistribution of social and economic power within the group, both power and autonomy become more evenly divided among the members. These more horizontal power relationships allow more cooperation among people in the group. (Cf. Helen E. Fisher, *Anatomy of Love*, 1992.)

The more closely the level of education and economic power of the client matches that of the doctor, the more collaborative the relationship between them. Level of education correlates with "access to" and "control of" information, and suggests the ability to be a learner and/or user of information. Economic power results from a combination of liquid assets, security, and community role, plus the autonomy to wield it without fear or restriction. As women acquire power and education they are much less likely to tolerate an authoritarian, traditional-style physician. The collaborative model of health care delivery requires that both the healer and the patient have access to all the information they can get, to help them choose a solution or course of action that is effective as well as acceptable to them both. In the process, the patient maintains power and so is able to recruit the impressive healing effects of his own activated psycho-neuro-immune system. The physician is relieved of unshared responsibility for the outcome, and therefore the need to be authoritarian. The process of the work becomes the healing process, as they create a path towards restored health together.

Sources of Health and Medical Information

There are many levels of information available, produced in many educational levels and languages, and targeted with many different purposes in mind. Health-related magazines and books abound, suggesting a very high market interest in stories and articles having to do with health issues. Unfortunately, many sources sensationalize or distort the medical information they contain. Many news weekly papers and magazines publish primarily positive articles about the products of their major advertisers. Objective, unbiased health information is rather the minority of that offered the general public. Worse, the popular press has a regrettable tendency to participate in and create disease "fads" in which large numbers of people may be misled into erroneous misdiagnosis or unnecessary treatments. Hypoglycemia, systemic candida, neurasthenia, hysteria, rheumatism, and mercury poisoning from dental amalgams are only a few of the conditions that, while occurring in a few people, have been widely overdiagnosed at different times.

Education and Cooperation

Public and private elementary schools frequently avoid teaching even basic anatomy, physiology or pharmacology, so many high school graduates are unable to locate their kidneys or their sinuses with any accuracy, let alone select an antibiotic for themselves. Information about health and medical matters is largely acquired from family members and friends. It has been estimated that one-third of medical clients are seeing and using alternative remedies for their problems, *along with* M.D.-prescribed modalities. Many do not tell their various practitioners about each other, despite potential adverse or positive effects. Clients want to get better, and will try almost anything that is marketed enthusiastically. Local practitioners must accept a wider educational role if they want to be useful and effective in their community, and develop a collaborative practice utilizing all effective methods. This cooperative role not only brings a variety of resources and ideas to the client, it also supports full disclosure by the client of methods and remedies tried in the past or being used currently.

Specific Resources

The mostly reliable information provided by local and national non-profit, self-help and support groups covers a wide range of general information, mostly "disease"-oriented, some examples of which are listed here.

Alcoholics Anonymous. P.O.Box 459, Grand Central Station, New York, NY 10163, (212) 686-1100

Alzheimer's Disease and Related Disorders Association. 70 East Lake Street, Suite 600, Chicago, IL 60601, (800) 621-0379, (800) 572-6037 in IL

American Association of Homes for the Aging. 1129 29th Street, NW, Washington, DC 20036

American Cancer Society. 1599 Clifton Road, NE, Atlanta, GA 30329, (800)-ACS-2345

American Council for the Blind. (800) 424-8666, (202) 393-3666 in Washington, DC

American Diabetes Association. P.O. Box 25757, 1660 Duke Street, Alexandria, VA 22313, (800) 232-3472

American Heart Association. 7320 Greenville Avenue, Dallas, TX 75231, (214) 373-6300

American Kidney Fund. (800) 638-8299, (800) 492-8361 in MD

American Liver Foundation. 1425 Pompton Avenue, Cedar Grove, NJ 07009, (800) 223-0179, (800) 857-2626 in NJ

American Lung Association. 1740 Broadway, New York, NY 10019-4374, (212) 315-8787

Arthritis Foundation. 1314 Spring Street, NW, Atlanta, GA 30309, (800) 283-7800

Asthma and Allergy Foundation of America. 1717 Massachusetts Avenue, Suite 305, Washington, DC 20036, (202) 265-0265

Asthma Information Line, American Academy of Allergy and Immunology. (800) 822-ASMA

Cancer Information Service. (800) 422-6237

Crohn's and Colitis Foundation of America. 444 Park Avenue South, New York, NY 10016-7374, (800) 343-3637

Cystic Fibrosis Foundation. 6931 Arlington Road, Bethesda, MD 20814, (800) 344-4823

Eczema Association for Science and Education. 1221 SW Yamhill, Suite 303, Portland, OR 97205, (503) 228-4430

Emphysema Anonymous. 7976 Seminole Blvd., Suite 6, Seminole, FL 33542

Epilepsy Foundation of America. 4351 Garden City Drive, Suite 406, Landover, MD 20785, (800) EFA-1000

Hospice Education Institute, Hospicelink. (800) 331-1620, (203) 767-1620 in CT

Huntington's Disease Society of America. (800) 345-4372, (212) 242-1968 in NY

Leukemia Society of America. 733 Third Avenue, New York, NY 10017, (212) 573-8484

Library of Congress National Library Services for the Blind and Physically Handicapped. (800) 424-8567

National Chronic Fatigue Syndrome Assn. 3521 Broadway, Suite 222, Kansas City, MO 64111, (816) 931-4777

National Digestive Diseases Information Clearinghouse. Box NDDIC, Bethesda, MD 20892, (301) 468-6344

National Head Injury Foundation. 333 Turnpike Road, Southboro, MA 01772

National Headache Foundation. 5252 N. Western Avenue, Chicago, IL 60625, (800) 843-2256, (800) 523-8858 in IL

The National Kidney Foundation. 30 East 33rd Street, New York, NY 10016, (800) 622-9010

National Mental Health Association. 1021 Prince Street, Alexandria, VA 22314-2971, (703) 684-7722

National Musculoskeletal and Skin Diseases Information Clearinghouse. Box AMS, Bethesda, MD 20892

National Multiple Sclerosis Society. 205 East 42nd Street, New York, NY 10017-5706, (800) 624-8236

National Organization for Rare Disorders. P.O. Box 8923, New Fairfield, CT 06812, (800) 447-NORD

National Osteoporosis Foundation. 2100 M Street NW, Suite 602, Washington, DC 20037, (202) 223-2226

National Parkinson Foundation. (800) 327-4545, (800) 433-7022 in FL, (305) 547-6666 in Miami

National Society to Prevent Blindness. 500 East Remington Road, Schaumberg, IL 60173, (708) 843-2020

National Stroke Association. 300 East Hampden Avenue, Suite 240, Englewood, CO 80110, (303) 762-9922

The Simon Foundation. P.O.Box 815, Wilmette, IL 60091, (800) 23-SIMON

United Cerebral Palsy Associations. 66 East 34th Street, New York, NY 10016, (800) USA-ICUP

United Ostomy Association. 36 Executive Park, Suite 120, Irvine, CA 92714, (714) 660-8624

United Parkinson Foundation. 360 West Superior Street, Chicago, IL 60610, (312) 664-2344

Consumer versions of disease-specific pamphlets and reprints are available nationally and locally. In addition, the local chapters often support self-help groups who exchange community-specific information on resources and interested and/or competent practitioners. Referring clients to these local resources can greatly assist them in becoming educated about a specific condition, and provide an opportunity for them to share the information they collect as they traverse their healing journey. Where local organizations do not exist, national offices can usually be accessed by such resource people as social workers, hospital discharge planners, librarians, the public health department, the local Area Agency on Aging, or the Social Security office. These organizations usually provide a living, proactive channel to the information stream, and their national organizations actively fish for new, or different, information about their particular cause.

Books

On the other hand, professional medical and health textbooks are written in dense medical English, are frequently out of date by the time they're in print, but can be useful as background, sometimes for therapy decisions, but not the last word. *The Merck Manual*, introduced in 1899, was expressly designed "to meet the needs of the general practitioner in selecting medication, noting that memory is treacherous. . ." New editions appear about every five years, a collaboration of hundreds of medical authorities, under the auspices of Merck (MSD), the pharmaceutical giant. Other medical updates, such as *Current Therapy* and *Current Diagnosis*, are published annually, but cannot, in one volume each, be specific enough to apply a particular method to a particular patient without some experience and further medical information. Standards of Practice are promulgated by many professional organizations and Public Health groups, and are generally published in the organization magazine. They are not distributed to the general public but can be ordered through their sponsoring groups. Patient care algorithms (e.g. *Patient Care Flowcharts*, Medical Economics Press) have also been developed, and though they are held in low regard by some academics, do represent good, basic diagnostic and treatment strategies for common diseases, problems and presentations. Nurses and others have been supported to deliver health care in rural or remote areas with the support of such devices, either on computer-based packages or via microwave transmission. Just recently computers have made full text, full color video consultations practicable between health care facilities over phone line systems to tertiary care centers. These information systems make independence from institutional locations possible, and make state-of-the art information transfer practical.

Pharmaceutical and Drug Information

Pharmaceutical information would at first glance seem to be easier to access, with Consumer Drug Information now mandated and "Package Inserts" available at all drug stores. But a knowledgeable person will often be frustrated, or even frightened, by the information they contain. Listings of side effects, without a discussion of incidence, seriousness, or placebo responses, can be alarming, particularly to older clients whose educational background may limit their understanding of physiology and molecular biochemistry. Medicines, plants, drugs, and information about them, are some of the most misunderstood areas in our society today.

Continuing Medical Education

Continuing Medical Education (CME) alone cannot be counted on to maintain the competence of the physicians and other health care workers in this country. And while many practitioner organizations have requirements for certification and updating, many others (especially the alternative practitioners) do not. Personal responsibility for the maintenance of professional competence is mandatory for the ethical health care worker. Commercial courses are available, often expensive, or combined with a vacation. These may be sponsored by universities, or by pharmaceutical companies with a product to describe and sell. Medical centers offer courses to update physicians, nurses, and other allopathic practitioners, but these may often be open to other health care workers. As well as being extremely up to date, these meetings can identify leading researchers in a particular field, and/or identify promising new areas or even clinical trials in progress. Pharmaceutical representatives can be a good source of information, and will usually provide scientific articles, if asked. They visit physicians' offices to inform and promote the use of their company's medications. They often leave informative pamphlets for patients and free samples of the medication, and complete drug information on the package insert. But they can request information from their company on particular questions if asked to do so. Drugs, pharmaceuticals, prescriptions, vitamins, additives, herbals, foods are all chemical substances that we feed ourselves. Each has specific and non-specific effects in our bodies. All are digested, absorbed, processed, metabolized and parts eliminated. ("We are not what we eat, but what we don't excrete.") Primate groups, in the wild, have been observed selecting certain plants, presumably for their medicinal properties. Unpleasant-tasting plants were nevertheless eaten for anti-helminthic properties by heavily infested monkeys, and plants with contraceptive properties selected by certain fertile females. Primate phytotherapeutics has a long, long history. But we presume that up until now, it has been memory-based, and the choices limited to what grew in the area. But like other major areas of our lives, accurate, appropriate action results from adequate information and multiple choices. Multiple choices arise from multiple information sources and delivery channels, and from many points of view.

Evaluating Information

Sorting through all these information sources, and limiting one's input to a manageable size, is a skill. The process of collecting and assimilating information these days has been likened to "Learning to Drink from a Fire Hose" (Robert Pool, Science, vol. 248, May 1990, pgs. 674-5). Factors to be considered include the reputation and reliability of the source, the intention, or agenda, of the article or writer, the source of funding behind the study, the date and place the information was gathered, whether this is a report of experimental findings, or a hypothesis, or a report of an observation, and is there any corroboration from another source? This is how we establish credibility; without such internal, automatic protocols, the data we gather is unsupported, and perhaps useless. Even so-called "non-scientific" information is useful, but it must be clearly labeled as an observation or hypothesis. Personal reports form the foundation of modern medicine and may as well form the basis for the alternative research and practices of the future. Both practitioners and clients should be encouraged to participate in the collection and sharing of their experiences. This is how the collaborative process expands. Electronic libraries and personal modems make it possible to recognize, store and retrieve reports of new and unusual experiences that point the way to discovery.

Chapter 3

Sources of Phytotherapeutic Information

Have you ever wondered how the authors of herb books or articles "know what they know"? What are their sources? Is it empirical knowledge based upon their experience, somebody else's experience, or did it just sound like a good idea at the time?

There are many valid forms of knowledge in addition to those that flow from the "scientific method," and herbalists celebrate this diversity of ways of knowing. However, there is a need for clarity about what basis is being used in any particular case. Questioning authority is not a denial of authority but an essential part of the educational process.

If the herbal renaissance is to flower into its full potential, there needs to be a empowering of U.S. herbalists with knowledge and skill so that their experience can grow. This will not happen if we simply do what we are told, no matter how authoritative the person doing the telling. Exploring the techniques of literature searching is an essential part of the modern herbalists' skills. Relevant information and insights can be found in many places other than the "herb books." This brief discussion will point the reader in directions that will prove useful, but by the nature of things it is an incomplete guide. As you explore the cornucopia of herbal knowledge please add your own insights and, of course, question this authority!

Types of Information

There are many ways—both written and oral—in which herbal wisdom takes form. While it may seem superfluous to list them, the following provides a "road map" for our more detailed subsequent explorations.

There are many types of written materials of value to herbalists, and by identifying such categories it makes finding relevant specifics a lot simpler. The main categories are:

- Published books
- Journals
- Magazines and periodicals
- Newspapers
- Not freely distributed manuscripts, dissertations etc.

Talking to knowledgeable people is another wonderful way of gaining herbal knowledge. There is an unfortunate tendency to bemoan the dearth of a living herbal tradition in North America. There is in fact a vibrant composite tradition made up of the many ethnic strands of herbalism, eclectic knowledge maintained by the Naturopaths, the phytotherapeutic medicine of Europe, the various medical systems of Asia as well as the scientific herbalism of modern medicine and pharmacology. Of course the ideal is to find an herbalist to talk to, but this is not always possible. However, there are many other people who have relevant information but may not describe themselves as herbalists. Consider the following groups:

Herbalists and Herbal Organizations—Organizations such as the AHG, AHA, HRF and AHPA (all described later) can supply lists of their members in your area.

Local Museums—Surprisingly rich sources of information and knowledgeable people.

University, College and School Botanists, Ethnobotanists and Historians

Recorded Accounts—These are often made by historians and anthropologists.

Tapes of Lectures

Libraries

Libraries are an incredible resource as long as the herbalist knows how to use them and, sometimes more importantly, how to relate to librarians! This is not the place to explore the intricacies of the Dewey decimal system or the subtleties of card indexes, but knowing such things can be as useful as knowing about garbling. Two primary matters are knowing of the existence of the library and knowing how to access the information it may contain. Bear in mind that not all you might be looking for is going to be under the heading of herbalism. Be willing to look up some very unherbal words. The various topic names might initially include those listed here, but each researcher will develop lists that relate to his main interests:

- name of a plant (in Latin and English)
- word herb and all its forms
- phytotherapy
- pharmacy
- pharmacology
- toxicology
- history of medicine
- agriculture
- horticulture
- ethnobotany
- medical botany
- botany
- folklore

A range of library types is relevant for the phytotherapist. These include public libraries (city, county or state), college and university libraries, school libraries, specialized libraries, libraries held by herb companies and even the private libraries of professional herbalists. A number of directories of libraries can guide the researcher:

American Library Directory, R.R. Bowker Co.
A massive work that is in all reference libraries, listing more than 30,000 libraries in the U.S. and 3,000 in Canada. The entries are arranged geographically by state and city with enough information to tell you whether they might be relevant to your interests.

Subject Collections, Lee Ash, R.R. Bowker Co., 5th ed. 1978
A more useful guide for the herbalist as it organizes libraries by subject and is then arranged alphabetically by geographical order. It also lists specialized collections within general libraries.

Directory of Special Libraries and Information Centers, Gale Research Co. A massive work that is in all reference libraries, listing more than 30,000 libraries in the US and 3,000 in Canada. The entries are arranged geographically by state and city with enough information to tell you whether they might be relevant to your interests.

The most helpful guide to specialized libraries is *Subject Collections*, which is available at all main libraries. In the following section is a listing of entries relevant to the herbalist. Of all the specialized libraries, the Lloyd Library is of paramount interest. This is the description given in the Lloyd Library's brochure.

The Lloyd Library, 917 Plum St., Cincinnati, OH 45202
The Lloyd Library is a scientific library which was originally the company library of the Lloyd Brothers, a pharmaceutical firm. Its collection excels in the literature of botany and pharmacy, and also contains substantial holdings in natural history, chemistry, zoology, and other sciences. The "Lloyd" refers to three brothers: John Uri Lloyd, Curtis Gates Lloyd, and Nelson Ashley Lloyd. They were manufacturing pharmacists and owners of the Lloyd Brothers pharmaceutical company. They were scholars, scientists, and researchers. They were writers, educators, and philanthropists; they were leaders, citizens, and neighbors. John Uri Lloyd was one of the first presidents of the American Pharmaceutical Association. As a leader in pharmaceutical education he served as professor at two local institutions. He authored eight books in pharmacy and chemistry, and several thousand research articles. He was also a renowned fiction writer of eight novels and numerous short stories. Curtis Gates Lloyd was a pharmacist-turned-mycologist who collected and described thousands of fungus specimens from all over the world. In the early 1920s, he impressed on his brothers the need to endow the library in order that it would carry on long after their lifetime. Nelson Ashley Lloyd was a pharmacist-turned-businessman, who ran the company, paid all the bills, and saw to it that the library lacked for nothing. He sent book agents to Europe to buy rare books, complete sets of scientific serials, and even complete libraries. Many of the treasures he obtained could scarcely be replicated today at any price.

The Lloyd Library has one of the finest collections of the literature of botany and pharmacy in the United States. Its holdings in plant chemistry, pharmacognosy, medicinal plants, and Eclectic Medicine are unexcelled. The periodicals collection is of particular value because it includes many rare journals hard to obtain elsewhere, and often in complete, unbroken sets. In botany, the library has extensive holdings in taxonomy, morphology, flora, and botanical museum publications. Also notable is its outstanding collection of herbals, Linnean literature, and lavishly illustrated botanical works. In pharmacy, the Lloyd Library has a unique collection of books and serials dating from 1493. The library boasts one of the world's largest and most complete collections of pharmacopoeias, formularies, and dispensatories. Many scientific organizations and libraries direct their patrons to the Lloyd Library for information not obtainable in any other institution.

The Lloyd Library provides reference and bibliographical services of a very high standard to all patrons. It maintains contact with other libraries by computer terminal, interlibrary cooperation, and by taking part in professional organizations. The library supports the scientific research of natural products through joint publication of the Journal of Natural Products (Lloydia) with the American Society of Pharmacognosy. The Lloyd Library often hosts meetings, lectures, and seminars for students and professors in the sciences, members of garden clubs, horticultural and herb societies, and other groups with an interest in our subject areas.

Anyone is welcome to use the library free of charge. Most of the library's patrons are students and faculty members of nearby colleges and universities. In addition, scholars and researchers from all over the country, and often abroad, consult the library's materials. Much information is also distributed by mail or provided over the phone. In the event that a question cannot be answered from the collection, the library staff will assist in finding another source where the information can be located. The Lloyd Library actively pursues a policy of purchasing new scientific books and serials of both current awareness and of permanent reference value.

The library is open to the public from 8:30 AM to 4:00 PM, Monday through Friday, and 9:00 AM to 4:00 PM the first and third Saturday of each month. Other hours may be scheduled for groups or classes by arrangement with the librarian at (513) 721-3707. The Lloyd Library is here to serve and has been serving the scientific community and the interested public for over a century.

The relevant headings and entries from *Subject Collections* are as follows:

Herbs and Herbals

Alaska
UNIVERSITY OF ALASKA, Museum Herbarium, 907 Yucan Dr., Fairbanks, AK 99701

California
UNIVERSITY OF SOUTHERN CALIFORNIA, School of Medicine, Norris Medical Library, 2025 Zonal Ave., Los Angeles, CA 90033 (Notes: *The Collection of American Indian Ethnopharmacology*)
HUNTINGTON BOTANICAL GARDENS LIBRARY, 1151 Oxford Rd., San Marino, CA 91108

Connecticut
YALE UNIVERSITY, Box 1603-A, Yale Station, New Haven, CT 06520
YALE UNIVERSITY, Medical Historical Library, Klebs Collection, 333 Cedar St., New Haven, CT 06520
UNIVERSITY OF CONNECTICUT LIBRARY, Special Collections Dept., Storrs, CT 06268

Delaware
UNIVERSITY OF DELAWARE, Hugh M. Morris Library, S. College Ave., Newark, DL 19711

Florida
FLORIDA STATE UNIVERSITY, Robert Manning Strozier Library, Special Collections Dept., Tallahassee, FL 32306

Illinois
UNIVERSITY OF ILLINOIS AT CHICAGO, Library of the Health Sciences, 1750 W. Polk St., PO Box 7509, Chicago, IL 60612
MORTON ARBORETUM, Sterling Morton Library, Lisle, IL 60532

Indiana
PURDUE UNIVERSITY LIBRARIES, Pharmacy, Nursing & Health Sciences Library, Pharmacy Bldg., West Lafayette, IN 47907

Kansas
UNIVERSITY OF KANSAS, Kenneth Spencer Research Library, Special Collections Dept., Lawrence, KS 66045

Massachusetts
HARVARD UNIVERSITY LIBRARY, Gray Herbarium Library, 22 Divinity Ave., Cambridge, MA 02138
HERB SOCIETY OF AMERICA, Library, 2 Independence Ct., Concord, MA 01742
SMITH COLLEGE, Library, Northampton, MA 01063

Michigan
UNIVERSITY OF MICHIGAN, Herbarium Library, University Herbarium, 2003 N. University Bldg., Ann Arbor, MI 48109

Minnesota
UNIVERSITY OF MINNESOTA, Owen H. Wangensteen Historical Library of Biology & Medicine, Diehl Hall, Minneapolis, MN 55455

Missouri
UNIVERSITY OF MISSOURI-COLUMBIA, Ellis Library, Special Collections Dept., 9th & Lowry, Columbia, MO 65201
MISSOURI BOTANICAL GARDEN LIBRARY. P.O. Box 299, St. Louis, MO 63166

New York
NEW YORK PUBLIC LIBRARY, Rare Books and Manuscripts Div., Fifth Ave. & 42 St., New York, NY 10018

Ohio
LLOYD LIBRARY & MUSEUM, 917 Plum St., Cincinnati, OH 45202
CLEVELAND MEDICAL LIBRARY ASSOCIATION/CASE WESTERN RESERVE UNIVERSITY, Cleveland Health Sciences Library, Historical Division, Allen Memorial Medical Library, 11000 Euclid Ave., Cleveland, OH 44106
CLEVELAND PUBLIC LIBRARY, Fine Arts & Special Collections Dept., 325 Superior Ave., Cleveland, OH 44114

KINGSWOOD CENTER, Library, 900 Park Ave. W., Mansfield, OH 41906

MASSILLON PUBLIC LIBRARY, 208 Lincoln Way E., Massillon, OH 44646

HOLDEN ARBORETUM, Warren H. Corning Library, 9500 Sperry Rd., Mentor, OH 44060

Oregon

UNIVERSITY OF OREGON LIBRARY. Special Collections Div., Eugene, OR 97403

Pennsylvania

PENNSYLVANIA HORTICULTURAL SOCIETY, Library, 325 Walnut St., Philadelphia, PA 19106

PENNSYLVANIA HOSPITAL, HISTORICAL LIBRARY, Eighth & Spruce Sts., Philadelphia, PA 19107

TEMPLE UNIVERSITY LIBRARIES, Special Collections Dept., Rare Books & Mss Section, Philadelphia, PA 19122

HUNT INSTITUTE FOR BOTANICAL DOCUMENTATION, Hunt Botanical Library, Carnegie-Mellon University, Pittsburgh, PA 15213

Rhode Island

UNIVERSITY OF RHODE ISLAND, Library, Special Collections, Kingston, RI 02881

Pharmacology, Primitive

Arizona

NORTHERN ARIZONA UNIVERSITY, Special Collection Library, Box 6022, Flagstaff, AZ 86011

California

UNIVERSITY OF S. CALIFORNIA, School of Medicine, Norris Medical Library, 2025 Zonal Ave., Los Angeles, CA 90033

Botany, Economic

Kentucky

UNIVERSITY OF KENTUCKY, Agriculture Library, Agricultural Science Center, North Lexington, KY 40546

Massachusetts

HARVARD UNIVERSITY LIBRARY, Botanical Museum Library, Cambridge 02138

Pennsylvania

CARNEGIE LIBRARY OF PITTSBURGH, Science & Technology Dept., 4400 Forbes Ave., Pittsburgh, PA 15213

Botany, Medical

California

UNIVERSITY OF S. CALIFORNIA, School of Medicine, Norris Medical Library, 2025 Zonal Ave., Los Angeles, CA 90033

Connecticut
YALE UNIVERSITY, Medical Historical Library, Klebs Collection, 333 Cedar St., New Haven, CT 06520
UNIVERSITY OF CONNECTICUT LIBRARY, Special Collections Dept., Storrs, CT 06268

Georgia
MEDICAL COLLEGE OF GEORGIA, Library, Laney Walker Blvd., Augusta, GA 30902

Illinois
UNIVERSITY OF ILLINOIS AT CHICAGO, Library of the Health Sciences, 1750 W. Polk St., P.O. Box 7509, Chicago, IL 60612

Kansas
UNIVERSITY OF KANSAS, Kenneth Spencer Research Library, Special Collections Dept., Lawrence, KS 66045

Massachusetts
MASSACHUSETTS COLLEGE OF PHARMACY & ALLIED SCIENCES, Sheppard Library, 179 Longwood Ave., Boston, MA 02115
HARVARD UNIVERSITY LIBRARY, Botanical Museum Library, Cambridge, MA 02138

Michigan
UNIVERSITY OF MICHIGAN, Herbarium Library, University Herbarium, 2003 N. University Bldg., Ann Arbor, MI 48109

Minnesota
UNIVERSITY OF MINNESOTA, Owen H. Wangensteen Historical Library of Biology & Medicine, Diehl Hall, Minneapolis, MN 55455
3M COMPANY, 3M Center, Riker Laboratories, St. Paul, MN 55101

New York
NEW YORK BOTANICAL GARDEN LIBRARY, Bronx, NY 10458

Ohio
LLOYD LIBRARY & MUSEUM, 917 Plum St., Cincinnati, OH 45202
CLEVELAND MEDICAL LIBRARY ASSOCIATION/CASE WESTERN RESERVE UNIVERSITY, Cleveland Health Sciences Library, Historical Division, Allen Memorial Medical Library, 11000 Euclid Ave., Cleveland, OH 44106
MIAMI UNIVERSITY, Walter Havighurst Special Collections, Library, Oxford, OH 45056

Pennsylvania
PENNSYLVANIA HOSPITAL, HISTORICAL LIBRARY, Eighth & Spruce Sts., Philadelphia, PA 19107

Other important libraries for the herbally oriented are:
National Agricultural Library—Lending Branch, U.S.D.A., Beltsville, MD 20705
Natural Gardening Research Center—Hwy. 48, Box 149, Sunman, IN 47041

United States National Arboretum—3501 New York Ave. NE, Washington, DC 20002

The Dewey Decimal System

The Dewey Decimal and Library of Congress classification systems have been developed in an attempt to facilitate access to the millions of books published in the English language. The Dewey Decimal System of Classification, commonly used in most local and school libraries to catalogue books, has the advantage of a limited number of general categories and short call-numbers. The system is based on ten classes of subject (000-999), which are then further subdivided. In the listing of number categories used in the Dewey system, shown below, it is clear that information relevant to the interests covered by the wide field of herbalism might be found in many sections:

000 Generalities
010 Bibliography
020 Library and information sciences
030 General encyclopedic works
040
050 General serials & their indexes
060 General organizations & museology
070 News media, journalism, publishing
080 General collections
090 Manuscripts & rare books

100 Philosophy & psychology
110 Metaphysics
120 Epistemology
130 Paranormal phenomena
140 Specific philosophical schools
150 Psychology
160 Logic
170 Ethics (Moral philosophy)
180 Ancient, medieval, Oriental philosophy
190 Modern Western philosophy

200 Religion
210 Natural theology
220 Bible
230 Christian theology
240 Christian moral & devotional theology
250 Christian orders & local church
260 Christian social theology
270 Christian church history
280 Christian denominations & sects
290 Other & comparative religions

300 Social sciences
310 General statistics
320 Political science
330 Economics
340 Law
350 Public administration

360 Social services; association
370 Education
380 Commerce, communications, transport
390 Customs, etiquette, folklore

400 Language
410 Linguistics
420 English & Old English
430 Germanic languages, German
440 Romance languages, French
450 Italian, Romanian, Rhaeto-Romanic
460 Spanish & Portuguese languages
470 Italic languages, Latin
480 Hellenic languages, Classical Greek
490 Other languages

500 Natural sciences & mathematics
510 Mathematics
520 Astronomy & allied sciences
530 Physics
540 Chemistry & allied sciences
550 Earth sciences
560 Paleontology, paleozoology
570 Life sciences
580 Botanical sciences
590 Zoological sciences

600 Technology (Applied sciences)
610 Medical sciences, medicine
620 Engineering & allied operations
630 Agriculture
640 Home economics & family living
650 Management & auxiliary services
660 Chemical engineering
670 Manufacturing

680 Manufacture for specific uses
690 Buildings

700 The arts
710 Civic & landscape art
720 Architecture
730 Plastic arts, sculpture
740 Drawing & decorative arts
750 Painting & paintings
760 Graphic arts, printmaking & prints
770 Photography & photographs
780 Music
790 Recreational & performing arts

800 Literature & rhetoric
810 American literature in English
820 English & Old English literatures
830 Literatures of Germanic languages

840 Literatures of Romance languages
850 Italian, Romanian, Rhaeto-Romanic
860 Spanish & Portuguese literatures
870 Italic literatures, Latin
880 Hellenic literatures, Classical Greek
890 Literatures of other languages

900 Geography & history
910 Geography & travel
920 Biography, genealogy, insignia
930 History of ancient world
940 General history of Europe
950 General history of Asia, Far East
960 General history of Africa
970 General history of North America
980 General history of South America
990 General history of other areas

Each of these sections can be further divided for accuracy in classification. For example, the numbers 500-599 cover the "pure" sciences, such as astronomy, chemistry, mathematics, paleontology, and physics. Each of these areas has its own division and section number. All books on botany are assigned numbers in the 580 to 589 range; botany is then broken down into types, which can then be subdivided through the use of decimal points to provide ten more categories. Additional digits can be added, creating an ever more precise categorization system. The examples given show the organization power of this system. Books are arranged alphabetically within each classification by the first letters of the author's last name. Therefore, a library that has several books on Herb Gardens will assign the same basic number (635.7) to all the books and shelve them alphabetically.

In the detailed guide to the system used by librarians around the world the following listings are given in the index that directly use the word herb:

Herb gardens	635.7
Herb teas	641.357
agriculture	635.7
commercial processing	663.96
cooking with	641.657
home preparation	641.877
Herbaceous flowering plants	582.13
Herbaceous plants	582.12
landscape architecture	716
Herbaceous shrubs	582.14
Herbaceous vines	582.14
Herbals	
pharmacognosy	615.321
Herbariums	580.742

Of course this is limiting the references to "herb," but if other relevant words are used a much richer array of references would become available. As examples consider the categories that are directly relevant in the major groupings of Botanical Science, Medical Science and Agriculture. Bear in mind that this does not include references that might be found in, for example, history or cooking.

580   Botanical Science

580.74	Museums, collections, exhibits
580.742	Herbariums
580.744	Botanical gardens
581	Botany
581.01-.09	Standard subdivisions
581.072	Research
581.0724	Experimental botany
581.074	Museums, collections, exhibits
581.075	Museum activities and services
581.09	Historical, geographical, person's treatment
581.1	Physiology of plants
581.2	Pathology of plants
581.3	Development and maturation of plants
581.4	Anatomy and morphology of plants
581.5	Ecology of plants
581.6	Economic botany
581.61	Beneficial plants
581.63	Edible and medicinal plants
581.632	Edible plants
581.634	Medicinal plants
581.64	Plants of industrial and technological value
581.65	Deleterious plants
581.652	Weeds
581.67	Allergenic plants
581.69	Poisonous plants
581.8	Tissue, cellular, molecular botany
581.9	Geographical treatment of plants
582	Spermatophytes (Seed-bearing plants)
583	Dicotyledons
584	Monocotyledons
585	Gymnospermae (Pinophyta)
586	Cryptogamia (Seedless plants)
587	Pteridophyta (Vascular cryptogams)
588	Bryophyta
589	Thallobionta (Thallophyta) and Prokaryotae

610   Medical Sciences

615	Pharmacology and therapeutics
615.1	Drugs (Materia medica)
615.11	Pharmacopeias
615.12	Dispensatories
615.13	Formularies
615.14	Posology

615.18	Drug preservation technique
615.19	Pharmaceutical chemistry
615.2	Inorganic drugs
615.3	Organic drugs
615.31	Synthetic drugs
615.32	Drugs of plant origin
615.321	Pharmacognosy
615.322	Drugs derived from bryophytes
615.323-.327	Drugs derived from specific plants
615.328	Vitamins
615.329	Drugs derived from thallophytes
615.34	Fish-liver oils
615.35	Enzymes
615.4	Practical pharmacy
615.42	Solutions and extracts
615.43	Pills, capsules, tablets, troches, powders
615.45	Ointments and emulsions
615.5	Therapeutics
615.53	General therapeutic systems, including eclectic, botanic medicine and Ayurveda
615.531	Allopathy
615.532	Homeopathy
615.533	Osteopathy
615.534	Chiropractic
615.535	Naturopathy
615.6	Methods of administering medication
615.7	Pharmacodynamics
615.8	Specific therapies and kinds of therapies
615.88	Empirical and historical remedies
615.882	Folk medicine
615.886	Patent medicines
615.9	Toxicology
615.952	Plant and plant-derived poisons

630	**Agriculture**
635	Garden crops (Horticulture), vegetables
635.04	Cultivation, harvesting, related topics
635.1	Edible roots
635.2	Edible tubers and bulbs
635.3	Edible leaves, flowers, stems
635.4	Cooking greens and rhubarb
635.5	Salad greens
635.6	Edible garden fruits and seeds
635.7	Aromatic and sweet herbs
635.8	Mushrooms and truffles
635.9	Flowers and ornamental plants

The Library of Congress Classification System

Dewey's aim was to create a system that would be simple enough for casual users to understand, but complex enough to meet a library's expanding needs. A second system was created to fit the requirements of a specific library, the Library of Congress. This system, now in wide use, is even more detailed and has the advantage of being able to accommodate growth of knowledge in unexpected areas. The Library of Congress was created in 1800 to provide "such books as may be necessary for the use of Congress." Over the succeeding years it has grown to become the national library of the United States, serving all government branches and the public at large. To cope with the vast range of topics covered it has developed a numerical system of subject classification.

The Library of Congress Classification System is used in most large public and university libraries today. A Library of Congress (LC) classification number contains three lines, a letter at the top, a number in the middle, and a letter/number combination at the bottom. The Library of Congress Classification System contains 20 classes:

A: General works
B: Philosophy and religion
C: History-auxiliary sciences
D: History and topography (except America)
E-F: American history
G: Geography, anthropology, folklore, manners and customs, recreation
H: Social sciences
J: Political sciences
K: Law of the United States
L: Education
M: Music and books on music
N: Fine arts
P: Language and literature
Q: Science
R: Medicine
S: Agriculture and plant and animal industry
T: Technology
U: Military science
V: Naval science
Z: Bibliography and library science

Each of these classes can be divided into a subclass with the addition of a second letter. By adding numbers, the category becomes even more specific. This is a very flexible system as the alphabet permits 26 subdivisions of any one class. Each of the subdivisions can be broken down further by using the numbers 1 to 9999. It is the flexibility and diversity of this system that leads librarians to recommend that herbal researchers turn to *Subject Headings in the Dictionary Catalog of the Library of Congress* for assistance. Because it groups related topics together, a researcher may discover unexpected, related avenues to pursue.

Newspaper & Periodical Indexes

From the explosion of printed media in the 19th century through to the staggering amount of newspapers and periodicals of today there is a cornucopia of material for the herbalist. With modern indexes and archives it is not too challenging to find the gems we seek.

Detailed indexes are available on microfiche and on-line databases for the major newspapers of the English-speaking world, including *The New York Times Index* and *The Times of London Index*. These can be invaluable for exploring the sociopolitical role of herbalism, for example, what was being said about the Flexner report at the time. A number of indexes deal with periodicals, helping the researcher find a range of perspectives on a topic.

Standard Periodical Directory, Oxbridge Communications Inc., 183 Madison Avenue, New York, NY 10016—Gives facts in over 68,000 American and Canadian periodicals, grouped by 230 subject categories.

Reader's Guide to Periodical Literature—The best single source from which to find references to magazine and journal articles. It indexes about 180 general and non-technical periodicals published in the U.S. starting from 1990. They also publish a smaller abridged *Reader's Guide*.

Popular Periodical Index, P.O. Box 739, Camden, NJ 08102—36 periodicals not in the *Reader's Guide*. From *Prevention* and *Mother Jones* to *Playboy*, *Conservative Review* and the *TV Guide*!

Alternative Press Index, P.O. Box 7229, Baltimore, MD 21218

More technical articles, not from peer review journals, are cited in a number of specialized periodical indexes.

Applied Science & Technology Index—Covers about 300 periodicals from 1958; before that date see *Industrial Arts Index*, started in 1913.

Biological & Agricultural Index—190 periodicals from 1964; its predecessor was *Agricultural Index* started in 1916.

Business Periodicals Index—270 periodicals from 1958.

General Science Index—Covers about 90 general science periodicals from 1978.

Index to Legal Periodicals—Covers about 375 periodicals, yearbooks and annual reviews from throughout the English-speaking world. Started in 1908.

Poole's Index to Periodical Literature—Articles indexed by subject. Volume 1—1802-81; Volume 2-6—1882-1906.

Author Index for Poole's—C.E. Wall ed., Pierian Press, 1970.

Nineteenth Century Readers' Guide to Periodical Literature.

General Reference Books

A number of general reference books can prove useful when starting to explore a field of study.

Reference Books: A Brief Guide, Enoch Pratt Free Library, 400 Cathedral Street, Baltimore, MD 21201

Subject Guide to Books in Print, R.R. Bowker Co., 1180 Avenue of the Americas, New York, NY 10036—Annually lists over 423,000 books, indexed under 62,000 headings.

Books In Print, R.R. Bowker Co., 1180 Avenue of the Americas, New York, NY 10036—Listed by subject or author.

National Directory of Newsletters and Reporting Services

Encyclopedia of Associations, Gale Research Co.—The best way to find specialists in thousands of specialized fields.

Public Relations Sources

PR companies and departments can be very helpful and are found in a variety of places, such as herb manufacturing companies, federal agencies or embassies. Places to start are:

O'Dwyer's Directory of Public Relations Firms, Jack O'Dwyer, ed.; J.R. O'Dwyer Co., 271 Madison Avenue, New York, NY 10016

Information Center of the Public Relations Society of America, 845 Third Avenue, New York, NY 10022

A partial list of herbal product manufacturing, importing or distributing companies includes:

Arkopharma Inc., 16-A Montesano, Fairfield, NJ 07006

Bioforce of America, Ltd., 21 West Mall, Plainview, NY 11803

Eclectic Institute, 11231 SE Market St., Portland, OR 97216

Frontier Cooperative Herbs, Box 299, Norway, IA 52318

Herbalist & Alchemist Inc., P.O. Box 553, Broadway, NJ 08808, (908) 689-9020

Herb-Pharm, 347 East Fork Road, Williams, OR 97544, (503) 846-7178

Herbs ETC., 1340 Rufina Circle, Santa Fe, NM 87501

McZand Herbal, P.O. Box 5312, Santa Monica, CA 90405

Nature's Apothecary, 997 Dixon Rd., Boulder, CO 80302, (303) 440-7422

Nature's Sunshine Products, Inc., P.O. Box 1000, Spanish Fork, UT 84660

Nature's Way Products, Inc., 10 Mountain Springs Parkway, P.O. Box 2233, Springville, UT 84663

Natureworks, Inc., 5341 Derry Ave., Suite F/G, Agoura Hills, CA 91301

Naturpharma, Inc. (Nature's Herbs), 1113 N. Industrial Park Dr., P.O. Box 336, Orem, UT 84059

Planetary Formulas, P.O. Box 533, Soquel, CA 95073

Rainbow Light Nutritional Systems, 207 Mc Pherson St., Santa Cruz, CA 95060

Simpler's Botanical, P.O. Box 39, Forestville, CA 95436, (707) 887-2012

Starwest Botanicals, Inc., 11253 Trade Center Dr., Rancho Cordova, CA 95742

Sunrider International, 3111 Lomita Blvd., Torrance, CA 90505

Traditional Medicinals, 4515 Ross Rd., Sebastopol, CA 95472

Turtle Island Herbs, Inc., Salina Star Route, Boulder, CO 80302

Wise Woman Herbals, Sharol Tilgner, MD., P.O. Box 328, Gladstone, OR 97027, (503) 239-6573

Government Sources

A number of federal agencies produce publications of relevance to the herbalist. The U.S.D.A. and F.D.A. are especially useful. The Government Publications Office produces a useful monthly guide and a bibliographic index that help navigate through the sea of paper.

Monthly Catalogue of U.S. Government Publications, Government Printing Office, Washington, DC

The Subject Bibliography Index—Contains a list of 270 subject bibliographies of GPO publications.

These are available in printed form or as CD-ROMs which most main libraries now have. Examples of the cornucopia of useful information that can be found courtesy of the federal government are:

McCarthy, Susan A.—***Ethnobotany and Medicinal Plants***. July 1990/July 1991. Quick bibliography series, QB 91-66, National Agricultural Library, 1991. Contains 591 citations from the AGRICOLA database.

McCarthy, Susan A.—***Ethnobotany and Medicinal Plants***. July 1991/July 1992. Quick bibliography series, QB 93-02, National Agricultural Library, 1992. Contains 546 citations from the AGRICOLA database.

Maclean, Jayne T.—***Culinary Herbs and Herbal Oils***. January 1979/May 1989. Quick bibliography series, QB 90-22, National Agricultural Library, 1990. Contains 331 citations from AGRICOLA.

Maclean, Jayne T.— ***Herb Gardening***. 1979-1986. Quick bibliography series, QB 87-09, National Agricultural Library, 1987. Contains 117 citations from AGRICOLA.

Maclean, Jayne T.—***Herb Gardening***. 1979-1985. Quick bibliography series, QB 86-26, National Agricultural Library, 1986. Contains 94 citations from AGRICOLA.

Maclean, Jayne T.—***Herb Gardening***. 1981-1989. Quick bibliography series, QB 89-76, National Agricultural Library, 1989. Contains 94 citations from AGRICOLA.

Maclean, Jayne T.—***Medical Botany and Herb Medicine, Books and Citations***. 1981-1989. Quick bibliography series, QB 87-15, National Agricultural Library, 1987. 271 citations.

Maclean, Jayne T.—***Medical Botany and Herb Medicine, Books and Citations.*** 1970-1984. Quick bibliography series, QB 85-27, National Agricultural Library, 1985. 270 citations.

Maclean, Jayne T.—*Sugar Substitutes and Alternative Sweeteners*. 1982-1985. Quick bibliography series, QB 86-68, National Agricultural Library, 1985. 165 citations.

Library of Congress—*Medical Botany*. Library of Congress, 1972. TB 72-19.

Gates, Jane—*Medical Botany and Herbal Medicine*. 1988-198 p. Quick bibliography series, QB 90-44, National Agricultural Library, 1990. 400 citations.

Much of the material published by federal agencies is now available through government computer bulletin boards. These government bulletin boards and how to access and use them are discussed later in the book.

Out-of-Print Books

As many of the primary source books in herbalism are out of print it is often necessary to use the services of Book-Search Specialists. Most bookstores can do a nationwide search but it is often cheaper and easier to go directly to the person doing the search. The Antiquarian Booksellers Association of America publish the Bookman's Weekly that is the leading guide to services and books offered. There are a few antiquarian book dealers that specialize in herbals and eclectic medicine material. One of these is Herbalist & Alchemist Books (P.O. Box 553, Broadway, NJ 08808, 908-689-9020), run by one of America's leading phytotherapists, David Winston. They publish a twice yearly catalogue of books and journals relating to herbalism, eclectic medicine, economic botany, pre-1920 pharmacy, ethnobotany, natural products chemistry and the history of medicine.

Computer Software

There are a number of software packages now available that include herbally relevant databases that can be used on personal computers. These are not the same as the massive on-line databases that are described in a later section, but are still large and useful sources of information for the phytotherapist.

Database of Phytochemical Constituents of Grass, Herbs, and Other Economic Plants—James A. Duke. 1992. CRC Press, 2000 Corporate Blvd. NW, Boca Raton, FL 33431

Database of Biologically Active Phytochemicals and Their Activities—James A. Duke. 1992. CRC Press, 2000 Corporate Blvd. NW, Boca Raton, FL 33431

GLOBALHERB—Steve Blake, FALCOR, 5831 S. Hwy. 9, Felton, CA 95018

The Herbalist CD-ROM—by David Hoffmann, Hopkins Technology, 421 Hazel Lane, Hopkins, MN 55343-7116

IBIS—AMR'TA, P.O. Box 14641, Portland, OR 97214

An Herbal Bibliography

The publishing world has discovered that there are profits to be made from books on herbs and healing, bringing with it the blessing of many wonderful books, some obscure gems, but unfortunately all too many volumes that do not justify the felling of the trees. As an author myself, that raises the question of whether any human writing can justify the current rape of the forests.

- It may prove useful to apply some guidelines in the seemingly endless search for that all too elusive "perfect" herbal. When considering a herbal new to you, consider these points:

- Is the author experienced in the area he is writing about? All too often the plethora of new herbals assailing the public is written by journalists commissioned by publishers to fill their subject catalogues. While they usually write better than herbalists, all they can write about will usually come from other books. On the whole, the bigger and glossier the book, the less likely it is to be of value, other than aesthetic.

- Is the author saying anything new about a specific herb? Is this new information correct? If it is the same material written about in a clear way, this may be very useful as herbalists tend not to be the best writers! If there are actual mistakes then avoid that book.

- Is the author saying anything new about the herbal treatment of an illness? Is the author's approach one that adds insight to that of other authors?

Herbals

An herbal is, strictly speaking, simply a book describing and listing the properties of herbs. The word is used more generally to cover books on not just herbs but also usage. There are a great number of excellent books on herbal gardening, identification, crafts, cosmetics, folklore and culinary use. I have left them out because of my lack of knowledge, *not* because they are of no interest.

History

Arber, Agnes. *Herbals: Their Origin and Evolution: A Chapter in the History of Botany 1470-1670.* 2nd ed. Cambridge, England: Cambridge University Press, 1953.

Anderson, Frank J. *An Illustrated History of the Herbals.* New York: Columbia University Press, 1977.

Boussel, Patrice, Henri Bonnemain, and Frank J. Bove. *History of Pharmacy and Pharmaceutical Industry.* Paris, Lausanne: Asklepios Press, 1983.

Griggs, Barbara. *Green Pharmacy.* Healing Arts Press, 1981.

Hamarenth, Sami K. and Ernst W. Stiev. **Pharmacy Museums and Historical Collections on Public View in the United States and Canada.** Madison, WI: American Institute of the History of Pharmacy in cooperation with the National Museum of American History, Smithsonian Institution, 1981.

Kremers, Edward, and George Urdang. **Kremers and Urdang's History of Pharmacy.** 4th ed. Philadelphia: J.B. Lippincott, 1976.

LaWall, Charles H. **Four Thousand Years of Pharmacy: An Outline History of Pharmacy and the Allied Sciences.** Philadelphia, PA: J. B. Lippincott, 1927.

Wootton, A. C. **Chronicles of Pharmacy.** London: Macmillan, 1910; repr. Boston, MA: Milford House for USV Pharmaceutical Corp., 1972.

Classic European Herbals

There are many tomes that would fit into this category, covering the ancient works of Dioscorides, Hippocrates and Galen through to Culpeper in the 17th century. Most can only be found in locked cabinets in well-endowed libraries, but some have been reprinted. Those that follow are available reprints but the selection reflects my handicap of only reading English!

Culpeper, N. **Culpeper's Complete Herbal & English Physician.** Glenwood: Meyerbooks, 1987.

Gerard, J. **The Herbal.** repr. of 1633, New York: Dover Press, 1975.

Strehlow & Hertzk. **Hildegard of Bingen's Medicine.** Santa Fe: Bear & Co., 1987.

Eclectic and Physiomedical and Other 19th Century U.S. Herbals

These are branches of medicine utilizing traditional herbal medicine and aspects of modern medicine popular in the 19th century and into the early twentieth century. These books are exceptionally relevant for the clinician but very expensive!

Bibliographical Contributions from the Lloyd Library. Cincinnati, OH: Lloyd Library, 1911-1918.

Ellingwood, Finley. **American Materia Medica, Therapeutics & Pharmacognosy.** 1898, repr. Eclectic Med. Pub., 1983.

Felter and Lloyd. **King's American Dispensatory Vol. 1 & 2.** repr. Eclectic Med. Pub., 1983.

Felter, Harvey W. **The Eclectic Materia Medica, Pharmacology & Therapeutics.** 1922, Eclectic Med. Pub., 1983.

Millspaugh, Charles F. **American Medicinal Plants: An Illustrated and Descriptive Guide to Plants Indigenous to and Naturalized in the United States Which Are Used in Medicine.** New York: Boericke, 1887; repr. New York: Dover, 1974.

Modern Herbals

Alstat, Edward. *Eclectic Dispensatory of Botanical Therapeutics, Vol 1.* Portland: Eclectic Med. Pub., 1989.

American Herbalist Guild. *American Herbalism: Essays on Herbs and Herbalism.* Freedom: The Crossing Press, 1992.

Castleman, Michael. *The Healing Herbs: The Ultimate Guide to the Curative Powers of Nature's Medicines.* Emmaus: Rodale Press, 1991.

Christopher, Dr. John R. *School of Natural Healing.* Springville: Dr. Christopher's Pub., Inc., 1991.

Conrow & Hecksel. *Herbal Pathfinders: Voices of the Herb Renaissance.* Santa Barbara: Woodbridge Press, 1983.

Duke, James A. *Handbook of Edible Weeds.* Boca Raton: CRC Press, 1992.

Duke, James A. *CRC Handbook of Medicinal Herbs.* Boca Raton: CRC Press, 1985.

Fluck, Hans. *Medicinal Plants: An Authentic Guide to Natural Remedies.* Garden City Park: Avery Pub. Group, 1988.

Foster, Steven. *Echinacea, Nature's Immune Enhancer.* Rochester: Inner Traditions, 1991.

Foster/Chongxi. *Herbal Emissaries: Bringing Chinese Herbs to the West.* Rochester: Inner Traditions, 1992.

Fulder & Blackwood. *Garlic: Nature's Original Remedy.* Rochester: Inner Traditions, 1991.

Gagnon & Morningstar. *Breathe Free.* Lotus: Lotus Press, 1990.

Gardner, Joy. *Healing Yourself During Pregnancy.* Freedom: The Crossing Press, 1987.

Gardner, Joy. *The New Healing Yourself.* Freedom: The Crossing Press, 1989.

Gosling, Nalda. *Successful Herbal Remedies.* San Francisco: Thorsons, 1985.

Graham, Judy. *Evening Primrose Oil.* Rochester: Inner Traditions, 1984.

Green, James. *The Male Herbal.* Freedom: The Crossing Press, 1991.

Grieve, Mrs. M. *A Modern Herbal, Vol. I and II.* New York: Dover Publications, 1971.

Hobbs, Christopher. *Ginkgo: Elixir of Youth.* Capitola: Botanical Press, 1991.

Hobbs, Christopher. *Foundations of Health: The Liver and Digestion Herbal.* Capitola: Botanica Press, 1992.

Hoffmann, David. *An Elder's Herbal.* Rochester: Inner Traditions, 1992.

Hoffmann, David. *Successful Stress Control.* Rochester: Healing Arts Press, 1986.

Hoffmann, David. *The Elements of Herbalism.* Shaftesbury: Element Books, 1990.

Hoffmann, David. *The Herbal Handbook.* Rochester: Inner Traditions, 1988.

Hoffmann, David. *The New Holistic Herbal.* Shaftesbury: Element Books, 1983.

Hoffmann, David. *Therapeutic Herbalism.* Sebastopol: Veritas Press, 1991.

Hutchens, Alma. *Indian Herbology of North America.* Acton: Shamballa Pub., 1991.

Hye Koo Yun. *Herbal Holistic Healing Approach to Arthritis.* Burnaby: Dominion Herbal College, 1988.

Keville, Kathi. *The Illustrated Herb Encyclopedia: A Complete Culinary, Cosmetic, Medicinal and Ornamental Guide to Herbs.* New York: Mallard Press, 1991.

Kloss, Jethro. *Back to Eden.* South Windsor: Lust, Benedict Pub., 1985.

Lust, John. *The Herb Book.* New York: Bantam Books, 1982.

Mabey, Richard. *The New Age Herbalist.* New York: Macmillan, 1988.

McIntyre, Anne. *Herbs for Mother and Child.* London: Sheldon Press, 1988.

McIntyre, Anne. *The Herbal for Pregnancy and Childbirth.* Shaftesbury: Element Books, 1992.

McIntyre, Michael. *Herbal Medicine for Everyone.* New York: Viking Penguin, 1989.

Meyer, C. *American Folk Medicine.* Glenwood: Meyerbooks, 1985.

Miller, Amy Bess Williams. *Shaker Herbs: A History and a Compendium.* New York: Clarkson N. Potter, 1976.

Mills, Simon. *Alternatives in Healing.* London: Marshall Editions, 1988.

Mills, Simon. *Dictionary of Modern Herbalism.* Rochester: Inner Traditions, 1985.

Mills, Simon. *Out of the Earth: The Science and Practice of Herbal Medicine.* New York: Viking Penguin, 1992.

Moore, Michael. *Medicinal Plants of the Mountain West.* Santa Fe: Museum of New Mexico Press, 1979.

Moore, Michael. *Medicinal Plants of the Desert & Canyon West.* Santa Fe: Museum of New Mexico Press, 1989.

Moore, Michael. *Los Remedios: Traditional Herbal Remedies of the Southwest.* Santa Fe: Museum of New Mexico Press, 1990.

Morton, Julia Frances. *Folk Remedies of the Low Country.* Miami: E.A. Seeman, 1974.

Mowrey, Daniel. *Next Generation Herbal Medicine: Guaranteed Potency Herbs.* New Canaan: Keats Pub., 1990.

Mowrey, Daniel. *The Scientific Validation of Herbal Medicine.* New Canaan: Keats Pub., 1990.

Murray, Michael. *The Healing Power of Herbs.* Rocklin: Prima Pub., 1992.

Parvati, Jeannine. *Hygieia, a Woman's Herbal.* Monroe: Freestone, 1979.

Potts, Billie. *Witches Heal.* Ann Arbor: Du Reve, 1988.

Priest & Priest. *Herbal Medications.* L. N. Fowler & Co. Ltd., 1982.

Riggs, Maribeth. *Natural Child Care.* New York: Harmony Books, 1989.

Roberts, Frank. *Modern Herbalism for Digestive Disorders.* San Francisco: Thorsons, 1978.

Rose, Jeanne. *Herbal Body Book.* New York: Putnam Pub., 1976.

Shauenberg & Paris. *Guide to Medicinal Plants.* New Canaan: Keats Publishing Inc., 1977.

Stary & Jirasek. *Herbs.* New York: Hippocrene Books, Inc., Ltd., 1973.

Steinmetz, E.F. *Codex Vegetabilis.* 2nd ed. Amsterdam, The Netherlands: E.F. Steinmetz, 1957.

Stuart, Malcom, ed. *The Encyclopedia of Herbs and Herbalism.* Guild Publishing, 1986.

Theiss, Peter & Barbara. *The Family Herbal.* Rochester: Inner Traditions, 1989.

Thomson, William. *Medicines From the Earth.* New York: McGraw-Hill, 1978.

Tierra, Michael. *Planetary Herbology.* Wilmot: Lotus Press, 1988.

Tierra, Michael. *The Way of Herbs.* Orenda/Unity Press, 1980.

Uphof, J .C. *The Dictionary of Economic Plants.* 2nd ed. Monticello, NY: Lubrecht and Cramer, 1968.

Usher, George. *A Dictionary of Plants Used by Man.* New York: Hafner Press, a division of Macmillan Publishing, 1974.

Weed, Susun. *Healing Wise.* Woodstock: Ash Tree Publishing, 1989.

Weed, Susun. *Wise Woman Ways for the Menopausal Years.* Woodstock: Ash Tree Publishing, 1992.

Weed, Susun. *Wise Woman Herbal for the Childbearing Years.* Woodstock: Ash Tree Publishing, 1985.

Weiner, M.A. *Earth Medicine, Earth Food.* New York: Fawcett, 1991.

Weiss & Weiss. *Growing and Using Healing Herbs.* Emmaus: Rodale Press.

Weiss, Rudolf. *Herbal Medicine.* Portland: Medicina Biologica, 1988.

Willard, Terry. *The Textbook of Modern Herbology.* Homosassa Springs: Progressive Publishing Inc., 1988.

Willard, Terry. *The Textbook of Advanced Herbology.* Calgary: Wild Rose College Ltd., 1992.

Wren, R.C. *Potter's New Cyclopedia of Botanical Drugs and Preparations.* C. W. Daniel, 1988

Pharmacognosy and Phytopharmacology Texts

Pharmacognosy is the study of the sources, identifying characteristics, constituents and uses of plants in their unprocessed states. Older editions of pharmacognosy books are filled with material about commonly used herbs, but modern books have more limited information but are nonetheless interesting and informative.

Baba, Akerele & Kawaguchi. *Natural Resources and Human Health—Plants of Medicinal and Nutritional Value.* New York: Elsevier Science Pub., 1992.

Dev, Sukh, Anubhav P. S. Narula, and Jhillu Singh Yadav. **CRC Handbook of Terpenoids: Monoterpenoids, 2 Vols.** Boca Raton: CRC Press, 1982.

Devon, T. K., and A. L. Scott. *Handbook of Naturally Occurring Compounds.* 1972.

Duke, J. A. *Handbook of Phytochemical Constituents of Grass, Herbs, and Other Economic Plants.* Boca Raton: CRC Press, 1992.

Duke, J. A. *Handbook of Biologically Active Phytochemicals and Their Activities.* Boca Raton: CRC Press, 1992.

Glasby, John S. *Encyclopedia of the Terpenoids.* New York: John Wiley and Sons, 1983.

Glasby, John S. *Encyclopedia of the Alkaloids.* New York: Plenum Publishing, 1983.

Glasby, John S. *Directory of Plants Containing Secondary Metabolites.* Bristol: Taylor & Francis, 1991.

Grundon, M. F. *The Alkaloids: A Review of the Literature.* London: The Chemical Society, 1969-1983.

Harborne, Jeffrey B. *Phytochemical Methods: A Guide to Modern Techniques of Plant Analysis.* 2nd ed. London: Chapman and Hall; Methuen, 1984.

Harborne and Baxter, eds. *Phytochemical Dictionary: A Handbook of Bioactive Compounds from Plants.* Bristol: Taylor & Francis, 1993.

Hartwell, Jonathan L. *Plants Used Against Cancer: A Survey.* Lawrence: Quarterman Publications, 1982.

Hocking, George MacDonald. *A Dictionary of Terms in Pharmacognosy and Other Divisions of Economic Botany.* Springfield: Charles C. Thomas, 1955.

Hudson, James B. *Antiviral Compounds from Plants.* Boca Raton: CRC Press, 1989.

Koji Nakansishi, Toshio Goto, Sho Ito, Shinsaku Natori, and Shigeo Nozoe. *Natural Products Chemistry.* Tokyo: Kodansha Ltd.; New York: Academic Press, 1974.

Leung, Albert Y. *Encyclopedia of Common Natural Ingredients Used in Food, Drugs, and Cosmetics.* New York: John Wiley and Sons, 1980.

Manitto, Paolo. *Biosynthesis of Natural Products.* Chichester, England: Ellis Horwood Ltd.; New York: John Wiley & Sons.

Manske, Rodrigo, Cordell, and Brossi. *The Alkaloids.* New York: Academic Press, 1950.

Pelletier, S. W., ed. *Alkaloids: Chemical and Biological Perspectives.* New York: John Wiley & Sons, 1983.

Pirson and Zimmerman. *Encyclopedia of Plant Physiology.* Berlin, Germany; New York: Springer Verlag, 1975.

Raffauf, Robert F. *A Handbook of Alkaloids and Alkaloid-Containing Plants.* Philadelphia: Wiley-Interscience, a division of John Wiley and Sons, 1970.

Robinson, T. *The Organic Constituents of Higher Plants.* North Amherst: Cordus Press, 1983.

Ross & Brian. *An Introduction to Phytopharmacy.* Pitman Medical Publishing, 1977.

Schultes, Richard E., and Albert Hofmann. *The Botany and Chemistry of Hallucinogens.* Springfield: Charles C. Thomas, 1980.

The Merck Index: An Encyclopedia of Chemicals, Drugs, and Biologicals. Edited by Martha Windholz. 10th ed. Rahway: Merck & Co., 1983.

Torssell, Kurt B.G. *Natural Product Chemistry: A Mechanistic and Biosynthetic Approach to Secondary Metabolism.* New York: John Wiley & Sons, 1983.

Trease & Evans. *Pharmacognosy.* 13th ed. London: Baillere Tindall, 1989.

Tyler, Brady & Robbers. *Pharmacognosy.* 8th ed. Malvern: Lea & Febiger, 1981.

Wagner, Bladt & Zgainski. *Plant Drug Analysis.* New York: Springer Verlag, 1984.

West, K. *How to Draw Plants: The Techniques of Botanical Illustration.* London: Herbert Press, 1983.

Womersley, J. S. *Plant Collecting and Herbarium Development: A Manual.* Rome: Food and Agriculture Organization of the United Nations; New York: Unipub, 1981.

Youngken. *A Textbook of Pharmacognosy.* Blakiston.

Pharmacopoeias and Extra Pharmacopoeias

British Herbal Pharmacopoeia. Bournemouth: British Herbal Medicine Assn., 1990.

British Pharmacopoeia. London: Her Majesty's Stationery Office, 1980.

British Pharmacopoeia (Veterinary). London: Her Majesty's Stationery Office, 1977.

The Merck Index. preferably 3rd ed. (1907); now on 10th ed. Rahway: Merck & Co.

United States Pharmacopoeias. eds. pre-WWII.

European Pharmacopoeia. 2nd ed. Sainte-Ruffine: Maisonneuve, 1980.

The Homeopathic Pharmacopoeia of the United States. 8th ed. Published under the direction of the Pharmacopoeia Convention of the American Institute of Homeopathy. Falls Church: American Institute of Homeopathy, 1979.

The International Pharmacopoeia. 3rd ed. Geneva: World Health Organization, 1977.

United States Pharmacopoeia. 21st rev. The National Formulary, 16th ed. United States Pharmacopoeial Convention, Inc., 1984.

Martindale: The Extra Pharmacopoeia. 28th ed. Edited by James E. F. Reynolds and Anne B. Prasad. London: The Pharmaceutical Press, 1982.

Pharmacy and Medicine Making

Green, James. *The Herbal Medicine Maker's Handbook.* Forestville: Simpler's Botanical Co. (Box 39, Forestville, CA 95436).

Cook & LaWall. *Remington's Practice of Pharmacy.* 8th ed. Philadelphia: J.B. Lippincott, 1936.

U.S. National Formulary. eds. pre-WWII.

Dittert, Lewis W., ed. *Sprowls' American Pharmacy: An Introduction to Pharmaceutical Techniques and Dosage Forms.* 7th ed. Philadelphia: J.B. Lippincott, 1974.

Remington's Pharmaceutical Sciences. 17th ed. Edited by Alfonso R. Gennaro. Easton: Mack Publishing Co., 1985.

Pharmaceutical Handbook: Incorporating the Pharmaceutical Pocket Book. 19th ed. Produced in the Department of Pharmaceutical Sciences, the Pharmaceutical Society of Great Britain. Edited by Ainley Wade. London: The Pharmaceutical Society, 1980.

The Pharmaceutical Recipe Book. 3rd ed. Washington, DC: American Pharmaceutical Association, 1943.

Pharmacological Research

Craker & Simon. *Herbs, Spices and Medicinal Plants.* Vol. 1-4. Oryx Press, 1987.

Funfgeld, E. W. *Rökan, Ginkgo biloba.* Springer Verlag, 1988.

Harborne, J.B. *Introduction to Ecological Biochemistry.* San Diego: Academic Press, 1982.

Wagner, Hikino & Farnsworth. *Economic & Medicinal Plant Research, Vol. 1.* San Diego: Academic Press, 1985.

Wagner, Hikino & Farnsworth. *Economic & Medicinal Plant Research, Vol. 2.* San Diego: Academic Press, 1988.

Wagner & Farnsworth. *Economic and Medicinal Plant Research, Vol. 4. Plants and Traditional Medicine.* San Diego: Academic Press, 1990.

Toxicology

Brinker, Francis. *An Introduction to the Toxicology of Common Botanical Medicines.* National College of Naturopathic Medicine, 1983.

De Smet, Keller, Hansel, Chandler. *Adverse Effects of Herbal Drugs, Vol 1.* New York: Springer Verlag, 1992.

Frohne, Dietrich, and Hans Jürgen Pfander. *A Colour Atlas of Poisonous Plants: A Handbook for Pharmacists, Doctors, Toxicologists, and Biologists.* London: Wolfe Publishing Ltd., 1984.

Fuller, T. *Poisonous Plants of California.* Berkeley: U. C. Press, 1987.

Handbook of Natural Toxins. Edited by Richard J. Keeler and Anthony T. Tu. New York: Marcel Dekker, 1983.

Mitchell, John, and Arthur Rook. *Botanical Dermatology: Plants and Plant Products Injurious to the Skin.* Vancouver: Greenglass, 1979.

Lampe, Kenneth F., and Mary Ann McCann. *AMA Handbook of Poisonous and Injurious Plants.* Chicago: American Medical Association; Chicago: Chicago Review Press, 1985.

Ethnobotany

Akerele, Heywood, Synge. *Conservation of Medicinal Plants.* New York: Cambridge Univ. Press, 1991.

Ayensu, Edward. *Medicinal Plants of West Africa.* Algonac: Reference Publications, 1978.

Bastien, Joseph. *Healers of the Andes: Kallawaya Herbalists and Their Medicinal Plants.* Salt Lake City: University Press of Utah, 1987.

Bhagwan Dash, Vaidya. *Materia Medica of Indo-Tibetan Medicine.* Delhi, Classics India Publication, 1987.

Boulos, Loufty. *Medicinal Plants of North Africa.* Algonac: Reference Publications, 1983.

Caius. *Medicinal and Poisonous Plants of India.* Jodhpur: Scientific Publishers, 1986.

Caius. *Medicinal and Poisonous Legumes of India.* Jodhpur: Scientific Publishers, 1988.

Cutler. *Uses of Plants by the Indians of the Missouri River Region.* Lincoln: University of Nebraska Press, 1977.

Gunther, Erna. *Ethnobotany of Western Washington: The Knowledge and Use of Indigenous Plants by Native Americans.* 4th ed. University of Washington Press, 1973.

Husain, Akhtar. *Major Essential Oil-Bearing Plants of India.* Lucknow: Central Institute of Medicinal and Aromatic Plants, 1988.

Hutchens, Alma. *Indian Herbology of North America.* Magnolia: Peter Smith Pub., 1992.

Jianzhe, Xiaolan, Qiming, Yichen, Huaan. *Icones of Medicinal Fungi from China.* Beijing: Science Press, 1987.

Moerman, Daniel. *Geraniums for the Iroquois.* Algonac: Reference Publications Inc., 1981.

National Institute for the Control of Pharmaceutical and Biological Products. *Colour Atlas of Chinese Traditional Drugs, Vol. 1.* Beijing: Science Press, 1987.

Ortiz de Montellano. *Aztec Medicine, Health & Nutrition.* New Brunswick: Rutgers Univ. Press, 1990.

Ott, Jonathan. *Hallucinogenic Plants of North America.* Oakland: Wingbow Press, 1976.

Prance, G. T. *Leaves: The Formation, Characteristics and Uses of Hundreds of Leaves Found in All Parts of the World.* New York: Crown Publishers, 1985.

Satyavati. *Medicinal Plants of India, Vol. 2.* New Delhi: India Council of Medical Research, 1987.

Schultes & Hofmann. *Plants of the Gods.* Hutchinson Publishing Group, 1979.

Soejarto & Gyllenhall. *Elements for a Caribbean Pharmacopoeia.* Santo Domingo: Enda-Caribe, 1988.

Train, Henrichs & Archer. *Medicinal Uses of Plants by Indian Tribes of Nevada.* Lincoln: Quarterman, 1990.

Vogel, Virgil. *American Indian Medicine.* Norman: University of Oklahoma Press, 1990.

Chinese, Ayurvedic, Unani Herbals

The cultural blinkers placed on us by the dominant culture have meant that, until recently, the profoundly holistic therapeutic systems of the rest of the world have been largely unknown in the West. There are now a number of excellent books available on these systems, but as neophytes in this aspect of herbal medicine, the author cannot give a meaningful book guide. Listed below are those that I personally use extensively, but there are many other excellent ones available.

Beinfield & Korngold. *Between Heaven and Earth: A Guide to Chinese Medicine.* New York: Ballantine, 1992.

Bensky & Gamble. *Chinese Herbal Medicine—Materia Medica.* Seattle: Eastland Press, 1986.

Frawley, David. *Ayurvedic Healing: A Comprehensive Guide.* Sandy: Morson Pub., 1990.

Hakim, Chishti. *The Traditional Healer's Handbook.* Rochester: Inner Traditions, 1988.

Kapoor. *CRC Handbook of Ayurvedic Medicinal Plants.* Boca Raton: CRC Press, 1990.

Lad/Frawley. *The Yoga of Herbs: An Ayurvedic Guide to Herbal Medicine.* Santa Fe: Lotus Press, 1986.

Tierra, Michael & Lesley. *Chinese-Planetary Herbal Diagnosis.* Santa Cruz: East West Herb School, 1988.

Vasant, Lad. *Ayurveda: The Science of Self-Healing—A Practical Guide.* Santa Fe: Lotus Press, 1984.

The Blue Poppy Press (1775 Linden Ave., Boulder, CO 80302, (303) 442-0796) is specializing in English translations of Chinese medical texts oriented to the practitioner.

Peer Review Journals

There are a number of scientific journals that focus on subjects that are often of immediate relevance to herbalists. These journals can be found in most university libraries, or abstracts can be found via on-line services such as Medline.

Advances in Economic Botany. Vol. 1. Bronx: New York Botanical Garden, 1984.

Current Topics in Medical Mycology. Vol. 1. New York: Springer Verlag, 1985.

Economic Botany. Vol. 1. New York: New York Botanical Garden, 1947.

Fitoterapia: The Journal of Research & Applications of Medicinal Plants. Inverni della Beffa.

Herb, Spice and Medicinal Plant Digest. Univ. of Mass. Coop. Ext., Stockbridge Hall, Univ. of Mass., Amherst, MA 01003

Herba Hungarica. Hungarian Research Institute for Medicinal Plants, Budapest, Hungary.

Journal of Ethnopharmacology. Vol. 1. Lausanne, Elsevier.

Journal of Natural Products (Lloydia). Vol. 1. Cincinnati: Lloyd Library and Museum and The American Society of Pharmacognosy, 1938.

Journal of Naturopathic Medicine. 54 Lafayette Place, Greenwich, CT 06830.

Phytochemistry. Vol. 1. Elmsford: Pergamon Press, 1962.

Phytotherapy Research. Heydon & Son Ltd., Spectrum House, Hillview Gardens, London, England NW 12 JQ.

Planta Medica. Vol. 1. Stuttgart: Thieme, 1953.

Via Ripamonti 99, 20141. Milan, Italy.

Zeitschrift für Phytotherapie. Thieme Medical Publishers, 381 Park Ave., South New York, NY 10016.

Many journals occasionally publish papers that relate to the field even though the focus of the journal is different. The following listing is very international in outlook and some of these journals are difficult to find in U.S. universities. However, they can all be found via interlibrary loan.

Acta Chimica Sinica (Beijing, China)
Acta Pharmaceutica Hungarica (Budapest, Hungary)
Acta Pharmaceutica Jugoslavica (Zagreb, Yugoslavia)
Acta Pharmaceutica Sinica (Beijing, China)
Acta Pharmaceutical Suecica (Stockholm, Sweden)
Acta Pharmaceutica Toxicoligia (Copenhagen, Denmark)
Acta Poloniae Pharmaceutica (Warsaw, Poland)
African Journal of Pharmacy and Pharmaceutical Sciences (Apapa, Nigeria)
Agents and Actions (Basel, Switzerland)
Agricultural and Biological Chemistry (Tokyo, Japan)
American Journal of Clinical Nutrition (Bethesda, MD, USA)
Anais de Farmacia E Quimica de Sao Paulo (Records of Pharmaceuticals and Chemicals of Sao Paulo) (Sao Paulo, Brazil)
Anales de Quimica, Serie C Bioquimica (Madrid, Spain)
Anales de la Real Academia de Farmacia (Madrid, Spain)
Ancient Science of Life (Coimbatore, India)
Annales Pharmaceutiques Françaises (Paris, France)
Antiseptic (Madras, India)
Archiv der Pharmazie (Weinheim) (Weinheim, Germany)
Archives of Dermatology (Chicago, IL, USA)
Archives Internationales de Pharmacodynamie et de Therapie (Ghent, Belgium)
Archives of Pharmaceutical Research (Seoul) (Seoul, Korea)
Arzneimittel Forschung (Aulendorf, Germany)
Atherosclerosis (Amsterdam, Netherlands)
Bangladesh Medical Journal (Dacca, Bangladesh)
Bangladesh Pharmaceutical Journal (Dacca, Bangladesh)
Biochemical and Biophysical Research Communications (New York, USA)
Biochemical Pharmacology (Oxford, England)
Boletim da Faculdade de Farmacia de Coimbra (Coimbra, Portugal)
Bollettino Chimico Farmaceutico (Milan, Italy)
Bollettino della Societa Italiana di Farmacia Ospedaliera (Turin, Italy)
British Medical Journal (London, England)
Bulletin of the Department of Medical Sciences (Bangkok, Thailand)
Bulletin of Faculty of Pharmacy, Cairo University (Cairo, Egypt)
Bulletin of Medico-Ethnobotanical Research (New Delhi, India)
Bulletin on Narcotics (Geneva, Switzerland)
Carbohydrate Research (Amsterdam, Netherlands)
Chemical and Pharmaceutical Bulletin (Tokyo, Japan)
Chemical and Druggist (London, England)
Chemistry and Industry (London, England)
Chemistry Letters (Tokyo, Japan)
Chinese Journal of Integrated Traditional and Western Medicine (Beijing, China)
Chinese Medical Journal (Beijing, China)

Clinical Pharmacology and Therapeutics (St. Louis, MO, USA)
Clinical Toxicology (New York, USA)
Clujul Medical (Cluj-Napoca, Romania)
Comptes Rendus de l'Académie Bulgare des Sciences (Sofia, Bulgaria)
Comptes Rendus de l'Académie des Sciences, Paris (Paris, France)
Contraception (California, USA)
Current Medical Practice (Bombay, India)
Current Science (Bangalore, India)
Deutsche Apotheker Zeitung (Stuttgart, Germany)
Drug and Cosmetic Industry (New York, USA)
Drug Information Bulletin (Maple Glen, USA)
East African Pharmaceutical Journal (Nairobi, Kenya)
Eastern Pharmacist (New Delhi, India)
Economic Botany (New York, USA)
Egyptian Journal of Chemistry (Cairo, Egypt)
Egyptian Journal of Pharmaceutical Sciences (Cairo, Egypt)
Egyptian Journal of Phytopathology (Cairo, Egypt)
Ethnomedizin (Hamburg, Germany)
Experimentia (Basel, Switzerland)
Farmatsevtichnyi Zhurnal (Ljubljana, Yugoslavia)
Farmacia (Bucharest) (Bucharest, Romania)
Farmacia (Pavia) (Pavia, Italy)
Farmaco, Edizione Practica (Milan, Italy)
Farmaco, Edizione Scientifica (Milan, Italy)
Farmatsevtichnyi Zhurnal (Kiev, USSR)
Farmatsiya (Moscow) (Moscow, USSR)
FEBS Letters (Amsterdam, Netherlands)
Fitoterapia (Milan, Italy)
Food and Chemical Toxicology (Oxford, England)
Gazzetta Chimica Italiana (Rome, Italy)
General Pharmacology (Oxford, England)
Geobios (Jodhpur) (Jodhpur, India)
Helvetica Chimica Acta (Basel, Switzerland)
Herba Hungarica (Budapest, Hungary)
Herba Polonica (Warsaw, Poland)
Heterocycles (Sendai, Japan)
Indian Drugs (Bombay, India)
Indian Drugs and Pharmaceuticals Industry (Bombay, India)
Indian Forester (Dehradun, India)
Indian Journal of Chemistry, Part B (New Delhi, India)
Indian Journal of Experimental Biology (New Delhi, India)
Indian Journal of Forestry (Dehradun, India)
Indian Journal of Medical Research (New Delhi, India)
Indian Journal of Nematology (New Delhi, India)
Indian Journal of Pharmaceutical Sciences (Bombay, India)
Indian Journal of Pharmacology (Varanasi, India)
Indian Medical Gazette (Calcutta, India)

Indian Perfumer (Jammu, India)
Indian Practitioner (Bombay, India)
International Journal of Crude Drug Research (Lisse, Netherlands)
Japanese Journal of Pharmacology (Kyoto, Japan)
Journal of African Medicinal Plants (Cairo, Egypt)
Journal of Agricultural and Food Chemistry (Washington, DC, USA)
Journal of the Association of Official Analytical Chemists (Washington, DC, USA)
Journal of Chemical Research (S) (London, England)
Journal of Chemical Society, Chemical Communications (London, England)
Journal of Chemical Society of Pakistan (Karachi, Pakistan)
Journal of Chemical Society, Perkin Transactions I (London, England)
Journal of Chromatography (Amsterdam, Netherlands)
Journal of Clinical Pharmacology (Connecticut, USA)
Journal of Drug Research (Cairo) (Cairo, Egypt)
Journal of Economic and Taronomic Botany (Jodhpur, India)
Journal of Ethnopharmacology (Lausanne, Switzerland)
Journal of Food Science (Illinois, USA)
Journal of Food Science and Technology (Mysore, India)
Journal of Indian Chemical Society (Calcutta, India)
Journal of Korean Pharmaceutical Sciences (Seoul, South Korea)
Journal of the National Integrated Medical Association (Mysore, India)
Journal of the National Research Council of Thailand (Bangkok, Thailand)
Journal of Natural Products (Lloydia) (Ohio, USA)
Journal of Organic Chemistry (Washington, DC, USA)
Journal of Pharmaceutical Sciences (Washington, DC, USA)
Journal of Pharmaceutical Society of Korea (Seoul, Korea)
Journal de Pharmacie de Belgique (Brussels, Belgium)
Journal of Pharmacy and Pharmacology (London, England)
Journal of Pharmacobio-Dynamics (Tokyo, Japan)
Journal of Pharmacology Experimental Therapeutics (Baltimore, USA)
Journal of Research in Ayurveda and Siddha (New Delhi, India)
Journal of Research Institute of Medical Sciences of Korea (Seoul, South Korea)
Journal of Food Science and Agriculture (London, England)
Journal of Scientific Research in Plants and Medicine (Hardwar, India)
Journal of Science Society of Thailand (Bangkok, Thailand)
Journal of Tropical Forestry (Jabalpur) (Jabalpur, India)
Khimiko-Farmatsevticheskii Zhurnal (Moscow, USSR)
Khimiya Prirodnykh Soedinenii (Tashkent, USSR)
Korean Journal of Internal Medicine (Seoul, South Korea)
Korean Journal of Pharmacognosy (Seoul, South Korea)
Korean Journal of Pharmacology (Seoul, South Korea)
Lancet (London, England)
Lawrence Review of Natural Products (Collegeville, PA, USA)
Lebensmittel-Wissenschaftlische und Technologie (Zurich, Switzerland)
Liebigs Annales Chemie (Weinheim, Germany)
Mahidol University Journal of Pharmaceutical Sciences (Bangkok,Thailand)
Medicina Traditional (Mexico)

Lipids (Champaign, IL, USA)
Nagarjun (Calcutta, India)
National Academy of Science Letters (New Delhi, India)
Naturwissenschaften (Heidelberg, Germany)
Naunyn-Schmiedeberg's Archives of Pharmacology (Heidelberg, Germany)
Nippon Nogeikagaku Kaishi (Tokyo, Japan)
Official Journal of Research Institute of Medical Sciences of Korea (Seoul, South Korea)
Pafai Journal (Bombay, India)
Pakistan Journal of Forestry (Peshawar, India)
Parfumerie und Kosmetik (Heidelberg, Germany)
Perfumer and Flavorist (Illinois, USA)
Parfums, Cosmetiques Aromes (Paris, France)
Parfums, Cosmetiques, Savons de France (Incorporating La France et ses Parfums) (Paris, France)
Pharmaceutica Acta Helvetica (Zurich, Switzerland)
Pharmaceutical Research Institute: Bulletin (Osaka, Japan)
Pharmaceutisch Weekblad (Amsterdam, Netherlands)
Pharmacological Research Communications (London, England)
Pharmacology (Basel, Switzerland)
Pharmazeutische Industrie (Aulendorf, Germany)
Pharmazeutische Rundschau (Heusenstamm, Germany)
Pharmazie in Unserer Zeit (Weinheim, Germany)
Pharmazeutische Zeitung (Frankfurt, Germany)
Pharmazie (Dresden, Germany)
Pharmindex (Portland, OR, USA)
Physicians' Drug Manual (New York, USA)
Phytochemistry (Oxford, England)
Plant Disease Reporter (Washington, DC, USA)
Plant Science Letters (Limerick, Ireland)
Planta Medica (Stuttgart, Germany)
Plantes Medicinales et Phytotherapie (Angers, France)
Polish Journal of Pharmacology and Pharmacy (Warsaw, Poland)
Rastitel'nye Resursy (Moscow, USSR)
Research Communications in Chemical Pathology and Pharmacology (New York, USA)
Revista de Ciencias Farmaceuticas (Sao Paulo, Brazil)
Revista Colombiana de Ciencias Quimica Farmaceuticas (Bogota, Columbia)
Revista Cubana de Farmacia (Havana, Cuba)
Revista Farmaceutica (Buenos Aires, Argentina)
Revista Latinoamericana de Quimica (Monterrey, Mexico)
Rheumatism (New Delhi, India)
Rivista Italiana Essenze Profumi, Piante Officinali, Aromi, Saponi, Cosmetici, Aerosol (Review of the Italian perfume essences, herbs, aromas, soaps, cosmetics and aerosol industries) (Milan, Italy)
Sachitra Ayurved (Patna, India)
Science and Culture (Calcutta, India)

Scientia Pharmaceutica (Vienna, Austria)
Scientia Sinica (Beijing, China)
Seoul University Journal (Seoul, South Korea)
Siriraj Hospital Gazette (Bangkok, Thailand)
Shoyakugaku Zasshi (The Japanese Journal of Pharmacognosy) (Tokyo, Japan)
Songklanaharian Journal of Science and Technology (Bangkok, Thailand)
Svensk Farmaceutisk Tidskrift (Stockholm, Sweden)
Taxon (Utrecht, Netherlands)
Tetrahedron (Oxford, England)
Tetrahedron Letters (Oxford, England)
Timisoara Medicala (Timisoara, Romania)
Toxicology (Amsterdam, Netherlands)
Toxicology and Applied Pharmacology (New York, USA)
Toxicology Letters (Amsterdam, Netherlands)
Toxicon (London, England)
Tropical Science (Surrey, England)
Vagbhata (Trivandrum, India)
Vastik Sel'skokhozyaistvennoi Nauki (Moscow, USSR)
Yakhak Hoeji (Seoul, South Korea)
Yakugaku Zasshi (Pharmaceutical Society of Japan Journal) (Tokyo, Japan)
Zeitschrift Naturforschungs Wissenschaftliche (Tubingen, Germany)
Zeitschrift für Phytotherapie (Munich, Germany)

Abstracts, Bibliographies, Indexes and Databases

To facilitate research and access to the information contained in such a vast sea of papers, a number of services have been established that index and abstract in specific fields of interest. Those most relevant for phytotherapeutic material include:

Andrews, Theodora, with the assistance of William L. Corya & Donald A. Stickel, Jr. *A Bibliography on Herbs, Herbal Medicine, "Natural" Foods, and Unconventional Medical Treatment.* Littleton: Libraries Unlimited, 1982.

Bibliography of Agriculture. Vol. 1. Phoenix, AZ: Oryx Press, 1942.

Biological Abstracts. Vol. 1. Philadelphia: BioSciences Information Service, 1927. Semimonthly. Appropriate Sections: Agronomy, Botany, Economic Botany, Pharmacognosy and Pharmaceutical Botany, Pharmacology, Plant Physiology, Biochemistry and Biophysics, and Toxicology.

Biological Abstracts/RRM (Reports, Reviews, Meetings). Vol. 18. Philadelphia: BioSciences Information Service, 1980.

Biological and Agricultural Index. Vol. 1. New York: H. W. Wilson, 1916.

Botanical Abstracts. Vols. 1-15. Baltimore, MD: Williams and Wilkins, 1918-26.

Bulletin Signaletique (Paris, France). Monthly. Appropriate Sections: Part 171: Chimie; Part 310: Genie Biomedicale Informatique Biomedicale; Part 330: Sciences Pharmacologique Toxicologie.

Chemical Abstracts. Vol. 1. Columbus, OH: Chemical Abstracts Service, 1907. Weekly. Appropriate Sections: 30: Terpenes & Terpenoids; 31: Alkaloids; 32: Steroids; 33: Carbohydrates; 34: Amino Acid Peptides & Proteins; 45: Industrial Organic Chemicals; Ethers, Fats and Waxes; 63: Pharmaceuticals; 64: Pharmaceutical Analysis, Pharmacology Plant Biochemistry, Biochemical Methods.

Current Advances in Plant Science (Oxford, England). Monthly. Relevant headings are secondary products: Terpenoids, Alkaloids, Flavonoids, Phenolics and Others.

Current Contents (Philadelphia, USA). Weekly. Editions: a. Agriculture, Biology and Environmental Sciences; b. Life Sciences; c. Physical, Chemical and Earth Sciences; and d. Clinical Practice.

Current Research on Medicinal and Aromatic Plants (Lucknow, India). Quarterly Abstracts divided into 10 subheadings.

Excerpta Medica (Amsterdam, Netherlands). Monthly. Section: Pharmacology and Toxicology.

Horticultural Abstracts (Slough, England). Monthly. Medicinal Plants mostly occur under Minor Temperate & Tropical Industrial Crops which are further subdivided under Condiments & Spice Plants; Essential Oil Plants; Insecticidal & Pesticidal Plants; Medicinal Plants.

Index Medicus (Bethesda, MD, USA). Monthly. Information on medicinal plants is mainly found under: Plant Extracts; Plant Poisoning; Plants, Medicinal; and Plants, Toxic.

International Pharmaceutical Abstracts (Washington, DC, USA). Bimonthly.

Lynn Index, A Bibliography of Phytochemistry. Vols. 1-5. Organized and edited by J. W. Schermerhorn & M. W. Quimby. Boston: Massachusetts College of Pharmacy, 1957-1962. Vol. 6 by Norman R. Farnsworth. Pittsburgh, PA: University of Pittsburgh, 1969. Vols. 7-8 by Norman R. Farnsworth. Chicago: University of Illinois at the Medical Center, 1972-74.

Medicinal and Aromatic Plants Abstracts. New Delhi, India: Publications and Information Directorate, 1979. Bimonthly. World literature on medicinal plants is covered under 16 subject headings.

Pharmaceutical Abstracts. Austin, TX: University of Texas College of Pharmacy, 1957-1969.

Pharmaceutical Abstracts. Washington, DC: American Pharmaceutical Association, 1935-1948.

Pharmacognosy Titles. Chicago, IL: Department of Pharmacognosy and Pharmacology, College of Pharmacy, University of Illinois at the Medical Center, 1966-1974.

Simon, James E., Alena F. Chadwick, and Lyle E. Craker. **Temperate Herbs: An Indexed Bibliography.** 1971-1980: The Scientific Literature on Selected Herbs, and Aromatic and Medicinal Plants of the Temperate Zone. Hamden, CT: Shoe String, 1984.

Zanoni, Thomas, and Eileen Schofield. *Dyes from Plants: An Annotated List of References.* New York: Council on Botanical and Horticultural Libraries, Library of the New York Botanical Garden, 1983.

Professional Phytotherapy Journals

The British Journal of Phytotherapy. Bucksteep Manor, Bodle St. Green, Nr. Hailsham, E. Sussex, U.K. BN 27 4RJ

The Canadian Journal of Herbalism. 181 Brookdale Ave., Toronto, Ontario, Canada M5M 1P4

Australian Journal of Medical Herbalism. P.O. Box 65, Kingsgrove, N.S.W. 2208, Australia

Journal of the Ontario Herbalists Association. 7 Alpine Ave., Toronto, Ontario, Canada M6P 3R6

Dittany: Journal of the Herb Federation of New Zealand. P.O. Box 20022, Glen Eden, Auckland, N. Z.

Newsletters and Magazines

American Ginseng Trends. P.O. Box 1982, Wausau, WI 54402-1982

American Herb Association, Quarterly Newsletter. P.O. Box 353, Rescue, CA 95672

Canadian Herbal Practitioners Newsletter. 302 Kensington Rd. N.W., Calgary, Alberta, Canada T2N 3P5

Coltsfoot. Rt. 1, P.O. Box 313A, Shipman, VA 22971

Foster's Botanical and Herb Reviews. P.O. Box 106, Eureka Springs, AR 72632

Herbal Review. The Herb Society Newsletter, 34 Boscobel Place, London, England SW 1W 9PE

*HerbalGram.** P.O. Box 201660, Austin, TX 78720

Herban Lifestyles. 84 Carpenter Rd., Apt. 78711-1, New Hartford, CT 06057

Homeopathic Research Reports. 5916 Chabot Crest, Oakland, CA 94618

It's Essential—Journal of Aromatherapy. c/o E-scentially Yours, 237-A East 53rd St., New York, NY 10022

Medical Herbalism. P.O. Box 33080, Portland, OR 97233

Quintessence Aromatherapy. P.O. Box 4996, Boulder, CO 80306

The Bu$iness of Herbs. Northwind Farm, Rt. 2, P.O. Box 246(G), Shevlin, MN 56676

The Herb Companion. Interweave Press, 201 East Fourth Street, Loveland, CO 80537

* HerbalGram also offers an exceptional series of reprints from other journals and historical sources. These are called the classical botanical reprint series.

The Herb Market Report. 525 SE H St., Grant's Pass, OR 97526

The Herb Quarterly. P.O. Box 548, Boiling Springs, PA 17007

The Herb Report. P.O. Box 95-3333, Stuart, FL 33495

The Ozark Herbalist. Rt. 4, P.O. Box 730, Oak Grove, AR 72660

Today's Herbs. Woodland Books, P.O. Box 1422, Provo, UT 84603

Classic Botanical Reprints

Volume I

#201 *Traditional Medicines: The Indian Scenario* by S. B. Goel. Reprinted with permission from the *International Traditional Medicine Newsletter*, Vol. 3, Issue 2, Spring 1989. 4 pages.

#202 *Introduction: Folk Lore and Folk Medicines* by John Scarborough, editor. Reprinted from *Folk Lore and Folk Medicines*, 1987, with permission of the American Institute of the History of Pharmacy. 8 pages.

#203 *John Uri Lloyd, Phr.M., Ph.D., 1849 - 1936,* by Varro E. Tyler and Virginia M. Tyler. Reprinted from the *Journal of Natural Products*, Vol. 50, No. 1, January/February 1987. 12 pages.

#204 *High Pharmaceutical Prices Call for Government-Sponsored Natural Drug Research* by James A. Duke, Ph.D. Reprinted from *HerbalGram*, Vol. 1, No. 4, Winter 1984. Rev. July 1989. 4 pages.

#205 *The Economic Significance of Herbs* by Portia Meares. Reprinted from *HerbalGram*, No. 13, Summer, 1987. Rev. July 1989. 8 pages.

#206 *Ethnobotany: Historical Diversity and Synthesis* by Richard I. Ford. Reprinted from *The Nature and Status of Ethnobotany*, Museum of Anthropology, University of Michigan, 1984. 20 pages.

#207 *Plant Drugs in the 21st Century* by Varro E. Tyler, Ph.D. Reprinted from *Economic Botany* 40(3), 1986, pp. 279-288. 12 pages.

#208 *Tropical Rain Forests: Potential Sources of New Drugs?* by D. D. Soejarto and N.R. Farnsworth. 1989. Reprinted with permission from *Perspectives in Biology and Medicine* 32(2):244-256. 16 pages.

#209 *The Present and Future of Pharmacognosy* by N. R. Farnsworth. Reprinted with permission from the *American Journal of Pharmaceutical Education* 43:239-243 (1979). 8 pages.

#210 *A New Look at Botanical Medicine* by Andrew Weil. Reprinted with permission from *Whole Earth Review*, No. 64, Fall 1989. 8 pages.

#211 *Higher Plants— Sleeping Giants of Drug Development* by Farnsworth & Morris. Reprinted with permission from the *American Journal of Pharmacy*. Vol. 147, No. 2, March/April 1976: 46-52. 8 pages.

#212 *Medicinal Plants in Therapy* from *Bulletin of the World Health Organization* 63(6):965-981 (1985). 20 pages.

#213 *Conservation, Ethnobotany, and the Search for New Jungle Medicines: Pharmacognosy Comes of Age . . . Again* by Mark J. Plotkin, Ph.D. Reprinted with permission from *Pharmacotherapy*, Vol. 8, No. 5, 1988. pp. 257-262. 8 pages.

#214 *Classic Botanical Reprints—Vol. I.* Complete set of reprints #201-213.

Volume II

#215 *What Is Herbal Medicine?* by R. F. Weiss. Reproduced from *Herbal Medicine* by R. F. Weiss, M. D., 1988. By permission of Beaconsfield Publishers, Ltd., Beaconsfield, England. Available from the publishers of, or from: *Medicina Biologica*, 2037 NE Flanders St., Portland, OR 97232. 12 pages.

#216 *Gifts of the Amazon Flora to the World* by R. E. Schultes. Reprinted with permission from *Arnoldia* 50(2):21-34. Copyright President & Fellows of Harvard College. 16 pages .

#217 *Information Gathering and Databases That Are Pertinent to the Development of Plant-Derived Drugs* by N. R. Farnsworth and W. D. Loub. Reprinted with permission from U. S. Congress, Office of Technology Assessment, *Plants: The Potential for Extracting Protein, Medicines, and Other Useful Chemicals*, pp. 178-195. Workshop Proceedings OTA-BP-F-23 (Springfield, VA: National Technical Information Service, September 1983). 16 pages.

#218 *Ginseng Research: The Root of the Issue* by Mark Blumenthal. Reprinted with permission of *Herbs!* March/April 1987. 4 pages.

#219 *The Need for Cooperation Between Modern and Traditional Medicine* by Ara Der Madersonian. Reprinted with permission of the author. *HerbalGram* #24. 12 pages.

#220 *Medicinal Plants and Primary Health Care: An Agenda for Action* by O. Akerele. *Fitoterapia* 59(5):355-63. Reprinted with permission from *Fitoterapia*. 12 pages.

#221 *Plant Pharmacy* by J. U. Lloyd. *American Journal of Pharmacy*, April 1922, pp. 1-7. Reprinted with permission from the *American Journal of Pharmacy*.

#222 *Medicine and Drugs in Colonial America* by Ara Der Madersonian and Mukund S. Yelvigi. *American Journal of Pharmacy*, July-August 1976, pp. 113-120. Reprinted with permission from the *American Journal of Pharmacy*. 8 pages.

#223 *Debunking the Ginseng Abuse Syndrome* by Mark Blumenthal. *Whole Foods*, March 1991. Reprinted with permission from *Whole Foods*. 12 pages.

#224 *Ginkgos and People—A Thousand Years of Interaction* by Peter Del Tredici. *Arnoldia*, Summer 1991, pp. 3 -15. Reprinted with permission from *Arnoldia*. 16 pages.

#225 **The Duke of Herbs** by Richard Leviton. *East West*, Sept./Oct. 1991, pp. 66-76. Reprinted with permission from *East West*. 12 pages.

#226 **Classic Botanical Reprints Vol. II.** Complete set of reprints #215-225.

#227 **Natural Products and Medicine: An Overview** by Varro E. Tyler. Presented at the symposium, "Tropical Forest Medical Resources and the Conservation of Biodiversity," sponsored by the Rainforest Alliance's Periwinkle Project and the New York Botanical Garden's Institute of Economic Botany, The Rockefeller University, New York City, January 24-25, 1992. 8 pages.

#228 **Natural Products and the Potential Role of the Pharmaceutical Industry in Tropical Forest Conservation** by C. Findeisen, Sarah Laird, ed. Report prepared by the Rainforest Alliance. 12 pages.

#229 **Ethnobotany and the Identification of Therapeutic Agents from the Rainforest** by M. J. Balick. D. J. Chadwick and J. Marsh, eds. 1990. Bioactive Compounds from Plants. Chichester & New York, John Wiley & Sons (Ciba Foundation Symposium 154). 16 pages.

#230 **Medicinal Plant Production: Breaking into the Marketplace** by Steven Foster. Reprinted from IHCMA Newsletter, September 1992. 8 pages.

#231 **Ancient and Medieval Chemotherapy for Cancer** by John Riddle. Reprinted from ISIS 76:319/330. 1985. 12 pages.

#232 **Oral Contraceptives in Ancient and Medieval Medicines** by John Riddle. Reprinted by permission of *American Scientist, Journal of Sigma Xi*, the Scientific Research Society. May/June 1992. 12 pages.

#233 **Tales from the Healing Forest** by John Simon. Reprinted from *World, Journal of the Unitarian Universalist Association*, Vol. VI, No. 3, May/June 1992, pp. 17-25. 12 pages.

#234 **WHO Guidelines for the Assessment of Herbal Medicines** by O. Akerele, M.D. Reprinted from *Fitoterapia*, Vol. LXII, No. 2, 1991, pp. 99-110. 12 pages.

#235 **The Materia Medica of Christopher Columbus** by George Griffenhagell. Reprinted by permission of *Pharmacy in History*. 1992. 16 pages.

#236 **Medicinal Ornamentals** by Steven Foster. Reprinted from *Fine Gardening*, September 1988. 4 pages.

#237 **World Aspects of Phytotherapy** by Barbara Steinhoff. Reprinted by permission of *European Phytotelegram*, No. 4, July 1992, pp. 5-9. 8 pages.

#238 **Materia Medica Americana: An Historical Review** by John Uri Lloyd. 1900. Reprinted by permission of *American Druggist and Pharmaceutical Record*. 12 pages.

Herbal Organizations

United States

Herbalism in the United States is in the paradoxical position of experiencing a flowering of interest in all its aspects, yet having few educational avenues to explore. This is one of the very few developed countries where Medical Herbalism is not legally recognized, making professional training a challenge! A move to change this anachronistic state of affairs has started with the launching of the American Herbalists Guild. A professional body dedicated to the promotion of excellence in herbalism, it is committed to the development of high educational and ethical standards in the practice and integration of herbalism into community health care. The guild provides a list of practitioners and herbal education around the country. For more information contact: **The American Herbalist Guild, P.O. Box 1683, Soquel, CA 95073.**

Other relevant organizations are:

American Aromatherapy Association. P.O. Box 606, San Rafael, CA 94915

American Herb Association. P.O. Box 353, Rescue, CA 96672

American Herb Product Association. 7353 El Tomaso Way, Buena Park, CA 90620

Herb Research Foundation. 1007 Pearl St., Suite 200, Boulder, CO 80302, (303) 449-2265

International Herb Growers & Marketers Association. P.O. Box 281, Silver Springs, PA 17575

Northeast Herbal Association. P. O. Box 146, Marshfield, VT 05658-0146

Rocky Mountain Herbalist Coalition. Salina Star Route, Boulder, CO 80302

South-West Herbalists Association. P.O. Box 74, Ojo Caliente, NM 87549

United Kingdom

British Herb Grower's Association. 17 Hooker St., London SW3

British Herbal Medicine Association. Field House, Lye Hole, Redhill, Avon BS18 7TB

British Holistic Medical Association. 179 Gloucester Place, London NW1 6DX

Council for Complementary and Alternative Medicine (CCAM). 10 Belgrave Square, London SW1X 8PH

Research Council for Complementary Medicine (RCCM). Suite 1A, Cavendish Square, London W1M 9AD

The National Institute of Medical Herbalists. 41 Hatherley Rd., Winchester, Hants SO22 6RR

The School of Phytotherapy. 148 Forest Rd., Tunbridge Wells, Kent TN2 5EY

Canada

The Ontario Herbalists Association. 181 Brookdale Ave., Toronto, Ontario, M5M 1P4

New Zealand

The College of Naturopathic Medicine. P.O. Box 4529, Christchurch, New Zealand

Australia

National Herbalists Association of Australia. P.O. Box 65, Kingsgrove, N.S.W. 2208, Australia

Chapter 4

The On-line Herbalist

I t might seem rather strange at first that the high tech of computers can contribute very much to the traditional field of herbalism. In fact, the burgeoning array of information databases that can be accessed via personal computers has much to offer the herbalist. With the increasing attention being given to herbal medicine by clinicians and researchers around the world, the simplest way of finding their research is via the on-line database services. Of course this only augments the core experience and material of herbal medicine, and in no way replaces it.

What are the on-line possibilities offered that might entice the herbalist? The information given here focuses on the medical research, but there is much relevant material in agricultural and biological databases as well. The field of building databases of medical information has been given its own name, Medical Informatics, so perhaps herbal database exploration might be called phyto-informatics!

All that is needed to gain access to the virtual world of databases is a computer, a modem, a telephone line and appropriate software. Modems are used to connect computers to telephone lines so that they can transmit data to one another at a distance. Data from a computer is fed to a modem. At the receiving end, another modem detects this data and produces a signal that is identical to the original. In this way, data can be transmitted rapidly over telephone lines. A detailed, comprehensive and readable guide to on-line services and the equipment needed to use them can be found in: Rittner, Don. *Ecolinking. Everyone's Guide to On-line Environmental Information.* Berkeley: Peachpit Press, 1992.

Electronic Bulletin Boards (BBS)

Bulletin board services (BBS) are operated by individuals, businesses, nonprofit organizations and government agencies for the purpose of sharing information—often at no cost or low cost to the user. Estimates on the number of private bulletin boards in the United States range from a few thousand to more than 100,000. Bulletin boards generally cater to people with a particular type of computer (for example, IBM PC, Amiga or Macintosh) or a particular interest (for example, botany or The Grateful Dead). Most bulletin boards are accessible around the clock, seven days a week, at no cost other than the cost of the telephone calls. There is an ever-changing array of BBSs so a current guide will facilitate finding one that is relevant. Each issue of Vulcan's *Computer Monthly* includes a state-by-state list of bulletin boards that are available to the public. To get a copy call (800) 874-2937. Many local computing newspapers also publish lists of bulletin boards. Some examples are:

Caduceus. An international computer bulletin board service for practitioners and others interested in natural medicine, preventive health care and alternative therapies. Their goal is to facilitate a worldwide network of health care practitioners connecting with each other and sharing in their healing work and professional development. IGC (Institute for Global Communications),

18 de Boom Street, San Francisco, CA 94107. Phone: (415) 442-0220 Fax: (415) 154-1794 E-mail: support@igc.org

Agriculture Library Forum. Provides an agricultural date book listing upcoming symposia, conferences and other events. The Agriculture Library Forum (ALF) maintains an excellent list on agricultural bulletin boards, as well as bibliographies and literature on agriculture, an information center, reference publications, a water quality dataline and information on using ALF and the National Agricultural Library. More than a dozen file libraries, whose contents range from agricultural alternatives to special reference briefs, are available on ALF. BBS Number: (800) 134-5575

F.D.A. (Food and Drug Administration) BBS. A good source of information: News releases, Drug and Device Product Approvals, Drug Bulletin texts, articles and consumer magazine index to FDA stories, Federal Register summaries, FDA testimony and speeches. BBS Number: (800) 222-0185; Login with "bbs," parameters 7E1.

NIST "FedWorld" BBS. Department of Commerce. This is the closest thing to a front-end government bulletin board service. FedWorld links dozens of government bulletin board services together. White House press releases are on line, as well as job information. Foreign broadcast news accounts and government statistics loaded daily. BBS Number: (703) 321-8020

Nutrition Databank (NHIS) BBS. Department of Agriculture. Provides up-to-date information about food composition, data releases, publications, and nutrition. BBS Number: (301) 436-5078

Office of the Assistant Secretary of Health (OASH). Health and Human Services. Message areas and files for many health programs including women's health issues, Office of Population Affairs, Surgeon General, Centers for Disease Control, Indian Health, F.D.A., NIH, and a major library of AIDS files. BBS Number: (202) 690-5423

Rutgers Cooperative Extension BBS. It is operated by the Rutgers University Cooperative Extension. Bulletins are available on topics including pathology, floriculture, farmer's markets, pesticides, horticulture, financial news, newsletters, and food technology. A door area contains the Alternative Farming Systems Literature database, which lists more than 6,000 citations, dating from the sixties to the mid-eighties, covering all aspects of organic growing and sustainable agriculture. BBS Number: (800) 722-0335 (New Jersey only) or (201) 383-8041.

On-line Databases

Before personal computers, creating bibliographies and finding reference material relevant to phytotherapy meant spending many hours in the library working through volumes of printed indexes and card catalogs, writing down each citation, finding the document and then photocopying it. On-line database retrieval companies now give the herbal researcher access to millions of articles at the touch of a keyboard 24 hours a day, seven days a week. For a low fee (usually less than the cost of gas to get to a library) anyone with a computer, modem, and communications software can conduct extensive bibliographical research.

A database is simply a large, complex list of facts and information such as telephone directories, airline flight guides, and bibliographic references. Databases are usually constructed on computers, but bear in mind that an elaborate paper filing system is a sort of database. They are distinguished from simple lists by the essential feature that upon request a specific group of diverse facts can be extracted from the full collection. An on-line database is an electronic database that is linked to telephone lines so that it can be reached by dialing through a modem and typing the appropriate commands. Two databases of primary importance to herbalism are NAPRALERT and MEDLINE (MEDLARS on LINE).

NAPRALERT (Natural Products Alert)

The largest and most comprehensive computerized database covering medicinal plants is NAPRALERT, short for Natural Products Alert, established by Professor Farnsworth and colleagues at the University of Illinois at Chicago. NAPRALERT also covers the world's literature on the chemistry and pharmacology, including human studies, of secondary metabolites of known structure, derived from natural sources.

The NAPRALERT team screen about 200 journals and record in the database any article containing information on the presence of secondary chemical constituents in living organisms. From this, they can prepare a wide range of printouts providing, for example, ethnomedical profiles, pharmacological profiles and phytochemical profiles for any given plant, animal or microbe. It is maintained by the Program for Collaborative Research in the Pharmaceutical Sciences, College of Pharmacy, University of Illinois at Chicago.

More than 75,000 articles and books, culled from about 200 journals and abstract services, cover all aspects of natural products and the use of plants and animals. Combined, the articles contain information on more than 87,000 chemicals and more than 38,000 plant and animal species and contain more than 426,000 records on biological activity associated with those species. Individual requests cost $10 per question, including up to three pages of computer output with bibliography. On-line access subscriptions range from $100 to $10,000. For subscription information, call (312) 996-2246.

National Library of Medicine

The National Library of Medicine on-line databases are geared for researchers in medicine and biology. MEDLARS, a biological database set, and TOXNET, a toxicological database set, are available 24 hours a day. More than 4,000 journals are covered in the databases.

The National Library of Medicine has Macintosh and IBM versions of its easy-to-use search software called Grateful Med. TOXNET, or Toxicology Data Network, contains a number of useful databases. These include:

The Hazardous Substance Databank (HSDB). This contains a wealth of information about individual chemicals and chemical compounds, their health and safety aspects, transport, health effects, physical and chemical properties, safety hazards, firefighting tips, typical environmental concentrations, sources, and manufacturers. It also includes a list of synonyms for each chemical, so you don't have to know its exact name.

The Integrated Risk Information System (IRIS). This is an EPA database containing numbers used in risk assessments.

The Toxic Release Inventory (TRI). This is a useful source of data on the release of chemicals into water, air, or soil. As part of the Community Right-to-Know Act, manufacturers must report such releases.

The Registry of Toxic Effects of Chemical Substances (RTECS). This provides a list of federal regulations applying to each chemical.

Cost: Each database has its own hourly charge, from $23.50 per hour to $171 per hour. There is no sign-up fee and no monthly minimum. Contact the MEDLARS service desk at (800) 638-8480.

MEDLINE (MEDLARS on LINE)

Produced by the U.S. National Library of Medicine, MEDLINE is a major source on biomedical literature. It contains over 6,500,000 biomedical references to articles published in 4,000 journals published in the United States and 70 other countries. It covers topics in pharmacology, medicine, surgery, dentistry, nursing, and health care management from 1966 to the present. MEDLINE is the source of the printed volumes of *Index Medicus, The Index to Dental Literature,* and *The International Nursing Index.*

Commercial On-line Services

A number of commercial ventures have developed on-line services to accommodate personal computer owners. These providers operate from one or more host computers, have multiuser capability, and charge a fee for access. Providers such as Knowledge Index, The WELL, and CompuServe cater to people with all types of computers. The nonprofit EcoNet caters specifically to the environmental community. Hundreds of services are offered by these on-line providers, from stock quotes, wire services such as UPI and AP, and airline ticket sales to E-mail. These services also provide libraries from which you can download and to which you can upload computer files, spreadsheets, and programs. Unlike private bulletin boards, these on-line providers charge an hourly fee for access. Some require a one-time sign-up fee or a monthly minimum. As examples of the potential for the herbalist consider CompuServe and Knowledge Index.

CompuServe

With over 500,000 members worldwide and over 1,200 on-line offerings, CompuServe Information Service is the largest of commercial on-line services. Every major personal computer format is supported, including IBM PC, Macintosh, Apple II, Commodore, and Atari, and CompuServe offers graphic software "interface" programs for ease of use. They offer an extensive range of services, including special interest groups and clubs, computing support for virtually every type of computer, financial and stock information, and a broad range of reference databases. CompuServe electronic mail has links to MCI Mail, fax, telex, and the Internet. One of the services they offer is access to PaperChase, perhaps the easiest way of entering the world of MEDLINE. This is explored in depth in the next section.

PaperChase

This is a service that provides convenient access to the National Library of Medicine's MEDLINE database. It is sponsored by Beth Israel Hospital, a major teaching hospital of the Harvard Medical School.

PaperChase is menu-driven and easy to use; search criteria can be by author, title, journal, or subject. You can order full-text articles on-line. Software is available for both PCs and Macintosh. An extensive user manual is included.

There is no subscription fee, no monthly minimum, and no start-up cost. You pay $2 per hour, plus 10 cents for each reference displayed. An average search costs around $6. Searching is available 24 hours a day, seven days a week. You can access PaperChase through CompuServe. Phone: (800) 722-2075, or (617) 732-4800.

Knowledge Index

Dialog Information Services, which offers Knowledge Index, is the largest on-line bibliographic company in the United States, with over 200 million items available for searching in 370 databases. To get information about subscribing to Knowledge Index, call Dialog Information Services at (800) 334-2564.

New subscribers pay a start-up fee of $35. The fee includes two hours of free time, a user manual containing a list of all Knowledge Index databases and their labels, sample searches, and other information, along with detailed explanations of the various search commands and shortcuts. On-line fees are $24 per hour, at off-peak times; the fee includes all connecting network phone charges. No fee is charged per citation. Instead of visiting a local library to make copies of articles, you can order the full text from Dialog for a fee of $7.50 per article plus 35 cents per photocopied page. You can also capture the text into your computer to print later.

Academic American Encyclopedia

A complete encyclopedia including over 34,000 articles written by 2,300 contributors who are experts in their fields. The articles average 300 words in length. Cross-references provide quick access to related subjects, and bibliographies are provided for longer articles.

Academic Index

Covers more than 400 scholarly and general interest publications, including the most commonly held titles in over 120 college and university libraries. Subjects covered include art, anthropology, economics, education, ethnic studies, government, history, literature, political science, general science, psychology, religion, sociology, and leisure.

Agribusiness USA

Provides controlled-vocabulary indexing and informative abstracts from approximately 300 industry-related trade journals and government publications.

Agricola

The database of the National Agricultural Library provides worldwide coverage of journals and monographs on agriculture and related subjects such as animal studies, botany, chemistry, entomology, fertilizers, forestry, hydroponics, and soils.

Agrochemicals Handbook

Provides information on the active components of agrochemical products used worldwide. For each substance, The Agrochemicals Handbook gives the following information: chemical name, including synonyms and trade names; CAS Registry Number; molecular formula; molecular weight; manufacturer's name; chemical and physical properties; toxicity; mode of action; activity; and health and safety concerns.

Books in Print

The major source of information on books currently in print in the United States. The database provides a record of forthcoming books, books in print, and books out of print. Scientific, technical, medical, scholarly, and popular works, as well as children's books, are included in the file.

CAB Abstracts

A comprehensive file of agricultural and biological information containing all the records from the 26 main abstract journals published by the Commonwealth Agricultural Bureau. Over 8,500 journals in 37 languages are scanned for inclusion, as are books, reports, theses, conference proceedings, patents, annual reports, and guides.

Consumer Drug Information Fulltext

The CDIF includes the complete text of the Consumer Drug Digest, published by the American Society of Hospital Pharmacists. CDIF contains in-depth descriptions of more than 260 drugs, including over 80 percent of all prescription drugs and a number of important nonprescription drugs. Information includes how the drugs work; possible side effects and how to manage them; precautions; instructions on dosage and use, including the foods and activities that are permitted during medication and what to do if a dose is missed and advice on storing drugs.

Dissertation Abstracts On-line

This is the definitive guide to virtually every American dissertation accepted at an accredited institution since 1861, when academic doctoral degrees were first granted in the United States.

Food Science and Technology Abstracts

FSTA provides access to research and new developments in food science and technology and allied disciplines such as agriculture, chemistry, biochemistry, and physics. Other related disciplines such as engineering and home economics are included when relevant to food science. Also included in the file is Vitis, a subfile on viticulture and enology. Information in this subfile covers grapes and grapevine science and technology. FSTA indexes over 1200 journals from over 50 countries, patents from 20 countries, and books in any language.

Government Printing Office

The GPO Publications Reference File indexes public documents currently for sale by the Superintendent of Documents, U.S. Government Printing Office, as well as forthcoming and recently out-of-print publications.

Heilbron

Hilbron is a chemical properties database which contains the complete text of the *Dictionary of Organic Compounds* (5th ed.), and the *Dictionary of Organometallic Compounds*. Also included are other source books: *Carbohydrates, Amino Acids and Peptides,* and *The Dictionary of Antibiotics and Related Compounds*.

Heilbron helps identify chemical substances based on their physical and chemical properties, compound variants, derivative names, synonyms, CAS Registry Numbers, molecular formulas and molecular weight, source statements, use and importance data, melting point, freezing point, boiling point, solubility, relative density, optical rotation, and dissociation constants. Chemical images can be displayed when you search with DialogLINK software.

Life Sciences Collection

This contains abstracts of information in the fields of animal behavior, biochemistry, ecology, endocrinology, entomology, genetics, immunology, microbiology, oncology, neuroscience, toxicology, virology and related fields. The collection is an on-line version of the 17 volumes of abstracts by the same name.

Magazine Index

Covers more than 435 popular magazines, providing extensive coverage of current affairs, the performing arts, business, sports, recreation and travel, consumer product evaluations, science and technology, leisure-time activities, and other areas.

The National Newspaper Index

Provides front-to-back indexing of the *Christian Science Monitor*, the *New York Times*, and the *Wall Street Journal*. All articles, news reports, editorials, letters to the editor, obituaries, product evaluations, biographical pieces, poetry, recipes, columns, cartoons and illustrations, and reviews are included. In addition, the *National Newspaper Index* covers national and international news stories written by the staff writers of the *Washington Post* and the *Los Angeles Times*.

Newsearch

A daily index of more than 2,000 news stories, articles, and book reviews from over 1,700 newspapers, magazines, and periodicals. In addition, Newsearch includes the Area Business Databank, which indexes old abstracts from over 100 local and regional business publications, and the complete text of PR Newswire.

Example of an On-line Search of MEDLINE

The MEDLINE database can be accessed in a variety of ways which require varying degrees of computer skills to navigate. One of the easiest and least intimidating ways of accessing the wealth of information contained in MEDLINE is to use the commercial service such as PaperChase. This is an on-line information service that helps you search both the continually updated MEDLINE database and the continually updated Health Planning and Administration (HEALTH) database.

MEDLINE contains over 6,500,000 biomedical references to articles published in 4,000 international journals, covering topics in medicine, surgery, dentistry, nursing, and health care management from 1966 to the present. MEDLINE is the source of the printed volumes of *Index Medicus*, *The Index to Dental Literature*, and *The International Nursing Index*. To give a sense of the tremendous scope of MEDLINE, an entire set of bound volumes of *Index Medicus* from 1966 to the present—which contains only a fraction of the information stored in MEDLINE—weighs about two and a half tons and takes up 60 feet of library shelving.

HEALTH contains over 500,000 references, covering topics in hospital administration, personnel, planning, budget matters, accreditation, organization, and other issues involving health care delivery. HEALTH is the source for the American Hospital Association's Hospital Literature Index.

PaperChase is available through the CompuServe Information System that makes accessing possible through a local phone call in almost all of North America. There is no need to memorize or look up special formats or terms to use PaperChase, as it also interprets whatever is typed and interacts with the user to define and direct the search with tips suggested on line. PaperChase monitors the search strategy being used and provides tailored help by suggesting ways to refine or expand the search in progress. The examples given below will clarify this, but are not a complete guide to the potential of this service. An excellent guide to the use of PaperChase is published by them and should be used and consulted by any herbalist going on line with them.

PaperChase isn't itself a medical database, but a program that searches MEDLINE, helping find references to articles on a specific subject, by specific authors, from specific journals. When an interesting reference is found, the abstract can be read on line, added to a list of references to print or download at the end of the search, or a photocopy of the full text of the article can be ordered.

Menus

PaperChase is menu-driven. This means that a set of commands is not needed to conduct a search as PaperChase shows a list of options from which to choose. To choose an option, type either the number to the left of the option, or the first letter of its first word, and press ENTER, which will be a specific key on the computer keyboard. The following options are those that appear when you connect to PaperChase.

PaperChase Options:

1 New Search
2 Old Search
3 Print From Old Search
4 Verify a Reference
5 Setup Custom Lists
6 Leave Comments
7 Instructions for Use
8 Reconfigure PaperChase for your Equipment
9 Exit PaperChase

CHOICE: *New//*

This menu of options varies depending on the previous use of PaperChase. For example, if this is the user's very first search, it will not have the options "Old Search" or "Print from Old Search." These menu choices will produce different results thus:

New Search

Choose the option "New Search" to start with a clean slate. This is the default—to select this option, press ENTER.

Old Search

"Old Search" tells the program to return to a previous search and continue with it. Users are shown a list of their old searches, most recent first, from which to choose. The list includes the date and time of the search, the first three lists that were created, and the update through which the search is current. All old searches are saved completely, including print and photocopy requests, for six months. Old searches are automatically updated weekly when new references are added to the database. About 8,000 new references are added each week.

Print from Old Search

This returns to an Old Search to print references or order photocopies previously selected.

Verify a Reference

"Verify a Reference" will confirm the existence of a known reference and display that reference on screen. This is useful for confirming references for a bibliography, viewing abstracts, and ordering photocopies.

Setup Custom Lists

If a certain series of lists is used repeatedly while doing different searches, use "Setup Custom Lists" and store these lists permanently, calling them up whenever needed by typing CUSTOM at LOOK FOR:. This option is particularly useful for the herbalist with the many MeSH terms applicable to medicinal plants.

LOOK FOR:

This is the core of the PaperChase program because it is at LOOK FOR: that the search specification is entered. This can be done in almost any format as PaperChase will either automatically translate the entry into a form that it can "read," or ask you questions so that the request can be clarified.

For example, suppose you enter "Herb" at LOOK FOR:

> **LOOK FOR: Herb**
>
> **1 Title Word or Medical Subject Heading**
> **2 Author Name**
>
> **CHOICE: 1**

Are there papers by Dr. Herb or is the term "Herb" meant? Once the user indicates that the term is meant, PaperChase then lists Medical Subject Headings (MeSH terms) that include the word herb. From these you can choose exactly what is wanted.

Title Word and *Medical Subject Headings	References
1 HERB	226
2 * HERBAL DRUGS, CHINESE	2,687
3 * HERBAL MEDICINE	700
4 * HERBICIDES	3,100
5 * HERBICIDES, CARBAMATE	195
6 * HERBICIDES, TRIAZINE	257
7 * HERBICIDES, UREA	255
8 * HERBS	1,212

CHOICES (MORE TO FOLLOW):
Display Related *Headings (Y/N)? Y // y

Related *Medical Subject Headings	References
1 * MEDICINE, CHINESE TRADITIONAL	3,326
2 * MATERIA MEDICA	242
3 * PLANTS, MEDICINAL	12,065
4 * BEVERAGES	2,028
5 * SIMAZINE	96
6 * 2,4,5-TRICHLOROPHENOXYACETIC ACID	531
7 * 2,4-DICHLOROPHENOXYACETIC ACID	883
8 * AMITROLE	461
9 * ATRAZINE	268

Related *Medical Subject Headings	References
1 * CHLORPROPHAM	73
2 * ALKALOIDS	10,867
3 * ALOE	200
4 * ARECA	375
5 * BELLADONNA	420
6 * CANNABIS	4,531
7 * CAPSICUM	183
8 * CINCHONA	119
9 * COCA	158

Related *Medical Subject Headings	References
1 * COLCHICUM	64
2 * DIGITALIS	3,047
3 * DRUGS	58,043
4 * ERYTHRINA	100
5 * EUCALYPTUS	111
6 * FERULA	37
7 * FRANGULA	19
8 * GARLIC	545
9 * GINSENG	645

Related *Medical Subject Headings	References
1 * LEGUMES	3,100
2 * MUSTARD	2,132
3 * PAPAVER	262
4 * PHARMACOGNOSY	459
5 * PLANTAGO	100
6 * PLANTS	31,833
7 * PODOPHYLLUM	239
8 * PROSCILLARIDIN	159
9 * RAUWOLFIA	616

Related *Medical Subject Headings	References
1 * RHAMNUS	54
2 * RHUBARB	157
3 * STRAMONIUM	264
4 * VALERIAN	143
5 * VERATRUM	209
6 * VISCUM	258
7 * DICAMBA	43
8 * ORTHODONTIC APPLIANCES, FUNCTIONAL	37

Users are thus offered a wide range of MeSH terms to choose from that might focus their search. To LOOK FOR: a topic, always type one thing at a time. Start by typing the most significant word or concept, leaving off all plurals and word endings. All PaperChase needs is a single word, or just the root of the word. It will then present you with a choice of words or phrases that match that root. LOOK FOR: can be seen as a way to browse through the index as one might look up something in a dictionary. The best way to LOOK FOR: a topic is to type just enough of the word to get to the right place in the index. Using word roots instead of whole words not only helps zero in on the topic of choice, but also facilitates a search for a term when the spelling is unsure. It also saves time if the word to enter is very long.

Pick from the menu by entering the number or numbers of the items on the menu. Select as many as wanted. For example, if you were interested in other terms for medicinal plants, you could start by entering plants, medicinal, and selecting the category Title Word or *Medical Subject Heading as shown on the following page.

```
LOOK FOR: plants, medicinal

*Medical Subject Headings                          References
  1   * PLANTS, MEDICINAL                          12,065
Related *Medical Subject Headings                  References
  2   * ALKALOIDS                                  10,160
  3   * DRUGS, CHINESE HERBAL                       2,687
  4   * DRUGS                                      55,102
  5   * MEDICINE, HERBAL                             700
  6   * PHARMACOGNOSY                                450
  7   * PROSCILLARIDIN                               155
CHOICE: 3


ENTRIES CHOSEN: 3      More Related *Headings (Y/N)? Y // y
```

Drugs, Chinese Herbal has been selected as another search term, but the program is offering other suggested MeSH terms as well. By responding yes more options appear that in turn lead to yet more options.

```
Related *Medical Subject Headings                  References
  1   * MEDICINE, CHINESE TRADITIONAL               3,158
  2   * MEDICINE, ORIENTAL TRADITIONAL              2,472
  3   * PLANT EXTRACTS                             10,616
CHOICES: 3


ENTRIES CHOSEN: 3      More Related *Headings (Y/N)? Y // y

Related *Medical Subject Headings                  References
  1   * BIOLOGICAL PRODUCTS                         2,559
  2   * PLANTS                                     30,927
CHOICE:
```

When none of the options are relevant and no more are offered or desired by the user, simply hit ENTER at the CHOICE: prompt. This will lead to the LIST menu.

Medical Subject Headings (MeSH terms)

Terms with an asterisk, like *PHARMACOGNOSY, are *Medical Subject Headings. Words without asterisks are Title Words, words used by the author in the title of an article. *Medical Subject Headings (also called MeSH terms) are carefully chosen, hierarchically organized terms defined and used by the National Library of Medicine to classify biomedical literature. Every reference in MEDLINE and in HEALTH is indexed under appropriate MeSH terms. Most articles are assigned four major MeSH terms and more than four minor ones. If you choose a Title Word instead of a MeSH term you will be offered a list of MeSH terms related to that Title Word that you can use instead of or in addition to your search term.

There are a number of reasons why *Medical Subject Headings are usually better than Title Words. Perhaps most important is that medical terminology contains many synonyms. Different authors may choose different Title Words for similar concepts. For example, the Title Word ALLERGY gives you about 7,000 references. However, the *Medical Subject Heading HYPERSENSITIVITY (which PaperChase offers if ALLERGY is entered) gives over 18,000 references. In contrast, *Medical Subject Headings are standardized. Additionally, not all topics discussed in a reference are explicitly mentioned in the title. The titles of many articles give an indication of their content, but in many instances a topic is implied rather than mentioned, or is not even mentioned at all. For example, it is not obvious that "The hospital that ate Chicago" is about hospital planning!

However, for the Phytotherapist it is often Title Words that are most useful for finding a particular reference that has a certain word in its title. For example, there are only a few herb genus names assigned as MeSH terms, but any herb discussed in a research paper will be accessible via its genus name. Title Words are also useful. Examples of MeSH terms relevant to phytotherapists include:

MeSH Terms That Directly Relate to Medicinal Plants

Plants, Medicinal—12,065 citations
Drugs, Chinese Herbal—2,687 citations
Herbs—1,212 citations
Plant Extracts—10,616 citations
Medicine, Herbal—700 citations

MeSH Terms That Relate to the General Field of Interest

History of Medicine
History of Medicine, Medieval
Legislation, Medicinal
Medicine, Primitive
Medicine, Traditional
African Medicine, Traditional
Traditional Medicine, African
Medicine, Arabic
Medicine, Ayurvedic
Medicine, Hindu
Chinese Traditional Medicine
Yang Deficiency

Yin Deficiency
Yin-Yang
Traditional Medicine, Chinese
Medicine, Chinese Traditional
Medicine, Oriental
Medicine, Oriental Traditional
Oriental Medicine, Traditional
Traditional Medicine, Oriental
Health Services, Indigenous
Indians, North American
Folklore
Ethnomedicine

Folk Medicine
Medicine, Folk
Medicine, Indigenous
Alternative Medicine

Herbs Listed in the Catalogue of MeSH Terms (*although many more are accessible as Title Words*)

Adonis	Cubeb	Polygonum
Aesculus	Echinacea	Rauwolfia
Aspidium	Gelsemium	Rosa
Castanea	Gentian	Salix
Chelidonium	Hydrastis	Sarsaparilla
Chenopodium	Lithospermum	Tamarind
Colchicum	Marrubium	
Colocynth	Myrica	
Crataegus	Oleander	

Other Relevant MeSH Terms

Alkaloids	Antilipemic agents	Astringents
Antiinfective agnets	Antineoplastic agents,	Clinical Trial
Antiinflammatory agents	phytogenic—1,292 cits.	Drugs
Anticarcinogenic agents	Antineoplastics, botanical	Food preservatives
Anticholesteremic agents	Antineoplastics, phytogenic	Human
Anticoagulants	Antioxidants	Pharmaceutic aids
Antidiarrheals	Antipruritics	Pharmacognosy—
Antiemetics	Antitussive agents	444 cits.
Antifungal agents	Antiviral agents	Review
Antihypertensive agents		

Human and all medicinal plant search terms—7,020
Clinical Trials and all medicinal plant search terms—456
Review and all medicinal plant search terms—891
Review, human and all medicinal plant search terms—564
Review, clinical trials and all medicinal plant search terms—10

Combining Lists

Once two or more lists have been created, they can be combined to create new lists that precisely address the area of interest. Specifically, you can:

- Find references common to 2 or more lists.
- Include (pool) references from 2 or more lists.
- Exclude references on one list from another list.

Find References Common to Two or More Lists

This option allows the creation of a new list of references that meet more than one search specification, such as references that discuss both PLANTS, MEDICINAL and HIV. This is the most frequently used option in PaperChase.

```
List                                    References
A) PLANTS, MEDICINAL                    12,065
B) HIV                                  10,253

OPTIONS:

1  Exit PaperChase
2  Display List
3  Look For Topic
4  Find References Common to 2 or More Lists
5  Include (Pool) References from 2 or More Lists
6  Put All References From a List on Print Queue

CHOICE: 4
```

Choose option 4, "Find References Common to Two or More Lists," by entering either F or 4, and when PaperChase asks "COMMON TO WHICH TWO OR MORE LISTS," respond AB <ENTER>. PaperChase creates a third list, List C, marked "*ON A & B," which contains references indexed under both PLANTS, MEDICINAL and HIV.

Include (Pool) References from 2 or More Lists

"Include (Pool) References from 2 or More Lists" gathers references from two or more lists into one list. This option is useful if you wish to expand your search to include related *Medical Subject Headings. For example, suppose you want to find all papers that might relate to "herbs."

```
List                                    References
A) DRUGS, CHINESE HERBAL                2,687
B) PLANT EXTRACTS                       10,616
C) PLANTS, MEDICINAL                    12,065
D) MEDICINE, HERBAL                     700

OPTIONS:

1  Exit PaperChase
2  Display List
3  Look For Topic
4  Find References Common to 2 or More Lists
5  Include (Pool) References from 2 or More Lists
6  Put All References From a List on Print Queue

CHOICE: 5
```

This creates List D, which PaperChase labels *SUM ABC.

List	References
A) DRUGS, CHINESE HERBAL	2,687
B) PLANT EXTRACTS	10,616
C) PLANTS, MEDICINAL	12,065
D) MEDICINE, HERBAL	700
F) *SUM ABDE	26,068

OPTIONS:

1 Exit PaperChase
2 Display List
3 Look For Topic
4 Find References Common to 2 or More Lists
5 Include (Pool) References from 2 or More Lists
6 Put All References From a List on Print Queue

CHOICE:

As an example of excluding references from a list consider a search of papers on the effects of pyrrolizidine alkaloid on humans. Rather than specifying no papers that relate to animal studies or veterinary research, it is best to use an additional MeSH term that relates. In this case it might be "human" or "clinical."

List	References
A) PYRROLIZIDINE ALKALOIDS	871
B) PLANTS, MEDICINAL	12,065
C) HUMAN	4,989,817
D) CLINICAL	205,903

OPTIONS:

1 Exit PaperChase
2 Display List
3 Look For Topic
4 Find References Common to 2 or More Lists
5 Include (Pool) References from 2 or More Lists
6 Put All References from a List on Print Queue

CHOICE: 4
Common to Which Two or More Lists? a c

In this case all papers with pyrrolizidine alkaloids and human will be searched for. However, additional search constraints can be added by specifying clinical papers only.

List	References
A) PYRROLIZIDINE ALKALOIDS	871
B) PLANTS, MEDICINAL	12,065
C) HUMAN	4,989,817
D) CLINICAL	205,903
E) *ON A&C	158

OPTIONS:

1 Exit PaperChase
2 Display List
3 Look For Topic
4 Find References Common to 2 or More Lists
5 Include (Pool) References from 2 or More Lists
6 Put All References from a List on Print Queue

CHOICE: *4*
Common to Which 2 or More Lists? *e d*

List	References
A) PYRROLIZIDINE ALKALOIDS	871
B) PLANTS, MEDICINAL	12,065
C) HUMAN	4,989,817
D) CLINICAL	205,903
E) *ON A&C	158
F) *ON D&E	FEW

OPTIONS:

1 Exit PaperChase
2 Display List
3 Look For Topic
4 Find References Common to 2 or More Lists
5 Include (Pool) References from 2 or More Lists
6 Put All References from a List on Print Queue

CHOICE: *3*

Lists That Are FEW

When lists are combined, PaperChase sometimes marks the resulting list FEW. This means that in the time it takes to write *ON D&E on the screen, PaperChase has not yet determined the final number or approximate number of references in the list. There is no need to wait for the word FEW to go away before displaying the list or combining it with another list. Until you touch the keyboard in some way, either by pressing <ENTER> or by choosing an option, the screen display is frozen, and the FEW note will not be updated with an estimate of the number of references found.

Viewing Lists On Line

There are two ways to view a list: DISPLAY and SCAN. To view a list of references on line, choose "Display List" from the Options Menu. (From LOOK FOR:, press <ENTER> to get the menu.) The first reference is always shown in the DISPLAY mode. DISPLAY shows each reference individually, on a full screen that includes the Unique Identifier Number of the reference, the last names and initials of all authors, the title of the article, the journal, year, volume, and page number, abstract note ("ABSTRACT ONLINE" or "NO ABSTRACT ONLINE"), the Major and Minor MeSH terms under which the reference is indexed, and the language of publication (if other than English). SCAN includes the title of the article, the abstract note, the last name of the first author, the journal, year, volume, and page numbers. Since only partial information on each reference is shown in SCAN, up to four references can be listed on one screen. From either DISPLAY or SCAN, an abstract can be displayed of any reference that has one.

A reference looks like this in DISPLAY:

```
92339978
Blesken R
[Crataegus in cardiology]
Crataegus in der Kardiologie.
[ABSTRACT ONLINE]
In: Fortschr Med (1992 May 30) 110(15):290-2

<Cardiotonic Agents> <Heart Failure, Congestive>
<Hemodynamics>

<Plant Extracts> <Plants, Medicinal> <English Abstract>
<Human>

Published in German

NEXT/BACK/EXITS/SCAN/ABSTRACT/PRINT/FOTOCOPY
(N/B/E/S/A/P/F) ? N//
```

The eight-digit number in the upper left corner is the reference's Unique Identifier Number. Each reference in MEDLINE has one, facilitating rapid referencing. The upper row of terms in brackets, like <Cardiotonic Agents>, are the Major *Medical Subject Headings. A Major *Medical Subject Heading is also called a Major Topic. Terms that are grouped separately underneath, like <Plants, Medicinal>, are Minor *Medical Subject Headings. These terms give an indication of the contents of the article, but from the herbalist's perspective they often reflect the inherent bias of orthodox medicine. Major Topics are used to describe the principal points discussed in the article. Minor *Medical Subject Headings are used as additional methods of finding a reference and describe the subject of an article to a lesser degree.

The horizontal menu on the bottom of the screen provides a range of options. These are the options available while you are viewing a list in either DISPLAY or SCAN mode:

The <ENTER> key gives you the default *NEXT*, which will display the next reference in your list.

B for *BACK-UP* backs up to the reference immediately preceding the one displayed. To go back to an earlier reference, type B followed by the number of the reference. Thus, to return to the first reference in the list, type B1.

E for *EXIT* stops the reference display and returns you to the Options Menu.

S for *SCAN* switches from DISPLAY to SCAN. SCAN is available when in the DISPLAY mode.

D for *DISPLAY* switches from SCAN to DISPLAY. DISPLAY is available when in the SCAN mode.

A for *ABSTRACT* will show the reference's abstract, assuming that there is an ABSTRACT ONLINE. When there is not an abstract available, you will not have this option.

P for *PRINT* puts the reference on a Print Queue for printing or downloading at the end of your search.

F for *FOTOCOPY* enables you to order a photocopy of the full text of the article.

The options to print or to photocopy a reference are presented again if you decide to look at a reference's abstract. There is also the opportunity to retract print or photocopy choices at the end of a search. The abstract is requested by entering A; the screen will look as follows:

```
92339978
Blesken R
[Crataegus in cardiology]
Crataegus in der Kardiologie.
In: Fortschr Med (1992 May 30) 110(15):290-2
```

The fact that the effectiveness of numerous phyto-preparations, so-called, has been demonstrated to the satisfaction of traditional medicine has led to increasing interest in phytotherapy. This also applies to Crataegus (whitethorn), the effects of which have been demonstrated in numerous pharmacological studies. These effects, produced mainly by the flavonoids, indicate a simultaneous cardiotropic and vasodilatory action, as confirmed clinically in controlled double-blind studies. This means that Crataegus can be employed for cardiological indications for which digitalis is not (yet) indicated. Prior to use, however, a Crataegus preparation must meet certain preconditions with respect to dosage, pharmaceutical quality of the preparation, and an accurate definition of the latter.

```
NEXT/BACK/EXITS/SCAN/ABSTRACT/PRINT/FOTOCOPY
(N/B/E/S/A/P/F) ? N//
```

In the SCAN mode, references look like this:

References to be Printed (1 OF 123)

1. Toxicity and activity of purified trichosanthin.
   [ABSTRACT ONLINE] Ferrari: AIDS (1991 Jul) 5(7):865-70

2. Modification of human immunodeficiency viral replication by pine cone extracts.
   [ABSTRACT ONLINE] Lai: AIDS Res Hum Retroviruses (1990 Feb) 6(2):205-17

3. Immunomodulatory effects of Panax Ginseng C.A. Meyer in the mouse.
   [ABSTRACT ONLINE] Jie: Agents Actions (1984 Oct) 15(3-4):386-91

4 Effect of salai guggal ex-Boswellia serrata on cellular and humoral immune responses and leucocyte migration.
   [ABSTRACT ONLINE] Sharma: Agents Actions (1988 Jun) 24(1-2):161-4

```
NEXT/BACK/EXITS/SCAN/ABSTRACT/PRINT/FOTOCOPY
(N/B/E/S/A/P/F) ? N//
```

The options are similar to the previous screen but with a few differences. Rather than moving ahead one reference at a time, pressing <ENTER> for the default option NEXT will bring up the next full screen of references, and entering B for BACK-UP will return to the previous screen of references. Since more than one reference is listed on the screen, if D for DISPLAY, A for ABSTRACT, P for PRINT, or F for FOTOCOPY is entered, PaperChase will ask which references are intended. From SCAN you can enter D for DISPLAY to switch back to the DISPLAY mode.

Finding Review Articles

Review Articles are an excellent way of getting an overview on the current research in a particular field or subject. To limit a list to Review Articles, LOOK FOR: REVIEW and choose the category "Review Articles." There are four different types of Review Articles:

Review. An article published after examination of published material on a subject. It may be comprehensive to various degrees and the time range of material scrutinized may be broad or narrow.

Academic Review. A more or less comprehensive review of the literature on a specific subject, with usually an extensive critical analysis and synthesis of the literature.

Multicase Review. A type of review literature giving demographic, laboratory, and clinical data on a group of persons or animals ranging over most of the known cases of a rare condition in large populations on whom the results of research will lead to the establishing of epidemiological analyses or predictions of the occurrence and natural history of diseases.

Tutorial Review. A type of review citing literature that will give the user a general and reasonably thorough coverage of a subject with which he may or may not be familiar.

For example:

LOOK FOR: Review

"Review Which Category Do You Have in Mind?
1 REVIEW ARTICLES
2 TITLE WORD or *MEDICAL SUBJECT HEADING
3 JOURNAL TITLE

CHOICE: *1*

Review Articles	References
1 REVIEW <ALL>	434,957
2 REVIEW, ACADEMIC	22,030
3 REVIEW, TUTORIAL	164,907
4 REVIEW, MULTICASE	3,086

CHOICE: *1*

Returning to the pyrrolizidine search we can now specify another selection criterion thus:

List	References
A) PYRROLIZIDINE ALKALOIDS	871
B) PLANTS, MEDICINAL	12,065
C) HUMAN	4,989,817
D) CLINICAL	205,903
E) *ON A&C	158
F) *ON D&E	2
G) REVIEW	434,957

OPTIONS:

1 Exit PaperChase
2 Display List
3 Look For Topic
4 Find References Common to 2 or More Lists
5 Include (Pool) References from 2 or More Lists
6 Put All References from a List on Print Queue

CHOICE: *4*
Common to Which 2 or More Lists? *a g*

List	References
A) PYRROLIZIDINE ALKALOIDS	871
B) PLANTS, MEDICINAL	12,065
C) HUMAN	4,989,817
D) CLINICAL	205,903
E) *ON A&C	158
F) *ON D&E	2
G) REVIEW	434,957
H) *ON A&G	FEW

OPTIONS:

1 Exit PaperChase
2 Display List
3 Look For Topic
4 Find References Common to 2 or More Lists
5 Include (Pool) References from 2 or More Lists
6 Put All References from a List on Print Queue

CHOICE: *4*
Common to Which 2 or More Lists? *e g*

List	References
A) PYRROLIZIDINE ALKALOIDS	871
B) PLANTS, MEDICINAL	12,065
C) HUMAN	4,989,817
D) CLINICAL	205,903
E) *ON A&C	158
F) *ON D&E	2
G) REVIEW	434,957
H) *ON A&G	80
I) *ON E&G	38

OPTIONS:

1 Exit PaperChase
2 Display List
3 Look For Topic
4 Find References Common to 2 or More Lists
5 Include (Pool) References from 2 or More Lists
6 Put All References from a List on Print Queue
7 Remove Lists in Display

CHOICE: 6
Which List Do You Want to Print? e

Printing and Downloading

As lists are displayed, they can be selected to print at the end of the search. All of the references on the list can be printed or downloaded as a continuous scroll. Because there are many different types of communications software and printers, PaperChase generally does not run your printer for you. Instead, PaperChase tells you when it is ready to transmit the information, and you simply activate your printer or capture (download) to disk in the way you normally do. There are two print formats from which to choose, as well as the option to include either abstracts and/or MeSH terms. Selection of references for printing is done by entering P for PRINT. All of the references on a particular list can also be printed without actually displaying the list on line.

There is the useful option of printing the selected references when the search is finished and the user is ready to sign off. This is a much faster method when large lists are wanted. Simply choose "Exit PaperChase to Print" from the Options menu. When you are printing a reference, the information from PaperChase is transmitted from the computer screen directly to the printer and is not stored on disk. Thus, you end up with a list of references on paper. However, if you want to store the references in your computer, you need to download the Print Queue. You will then be able to print from your disk.

Once you have downloaded a list, you may choose to manipulate the references using a word-processing program.

Formats

PaperChase offers two print formats, PaperChase Format and the National Library of Medicine Format, which can be used with reprint management software. When the search is finished and exit to print is chosen a menu gives the following options:

OPTIONS:

1 **PaperChase Format**
2 **National Library of Medicine Format**
3 **Hold for Later Printout**
4 **Offline Printout (PaperChase Mails List to You)**

CHOICE:

After telling PaperChase which format to use (see below), a number of options are offered that vary the amount of detail downloaded. References can be printed with or without abstracts, with or without *Medical Subject Headings.

All references include Authors, Title, and Journal citation.

WOULD YOU LIKE:

1 **Just the References**
2 **References plus Abstracts**
3 **References plus *Medical Subject Headings**
4 **References plus Abstracts and *Medical Subjects Headings**

CHOICE:

PaperChase Format

This format is similar to that seen when a reference is displayed on screen. It also includes the user's name, date, the lists created, numbers of references in each list, the institutional address where reprint requests can be sent, and the charges. This is how a reference appears in the PaperChase Format, including an abstract and *Medical Subject Headings:

88068428
Kendler BS
Garlic (*Allium sativum*) and onion (*Allium cepa*): a review of their relationship to cardiovascular disease.
[ABSTRACT ONLINE]
In: Prev Med (1987 Sep) 16(5):670-85

<Allium> <Cardiovascular Diseases> <Garlic> <Plants, Medicinal>
<Animal> <Fibrinolysis> <Human> <Hyperlipidemia> <Hypertension> <Plant Extracts> <Platelet Aggregation> <Rabbits> <Rats> <Review> <Review, Tutorial>

Garlic and onion have been used for millennia in the traditional medical practice of many cultures to treat cardiovascular and other disorders. Both Allium species, their extracts, and the chemical constituents of these plants have been investigated for possible effects on cardiovascular disease risk factors—both definite (hyperlipidemia, hypertension and hyperglycemia) and suspected (platelet aggregation and blood fibrinolytic activity). Action of these Allium species on blood coagulability is more clearly defined than their effect on the other risk factors. While many of the studies have serious methodological shortcomings, there is some evidence to suggest that use of certain formulations of garlic and/or onion is accompanied by favorable effects on risk factors in normal subjects and in patients with atherosclerotic disease. The possibility of toxicity resulting from acute and chronic ingestion of large amounts of these plants or their extracts is unresolved. Accordingly, further clinical and epidemiological studies are required before the role of these plants in the prevention and control of cardiovascular disorders is understood and can be realized. Additional research in this area is recommended.

National Library of Medicine Format

Each item is listed separately and labeled with a code. This makes it easier to use some reprint management programs that sort the references according to descriptor, such as subject or author. The National Library of Medicine Format can be used for printing, but is primarily used for downloading into bibliographic management software. The codes used to identify the fields in this format are:

AU: Author

TI: Title

AB: Abstract

MH: *Medical Subject Heading

AD: Address where reprint request can be sent, addressed to first author

SO: Source (journal name)

DP: Date Published

TA: Title Abbreviation

PG: Pages

IP: In Part

VI: Volume Issue

PT: Publication Type

UI: Unique Identifier Number

LA: Language

The following is an example of the National Library of Medicine Format:

AU: KreisW; KaplanMH; FreemanJ; SunDK; SarinPS

TI: Inhibition of HIV replication by Hyssop officinalis extracts.

AB: Crude extracts of dried leaves of Hyssop officinalis showed strong anti-HIV activity as measured by inhibition of syncytia formation, HIV reverse transcriptase (RT), and p17 and p24 antigen expression, but were non-toxic to the uninfected Molt-3 cells. Ether extracts from direct extraction (Procedure I), after removal of tannins (Procedure II), or from the residue after dialysis of the crude extract (Procedure III), showed good antiviral activity. Methanol extracts, subsequent to ether, chloroform and chloroform ethanol extractions, derived from procedure I or II, but not III, also showed very strong anti-HIV activity. In addition, the residual material after methanol extractions still showed strong activity. Caffeic acid was identified in the ether extract of procedure I by HPLC and UV spectroscopy. Commercial caffeic acid showed good antiviral activity in the RT assay and high to moderate activity in the syncytia assay and the p17 and p24 antigen expression. Tannic acid and gallic acid, common to other teas, could not be identified in our extracts. When commercial products of these two acids were tested in our assay systems, they showed high to moderate activity against HIV-1. Hyssop officinalis extracts contain caffeic acid, unidentified tannins, and possibly a third class of unidentified higher molecular weight compounds that exhibit strong anti-HIV activity, and may be useful in the treatment of patients with AIDS.

MH: Antiviral Agents

MH: HIV [drug effects]

MH: Plant Extracts [pharmacology]

MH: Plants, Medicinal

MH: Virus Replication [drug effects]

MH: Caffeic Acids [pharmacology]

MH: Cell Fusion

MH: Cells, Cultured

MH: Chromatography, High Pressure Liquid

MH: HIV Antigens [analysis]; HIV [analysis]

MH: Plant Extracts [analysis]

MH: Plants, Medicinal [analysis]

MH: Reverse Transcriptase [analysis]

MH: Spectrophotometry, Ultraviolet

MH: Tannins [analysis]

AD: Department of Medicine, North Shore University Hospital, Manhasset, NY 11030.

SO: Antiviral Res (Netherlands), Dec 1990, 14(6) p323-37

PT: JOURNAL ARTICLE

UI: 91207058

LA: English

A Sample Search

It is important to think through the parameters of a search as there is a wealth of information concerning medicinal plants in MEDLINE, but it is not always easy to find.

Consider the example of looking for published journal papers concerning herbs and immunity. The first question is what MeSH terms to use in searching for "herbs." Here are a list of possible terms used and the number of citations that they would produce:

Term	# of Citations
BOTANY	295
DRUGS, CHINESE HERBAL	2,687
HERBS	1,212
MATERIA MEDICA	215
MEDICINE, HERBAL	700
PHARMACOGNOSY	444
PLANT EXTRACTS	10,616
PLANTS	30,338
PLANTS, MEDICINAL	12,065
MEDICINE, TRADITIONAL	3,485
MEDICINE, CHINESE TRADITIONAL	3,104
MEDICINE, ORIENTAL TRADITIONAL	2,465

It may seem that "plants" would be the most useful, but this term also covers electricity generating plants! The single most useful term is "plants, medicinal," acting as an umbrella for most of the rest. However, there are some situations where there is no overlap, so a grouping of terms can be done:

DRUGS, CHINESE HERBAL + PLANT EXTRACTS + PLANTS, MEDICINAL + MEDICINE, HERBAL = 26,068

Selecting the search term for immunity can be a challenge, necessitating the herbalist to clearly think through the real goal. Using Immunity as the search term will prompt the system to offer many options to focus the search:

Term	# of Citations
IMMUNITY	23,414
IMMUNITY <ALL>	412,669
IMMUNITY, ACTIVE	2,319
IMMUNITY, CELLULAR	29,747
IMMUNITY, MATERNALLY-ACQUIRED	3,540
IMMUNITY, NATURAL	5,223
IMMUNE SYSTEM	3,516
IMMUNE TOLERANCE	12,940
IMMUNOCOMPETENCE	1,442
IMMUNOCOMPROMISED HOST	607
IMMUNOGENETICS	1,802
IMMUNOLOGIC DEFICIENCY SYNDROMES	8,363
IMMUNOLOGIC MEMORY	3,272
IMMUNOLOGIC TECHNIQUES	9,553
IMMUNOSUPPRESSION	16,463

However, it may be that what is desired has nothing to do with these aspects of immunity. By clarifying the concepts embraced by the term IMMUNITY, a search direction should become clear. MEDLINE provides suggestions of terms related to the initial word used. Below is the complete list of suggestions, with the number of citations in the database, that followed from IMMUNE:

Term	# of Citations
ANTIBODY DIVERSITY	643
ANTIBODY FORMATION	41,820
ANTIBODY SPECIFICITY	20,862
ANTIBODY-DEPENDENT CELL CYTOTOXICITY	3,908
ANTIGEN-ANTIBODY REACTIONS	19,342
ANTIGEN-PRESENTING CELLS	3,159
ANTIGENS, DIFFERENTIATION, T-LYMPHOCYTE	5,692
AUTOANTIBODIES	21,276

AUTOIMMUNITY	2,278
BLOOD GROUPS	9,899
BLOOD PLATELETS	36,741
BONE MARROW	51,801
CD4-CD8 RATIO	396
COMPLEMENT ACTIVATION	4,600
CYTOTOXICITY, IMMUNOLOGIC	17,190
DESENSITIZATION, IMMUNOLOGIC	3,582
DOSE-RESPONSE RELATIONSHIP, IMMUNOLOGIC	6,592
HELPER CELLS	1,043
HISTAMINE LIBERATION	6,993
HYPERSENSITIVITY, DELAYED	13,065
IMMUNIZATION	26,146
IMMUNOSUPPRESSIVE AGENTS	12,307
IMMUNOTHERAPY	10,635
IMMUNOTHERAPY, ACTIVE	385
KILLER CELLS	4,944
KILLER CELLS, LYMPHOKINE-ACTIVATED	1,454
KILLER CELLS, NATURAL	8,767
LEUKOCYTES	35,973
LYMPHATIC SYSTEM	6,373
LYMPHOCYTE COOPERATION	1,919
LYMPHOCYTE DEPLETION	1,797
LYMPHOCYTE TRANSFORMATION	44,547
LYMPHOCYTES	80,441
LYMPHOCYTES, TUMOR-INFILTRATING	463
LYMPHOKINES	7,065
LYMPHOMA, T-CELL	2,477
LYMPHOMA, T-CELL, PERIPHERAL	171
MACROPHAGE ACTIVATION	3,853
MAST CELLS	10,035
NEUROIMMUNOMODULATION	280
PHAGOCYTES	3,873
RECEPTORS, IMMUNOLOGIC	7,780
RETICULOENDOTHELIAL SYSTEM	3,864
SUPPRESSOR CELLS	2,511
T-LYMPHOCYTES, HELPER-INDUCER	5,711
T-LYMPHOCYTE SUBSETS	2,479
T-LYMPHOCYTES	64,533
T-LYMPHOCYTES, CYTOTOXIC	7,237
T-LYMPHOCYTES, REGULATORY	346
T-LYMPHOCYTES, SUPPRESSOR-INDUCER	3
T4 LYMPHOCYTES	2,643
TRANSFER FACTOR	1,559

By looking for citations that are common to two or more search terms, relevant information can be identified rapidly. In our search for research on herbs and the immune system, the steps are as follows:

1. **Decide on the herbal MeSH term.** In the case of a broad search such as this use a summation of all the terms that might relate to herbs in general. Thus:

DRUGS, CHINESE HERBAL + PLANT EXTRACTS + PLANTS, MEDICINAL + MEDICINE, HERBAL
SUM (F) = 26,068

If the query concerns a specific herb, then use its genus name as the search term. An example might be *Echinacea* or *Astragalus*. The letter F in this particular search example simply resulted from the sum of terms being the sixth entry in the search list.

2. **Decide upon the medical MeSH term.** Be as specific as possible but do not compromise on meaning.

3. **Run the search looking for citations that share both search terms.** The results were as follows:

ON F& IMMUNE SYSTEM	5
ON F& IMMUNITY	54
ON F& AUTOIMMUNITY	1
ON F& KILLER CELLS, NATURAL	46
ON F& IMMUNOSUPPRESSION	16
ON F& IMMUNOTHERAPY	11
ON F& T-LYMPHOCYTES	75

These references relate to specific issues or are so broad that phytotherapy has not been applied to them in a research setting. The much more general concept of "boosting the immune system" is now covered in MEDLINE by the MeSH term "adjuvant, immunological." This is not an immediately obvious term(!), but was found by consulting the latest published guide to MeSH terms. A search gave the following results:

F& ADJUVANTS, IMMUNOLOGIC	43

As examples of the information found this way, here is the download for the sum of all herb terms plus immune system:

87171361 (REFERENCE 1 OF 5)
Atal CK Sharma ML Kaul A Khajuria A
Immunomodulating agents of plant origin. I: Preliminary screening.
J Ethnopharmacol (1986 Nov) 18(2):133-41

The immunobiological activity was investigated of certain medicinal plants widely used in the Ayurvedic and Unani systems of medicine for treatment of chronic infections and immunological disorders. The effect of an ethanolic extract of each drug was studied on delayed type hypersensitivity, humoral responses to sheep red blood cells, skin allograft rejection, and phagocytic activity of the reticuloendothelial system in mice. Picrorhiza kurroa was found to be a potent immunostimulant, stimulating both cell-mediated and humoral immunity. Tylophora indica, Aconitum heterophyllum and Holarrhenaantidysenterica appeared to stimulate phagocytic function while inhibiting the humoral component of the immune system. Tinosporacordifolia and Ocimum gratissimum appeared to improve the phagocytic function without affecting the humoral or cell-mediated immune system. Hemidesmus indicus suppressed both the cell-mediated and humoral components of the immune system.

82211553 (REFERENCE 2 OF 5)
Bernal-Madrazo MA Ham-Carrillo MS
[Effect of tobacco on the immune system. I. Production of the cell migration inhibition factor in the presence of tobacco extract as an antigen in smokers and non-smokers]
Gac Med Mex (1981 Oct) 117(10):412-4

91301916 (REFERENCE 3 OF 5)
Li SY Teh BS Seow WK Liu YL Thong YH
In vitro immunopharmacological profile of the plant flavonoid baohuoside-1.
Int J Immunopharmacol (1991) 13(2-3):129-34

A novel flavonoid compound baohuoside-1 (3,5,7-trihydroxy-4'-methoxyl-8-prenylflavone-3-O-alpha-L-rhamnopy ranoside) was investigated for immuno-pharmacological properties in vitro. The results show that baohuoside-1 has significant suppressive effects on neutrophilchemotaxis, mitogen-induced lymphocyte transformation, mixed-lymphocyte culture, NK-cell cytotoxicity and IL-2 production. These dose-dependent inhibitory effects were found to be significant at concentrations of less than 1 microgram/ml, compared with greater than 94% cell viability at concentrations of 10 micrograms/ml. These results suggest that baohuoside-1 may have potential as an anti-inflammatory/immunosuppressive agent.

86006106 (REFERENCE 4 OF 5)
Bernal-Madrazo MA Casales-Ortiz G Ham-Carrillo MS
[Tobacco addiction and the immune system: II. Production of the cellular migration inhibitory factor in the presence of tobacco extract as an antigen, in patients with extrinsic bronchial asthma]
Gac Med Mex (1985 May-Jun) 121(5-6):195-8

92322148 (REFERENCE 5 OF 5)
Dai Y Hang B Huang Z Li P
[Anti-inflammatory activities and effect of Rhizoma Alismatis on immune system]
Chung Kuo Chung Yao Tsa Chih (1991 Oct) 16(10):622-5, inside back cover

10 and 20 g/kg of Rhizoma Alismatis (RA) markedly decrease the clearance rate of charcoal particles in mice, but have no significant effect on the weight of immune organs, or on the content of serum antibody hemolysin and immunoglobulin G and the delayed footpad edema induced by sheep red blood cell. The contact dermatitis of mouse pinnae immunized with dinitrochlorobenzene is inhibited by RA when it is given before challenge. In addition, RA 20g/kg suppresses the swelling of mouse pinnae induced by xylene and the proliferation of granuloma induced by cotton-pellet in rats. However, the content of vitamin C in the adrenal of rats is not clearly affected by RA.

Here are selections from the download of the list that is the sum of all herb terms plus killer cells, natural.

93060412
Won SJ Lin MT Wu WL
Ganoderma tsugae mycelium enhances splenic natural killer cell activity and serum interferon production in mice.
Jpn J Pharmacol (1992 Jun) 59(2):171-6

Effects of the water-soluble extract of Ganoderma tsugae mycelium (GT), its alcohol-insoluble subfraction (GTI), and its alcohol-soluble subfraction (GTS) on splenic natural killer (NK) cell activity and serum interferon (IFN) production were assessed in mice. Intraperitoneal administration of GT (4-200 mg/kg) or GTI (1-50 mg/kg), but not GTS, augmented the NK cytotoxic activity in a dose-dependent manner in C3H/HeN mice. This augmentation of splenic NK cytolytic activity was not mouse-strain-dependent. The serum IFN titers of mice were also elevated after i.p.-doses of GTI. The GTI-induced serum IFN was reduced by either IFN-(alpha+beta) antiserum or IFN-gamma monoclonal antibody in vitro. The treatment with antiserum neutralizing IFN-(alpha+beta) resulted in a 70% reduction of GTI-induced IFN, while monoclonal antibody against mouse IFN-gamma moderately neutralized the GTI-induced IFN (50%). These results demonstrated that both the splenic NK activity and serum IFN [IFN-(alpha+beta) and IFN-gamma] titers are elevated by Ganoderma tsugae mycelium extracts in mice.

93005449
Liu C Lu S Ji MR
[Effects of Cordyceps sinensis (CS) on in vitro natural killer cells]
Chung Kuo Chung Hsi I Chieh Ho Tsa Chih (1992 May) 12(5):267-9, 259

The effects of Cordyceps sinensis (CS) on peripheral NK cells from healthy persons and leukemia patients were studied. The results showed that CS could augment the NK cell activity, meanwhile, the dose-dependent effect was found within the range of dosage adopted (r= 0.984, P less than 0.01; r = 0.988, P less than 0.01). Furthermore, CS could also improve the CD16 marker expression on lymphocytes and the binding capacity to K562 cells. Cytotoxicity could not be present when the PBNCs were co-incubated with CS. These results suggested that CS could be exploited and utilized as an approach of biological responsive modifier therapy (BRMT) in the treatment of leukemia.

93013938
Kuttan G Kuttan R
Immunomodulatory activity of a peptide isolated from Viscum album extract (NSC 635 089).
Immunol Invest (1992 Jul) 21(4):285-96

A peptide isolated from Viscum album extract (Iscador) has been earlier reported to have cytotoxic and tumor reducing activity. Administration of the peptide (2 micrograms/ml) was found to produce increased natural killer cell activity (NK-activity) in the normal animals and tumor bearing animals. The peak activity was observed on the 3rd day after the administration of the peptide. Administration of the peptide also stimulated antibody dependent cellular cytotoxicity (ADCC) which was expressed maximally on the fourth day. There was also an increase in antibody forming cells in the spleen, and antibody titers were increased in the animals treated with the peptide. Activity of the crude plant extract coincided with the activity of the peptide, indicating that the isolated peptide is mainly responsible for the immunostimulatory activity present in Viscum album extract.

85118751
Jie YH Cammisuli S Baggiolini M
Immunomodulatory effects of Panax Ginseng C.A. Meyer in the mouse.
Agents Actions (1984 Oct) 15(3-4):386-91

An aqueous extract of Panax Ginseng C.A. Meyer (G.S.) was prepared by boiling crushed G.S. roots in water. The extract obtained was adjusted to 125 mg G.S. per ml and was administered orally to mice for 5 to 6 days at the daily dose of 10, 50 and 250 mg G.S. per kg or was added to cultures of mouse spleen cells at concentrations varying between 0.25 and 8 mg G.S. per ml. The average total ginsenoside content of the G.S. roots used was determined by HPLC analysis and found to be 0.58% (w/w). Treated mice responded with enhanced antibody formation to either a primary or a secondary challenge with sheep red cells. The effects were dose-dependent. At the highest dose regimen, the primary IgM response was increased by 50% and the secondary IgG and IgM responses were increased by 50 and 100%, respectively. An even more pronounced effect was obtained with natural killer cell activity which was enhanced between 44 and 150% depending on the effector-to-target cell ratios used in the assay. In vitro, G.S. showed two main effects, an inhibition of stimulated and spontaneous lymphocyte proliferation at high, but not cytotoxic, concentrations and an enhancement of interferon production particularly in non-stimulated spleen cells. The immunostimulating effects obtained in vivo are in agreement with the stimulation of interferon production observed in vitro. The inhibition of lymphocyte proliferation, however, cannot be reconciled with the immunostimulatory action of G.S. observed in vivo.

87221090
Hamprecht K Handgretinger R Voetsch W Anderer FA
Mediation of human NK-activity by components in extracts of Viscum album.
Int J Immunopharmacol (1987) 9(2):199-209

Viscum album extracts (Iscador) were investigated for their potency to influence NK cytotoxicity in vitro. In vitro short-term cytotoxicity assays (4 h) with human peripheral mononuclear cells (PMNC) and human K 562 tumor cells showed a drastic enhancement of NK cytotoxicity in the presence of V. album extracts. The presence of the V. album components during tumor cell lysis was essential since preincubation of PMNC with V. album extract followed by thorough washing did not lead to enhancement of NK cytotoxicity. One responding effector cell was identified as a member of the large granular lymphocyte (LGL) family carrying both Leu 7 and Leu 11 surface markers. Furthermore, monocytes depleted of LGL, but not differentiated macrophages, showed a weak enhancement of their cytolytic activity in the presence of V. album extract. Fractionation of V. album extracts revealed two active fractions, one (C1) with about 3-4000 D and the other (C2) less than 1000 D. Both components enhanced NK cytotoxicity of LGL (Leu 7+, Leu 11+) as well as of monocytes showing enhancing effects also against moderately NK-sensitive tumor cell lines.

92298813
Yan YS
[Effect of Chinese tea extract on the immune function of mice bearing tumor and their antitumor activity] Chung Hua Yu Fang I Hsueh Tsa Chih (1992 Jan) 26(1):5-7

The dynamic changes of cellular immune function and antitumor effect of GTE (green tea extract) in the BALB/c mice bearing EAC, HAC and S-180 tumor were investigated. Results showed that intraperitoneal injection GTE daily dose of 80 mg/kg stimulates the proliferation of T-Lymphocyte S-180 tumor bearing mice, the 125-IudR incorporation value (cpm) of control group was 932 & that of GTE treated group increased to 2988. The Natural Killer cell's activity (cpm) of treated group was raised from 10.7% of control group to 41%. Daily dose 50 mg/kg inhibited the EAC, HAC and the lifespan of GTE mice bearing EAC ascites tumor prolonged 128%. The GTE were effective on growth activity against mouse Ehrlich tumor at a dose of 500 mg/kg by oral administration (P less than 0.05), the inhibition ratio being about 32%. The authors suggested the mechanism of antitumor effects of GTE possible included both cellular immune function and the inhibition of tumor growth.

The list for the sum of all herb terms plus t-lymphocytes found 123 references. As this would take quite some time to download screen by screen, the faster method of downloading at the end of the search was chosen. PaperChase sorts the citations by journal as shown below.

<IN PaperChase Core Journals>

AIDS
(REFERENCE 1 OF 123)
91369520
Ferrari P Trabaud MA Rommain M Mandine E Zalisz R Desgranges C Smets P
Toxicity and activity of purified trichosanthin.
AIDS 1991 Jul;5(7):865-70

Trichosanthin was purified from fresh Chinese root tubers of Trichosanthes kirilowii and evaluated for anti-HIV activity. Trichosanthin inhibited syncytium formation between infected H9 cells and uninfected Sup-T1 cells from 0.5 to 4 micrograms/ml. Trichosanthin also inhibited HIV replication in H9 and CEM-SS cells at 1 microgram/ml, but was toxic for MT-4 cells (HTLV-I-positive), at doses greater than 0.25 microgram/ml. This new purification procedure confirms the anti-HIV activity of trichosanthin on some cell lines in different biological assays.

ANNUAL REVIEW OF MEDICINE
(REFERENCE 2 OF 123)
75203746
Norman PS
Immunotherapy (desensitization) in allergic disease.
Annu Rev Med 1975;26:337-44
[No Abstract Available]

ARTHRITIS AND RHEUMATISM
(REFERENCE 3 OF 123)
92029100
Tao X Davis LS Lipsky PE
Effect of an extract of the Chinese herbal remedy Tripterygium wilfordii Hook F on human immune responsiveness.
Arthritis Rheum 1991 Oct;34(10):1274-81

Tripterygium wilfordii Hook F (TWH) is a vine-like plant that grows in a wide area of south China. An alcohol extract of this plant known as T2 has been suggested to be effective in the treatment of rheumatoid arthritis (RA). To examine the mechanism by which this herbal remedy might be effective in RA, the capacity of T2 to alter human immune responsiveness in vitro was investigated. Human peripheral blood mononuclear cells were obtained from normal adults and separated into purified populations of monocytes, T cells, and B cells. T2 at 0.1-1 micrograms/ml inhibited antigen- and mitogen- stimulated proliferation of T cells and B cells, interleukin-2 (IL-2) production by T cells, and immunoglobulin production by B cells. T2 did not affect

IL-2 receptor expression by T cells, IL-1 production by monocytes, or the capacity of monocytes to present antigen. Inhibition could not be accounted for by nonspecific toxicity. These results support the conclusion that T2 exerts a powerful suppressive effect on human immune responses. This action might account for its therapeutic effectiveness in RA.

BRITISH JOURNAL OF RHEUMATOLOGY
(REFERENCE 4 OF 123)
90002068
Rantapaa Dahlqvist S Norberg B Sondell K Nordenson I Holmgren G
The effect of CPH 82 on the growth of human lymphocytes in vitro. Definition of cytobiological action.
Br J Rheumatol 1989 Oct;28(5):418-21

A drug composed of two semisynthetic podophylline derivatives, CPH 82, has recently been launched for the treatment of severe rheumatoid arthritis. The present in vitro study of PHA-stimulated human T-lymphocytes showed that CPH 82 arrested cell division in a metaphase- like configuration. The cell cycle effects of CPH 82 were indistinguishable from the cell cycle effects of the classical microtubule depolymerizers, Colcemid (a colchicine derivative) and podophyllotoxin. A CPH 82 concentration of 1 microgram/ml, which is close to therapeutic serum concentrations, had an almost maximal effect on cell division. It is suggested that at least part of the anti-inflammatory effect of CPH 82 is due to a colchicine-like activity on, for example, proliferating lymphocytes.

CANCER
(REFERENCE 5 OF 123)
89106063
Sun Y Hersh EM Talpaz M Lee SL Wong W Loo TL Mavligit GM
Immune restoration and/or augmentation of local graft versus host reaction by traditional Chinese medicinal herbs.
Cancer 1983 Jul 1;52(1):70-3

The in vitro restorative effect of aqueous extracts from two traditional Chinese medicinal herbs were studied in 19 cancer patients and in 15 normal healthy donors. Using the local graft versus host (GVH) reaction as a test assay for T-cell function, the extract from astragalus membranaceus (10 microgram/ml) induced a restored reaction in nine of ten patients with an increase in local GVH reaction from 18.2 plus/minus 15.8 mm3 to 112.9 plus/minus 94.2 mm3 (P less than 0.01). The extract from ligustrum lucidum likewise effected an immune restoration in nine of 13 cancer patients with an increase in local GVH reaction from 32.3 plus/minus 36.1 mm3 to 118 plus/minus 104.9 mm3 (P less than 0.01). This degree of immune restoration appears to be complete as it equals the local GVH reaction observed among untreated mononuclear cells from normal healthy donors (82.8 plus/minus 41.1 mm3, P greater than 0.1). These results suggest that both extracts of the traditional Chinese medicinal herbs contain potent immune stimulants which may provide the rational basis for their therapeutic use as biological response modifiers.

CLINICAL AND EXPERIMENTAL IMMUNOLOGY
(REFERENCE 6 OF 123)
74101513
Asherson GL Ferluga J Janossy G
Non-specific cytotoxicity by T cells activated with plant mitogens in vitro and the requirement for plant agents during the killing reaction.
Clin Exp Immunol 1973 Dec;15(4):573-89
[No Abstract Available]

IMMUNOLOGY

(REFERENCE 7 OF 123)
83005598
Kumazawa Y Mizunoe K Otsuka Y
Immunostimulating polysaccharide separated from hot water extract of Angelica acutiloba Kitagawa (Yamato tohki).
Immunology 1982 Sep;47(1):75-83

Separation of immunostimulating polysaccharide (ATP) from Angelica and its biological activities were investigated. AIP was separated as an acetone-insoluble and non-dialysable fraction from hot water extract obtained by heating the root of Angelica acutiloba in water at 95 degrees—98 degrees for 30 min. It is a water-soluble heteropolymer(s) consisting of uronic acid, hexose and peptide. The anti-tumor activity of AIP was observed in terms of prolongation of the survival period of mice bearing Ehrlich ascites cells. The uptake of tritiated thymidine into murine and human spleen cells could be stimulated by AIP in a dose-dependent manner. Murine B cells were activated polyclonally by AIP and differentiated to antibody-forming cells even in the absence of either helper T cells or macrophages. The possibility that the biological activity of AIP might be due to contamination by bacterial lipo-polysaccharides (LPS) or lipid A-associated protein (LAP) was ruled out for the following reasons: (i) polyclonal B-cell activation by AIP was shown in spleen cell cultures of C3H/HeJ mice, a low responder strain to LPS; (ii) the activity of AIP disappeared completely after a mild periodate oxidation whereas that of LPS containing LAP was not lost by similar treatment. In addition, the primary antibody response to sheep-erythrocytes was markedly augmented by an intraperitoneal injection of AIP. This result shows that AIP is a potent adjuvant.

INTERNATIONAL ARCHIVES OF ALLERGY AND APPLIED IMMUNOLOGY

(REFERENCE 8 OF 123)
83159926
Anfosso FJ Guillard PM Charpin JP
Studies on a new lymphocyte mitogen from pollen aqueous extract: induction of proliferation in human and rodent lymphocytes.
Int Arch Allergy Appl Immunol 1983;71(1):6-14

Fraction III (Fr III) mitogen was isolated from the whole aqueous extract (WAE) of plane-tree pollen by Con A-Sepharose chromatography and gel filtration. It stimulated mouse spleen cells, and peripheral blood lymphocytes from plane-tree non-sensitive patients or from cord blood. A 6-day culture gave the best response. The proliferation was not abolished by washing the cells after a short pulse of Fr III given in the initial step but was inhibited by alpha-D-methylmannoside. These results suggested that Fr III bound to a specific site onto spleen cells. This mitogen was not immunogenic in mice and did not bind to human IgE. It induced the proliferation of T lymphocytes in presence of accessory cells and was a polyclonal activator.

(REFERENCE 9 OF 123)
88226997
Wheeler AW Spackman VM Cottam GP Moran DM
Retained T-cell reactivity of rye grass pollen extract following cleavage with cyanogen bromide and nitrothiocyanobenzoic acid.
Int Arch Allergy Appl Immunol 1988;86(1):1-8

Rye grass pollen extract was fragmented by sequential treatments with cyanogen bromide and 2-nitro-5-thiocyanobenzoic acid, and a fraction containing fragments of molecular weight greater than 10,000 Mr was isolated. The in vitro reactivity of the extract with specific IgE was extensively reduced by fragmentation. Less reduction in activity was shown either by skin testing or by inhibition of an extract-specific IgG-binding assay. Reactivity with, and ability to induce, extract-specific mouse T cells were retained by the fragment preparation, and the ability to cause transformation of lymphocytes from atopic donors was unchanged. Fragments did not induce extract-specific IgG antibody in mice, were unable to stimulate the production of T-helper cells which could collaborate in an adoptive cell-transfer system, and did not induce delayed hypersensitivity reactions in guinea pigs. The possibility that such T-cell-reactive modified allergens (T'allergoids) might be used to stimulate selectively T-cell subsets and, therefore, could be used to advantage in immunotherapy is discussed.

INTERNIST
(REFERENCE 10 OF 123)
92064427
[The role of natural substances in modern drug therapy. Satellite symposium of the 2nd German Physician's Congress. Dresden, 15 June 1991]
Internist (Berl) 1991 Sep;32(9 Suppl [WERT]):1-8 (Published in German)
[No Abstract Available]

JOURNAL OF THE AMERICAN ACADEMY OF DERMATOLOGY
(REFERENCE 11 OF 123)
86169091
Baadsgaard O
Circulating and in situ lymphocyte subsets and Langerhans cells in patients with compositae oleoresin dermatitis and increased ultraviolet A sensitivity during treatment with azathioprine.
J Am Acad Dermatol 1986 Apr;14(4):577-81

Circulating and in situ lymphocyte subsets and Langerhans cells in four patients with compositae oleoresin dermatitis and increased ultraviolet A sensitivity before and during treatment with azathioprine were estimated. It was found that the number of Leu 6+ Langerhans cells decreased during therapy. This decrease was accompanied by a reduction in the number of Leu 2a+, Leu 3a+, Leu 4+, DR+, and Leu M2+ cells in the blood and a reduction in the number of Leu 2a+, Leu 3a+, Leu 4+, and DR+ cells in the skin. Concomitantly with the changes in the number of immuno-competent cells, the eczema cleared.

JOURNAL OF CLINICAL INVESTIGATION
(REFERENCE 12 OF 123)
80050143
Byers VS Castagnoli N Jr Epstein WL
In vitro studies of poison oak immunity. II. Effect of urushiol analogues on the human in vitro response.
J Clin Invest 1979 Nov;64(5):1449-56
[No Abstract Available]

(REFERENCE 13 OF 123)
80050142
Byers VS Epstein WL Castagnoli N Baer H
In vitro studies of poison oak immunity. I. In vitro reaction of human lymphocytes to urushiol.
J Clin Invest 1979 Nov;64(5):1437-48

Poison oak, ivy, and sumac dermatitis is a T-cell-mediated reaction against urushiol, the oil found in the leaf of the plants. This hapten is extremely lipophilic and concentrates in cell membranes. A blastogenesis assay employing peripheral blood lymphocytes obtained from humans sensitized to urushiol is described. The reactivity appears 1 to 3 weeks after exposure and persists from 6 weeks to 2 months. The dose-response range is narrow, with inhibition occurring at higher antigen concentrations. Urushiol introduced into the in vitro culture on autologous lymphocytes, erythrocytes and heterologous erythrocytes produces equal results as measured by the optimal urushiol dose, the intensity of reaction, and the frequency of positive reactors. This suggests that the urushiol is passed from introducer to some other presenter cell. Although the blastogenically reactive cell is a T cell, there is also a requirement for an accessory cell, found in the non-T-cell population, for reactivity. Evidence is presented that this cell is a macrophage.

(REFERENCE 14 OF 123)
75133810
Woody JN Ahmed A Knudsen RC Strong DM Sell KW
Human T-cell heterogeneity as delineated with a specific human thymus lymphocyte antiserum. In vitro effects on mitogen response mixed leukocyte culture, cell-mediated lymphocytotoxicity, and lymphokine production.
J Clin Invest 1975 May;55(5):956-66

Human peripheral blood lymphocytes (PBL) were evaluated by their responses to phytohemagglutinin (PHA-P), concanavalin A (con-A), and pokeweed mitogen (PWM), both before and after treatment with an antiserum against human thymic lymphocyte antigens (HTLA) that had been made T-cell-specific by multiple absorptions with immunoglobulin EAC-positive lymphoblast cell lines (B cells). Cells treated with HTLA were examined for their ability to react in a mixed lymphocyte culture (MLC) and to form killer cells in a cell-mediated lymphocytotoxicity (CML) system. Sensitized cells were also examined for their ability to respond to purified protein derivative (PPD) by blastogenesis, migration inhibitory factor release (MIP), and lymphotoxin (LT) production, both before and after treatment with HTLA and complement. The HTLA was in itself highly stimulatory to PBL. However, with the addition of complement and subsequent cell destruction, a marked decrease in its stimulatory response was noted. PBL treated with HTLA and complement exhibited marked inhibition of responsiveness to con-A with little decrease in PHA-P or PWM stimulation except at very high concentrations of HTLA. MLC reaction was inhibited only when responder cells were treated with HTLA + C'. Treatment of stimulator cells with HTLA + C' did not significantly alter the MLC response. The HTLA + C'-treated cells failed to form killer cells in the CML reaction and inhibited PPD-induced blastogenesis from PPD-sensitized individuals; however, treatment of sensitized cells with HTLA + C' had little effect on the release of MIF and LT. It is suggested that subpopulations of T-cells carry surface antigens that bind with this specific antisera, and that the con-A-responsive cells, the responder cells in the MLC, and killer T-cells comprise a separate subset from cells responding to PHA-P or PWM, or the MIF- and LT-producing cells.

JOURNAL OF EXPERIMENTAL MEDICINE
(REFERENCE 15 OF 123)
69236892
Marshall WH Valentine FT Lawrence HS
Cellular immunity in vitro. Clonal proliferation of antigen-stimulated lymphocytes.
J Exp Med 1969 Aug 1;130(2):327-43
[No Abstract Available]

JOURNAL OF IMMUNOLOGY
(REFERENCE 16 OF 123)
77052516
Fairchild SS Malley A

Mouse B and T lymphocyte responses to purified timothy pollen antigens in vitro.
J Immunol 1976 Dec;117(6):2137-42

Purified populations of splenic B and T lymphocytes from LAF mice immunized with a crude extract of timothy pollen (WST) responded specifically to pollen antigens in an in vitro lymphocyte transformation system. The peak lymphocyte transformation response occurred 5 days after a secondary immunization and was the result of T-B cell cooperation in vitro. With two purified pollen antigens as in vitro stimulants we were able to define at least two antigen-specific populations of B cells and one population of T cells. These results were confirmed by inhibition studies with a monovalent hapten from WST, Antigen D.

JOURNAL OF INFECTIOUS DISEASES
(REFERENCE 17 OF 123)
92166420
Baylor NW Fu T Yan YD Ruscetti FW
Inhibition of human T cell leukemia virus by the plant flavonoid baicalin (7-glucuronic acid, 5,6-dihydroxyflavone).
J Infect Dis 1992 Mar;165(3):433-7

The ability of baicalin (7-glucuronic acid, 5,6-dihydroxyflavone), a flavonoid compound purified from the Chinese medicinal herb, Scutellaria baicalensis georgi, to inhibit human T cell leukemia virus type I (HTLV-I) was examined. Baicalin produced concentration-dependent inhibition of HTLV-I replication in productively infected T and B cells. Moreover, baicalin treatment selectively reduced the detectable levels of HTLV-I p19 gag protein in infected cells by greater than 70% at concentrations that produced insignificant effects on total cellular protein and DNA synthesis with no loss in cell viability. Resistance to HTLV-I infection and virus-mediated transformation was noted in uninfected peripheral blood lymphocytes pretreated with baicalin before cocultivation with lethally irradiated chronically infected cells. Baicalin inhibited reverse transcriptase activity in HTLV-I-infected cells as well as the activity of purified reverse transcriptase from Moloney murine leukemia virus and Rous-associated virus type 2. These results suggest that baicalin may be a potential therapeutic agent against HTLV-I-associated T cell diseases.

NATURE
(REFERENCE 18 OF 123)
68005267
Fujiwara M Natata T
Induction of tumor immunity with tumor cells treated with extract of garlic (Allium sativum).
Nature 1967 Oct 7;216(110):83-4
[No Abstract Available]

PROCEEDINGS OF THE SOCIETY FOR EXPERIMENTAL BIOLOGY AND MEDICINE
(REFERENCE 19 OF 123)
75196774
Furusawa E Suzuki N Furusawa S Lee JY
Combination chemotherapy of Rauscher leukemia and ascites tumors by narcissus alkaloid with standard drugs and effect on cellular immunity.Proc Soc Exp Biol Med 1975 Jul;149(3):771-8

The therapeutic activity of the narcissus residual alkaloid A-2 against Rauscher leukemia has been compared with 10 standard anticancer drugs, and synergistic or additive combination pairs have been selected using a viral leukemia and two transplantable tumor systems. An increased beneficial effect has been demonstrated by a combination of the alkylating and DNA-binding agents and the alkaloid against the three malignant tumors, while a beneficial effect by combining the alkaloid and the anti-metabolites (either 6-MP or 5-azacytidine) was seen only against the viral leukemia. The alkaloid has no suppressive activity against cellular immunity as tested by PHA reactivity and allogeneic tumor rejection systems.

<NOT IN PaperChase Core Journals>

AIDS RESEARCH AND HUMAN RETROVIRUSES
(REFERENCE 20 OF 123)
90226890
Lai PK Donovan J Takayama H Sakagami H Tanaka A Konno K Nonoyama M
Modification of human immunodeficiency viral replication by pine cone extracts.
AIDS Res Hum Retroviruses 1990 Feb;6(2):205-17

We have shown previously that two fractions (PC6 and PC7) extracted from cones of the Japanese white pine Pinus parvifloria Sieb. et Zucc have potent immunopotentiating effects. Here, we show that PC6 and PC7 inhibited HIV-1 repli-cation (greater than 95%), in a dose-dependent manner, in chronically infected CR10/HIV-1 cells and in acute cytolytic HIV-1 infection of CEM cells. Treatment of CEM cells, prior to or after acute infection with HIV-1, reduced subsequent viral produc-tion, but the best inhibitory effect was obtained with treatment before and after in-fection: an 80% inhibition was achieved with as little as 3 micrograms/ml of PC6. Comparable results were also obtained when PC6 was used to inhibit HIV-1 replica-tion in the U937 human histiocytic lymphoma cell line. Both PC6 and PC7 were relatively nontoxic to cells. The anti-HIV-1 effect of PC6 and PC7 we observed in this report, coupled with earlier reports of their immunopotentiating properties, suggest their potential as ideal therapeutic agents for the treatment of AIDS.

AGENTS AND ACTIONS
(REFERENCE 21 OF 123)
85118751
Jie YH Cammisuli S Baggiolini M
Immunomodulatory effects of Panax Ginseng C.A. Meyer in the mouse.
Agents Actions 1984 Oct;15(3-4):386-91

An aqueous extract of Panax Ginseng C.A. Meyer (G.S.) was prepared by boiling crushed G.S. roots in water. The extract obtained was adjusted to 125 mg G.S. per ml and was administered orally to mice for 5 to 6 days at the daily dose of 10, 50 and 250 mg G.S. per kg or was added to cultures of mouse spleen cells at concentrations varying between 0.25 and 8 mg G.S. per ml. The average total ginsenoside content of the G.S. roots used was determined by HPLC analysis and found to be 0.58% (w/w). Treated mice responded with enhanced antibody formation to either a primary or a secondary challenge with sheep red cells. The effects were dose-dependent. At the highest dose regimen, the primary IgM response was increased by 50% and the sec-ondary IgG and IgM responses were increased by 50 and 100%, respectively. An even more pronounced effect was obtained with natural killer cell activity which was enhanced between 44 and 150% depending on the effector-to-target cell ratios used in the assay. In vitro, G.S. showed two main effects, an inhibition of stimulated and spontaneous lymphocyte proliferation at high, but not cytotoxic, concentrations and an enhancement of interferon production particularly in non-stimulated spleen cells. The immunostimulating effects obtained in vivo are in agreement with the stimula-tion of interferon production observed in vitro. The inhibition of lymphocyte prolif-eration, however, cannot be reconciled with the immunostimulatory action of G.S. observed in vivo.

(REFERENCE 22 OF 123)
88307095
Sharma ML Khajuria A Kaul A Singh S Singh GB Atal CK
Effect of salai guggal ex-Boswellia serrata on cellular and humoral immune responses and leucocyte migration.
Agents Actions 1988 Jun;24(1-2):161-4

Effect of alcoholic extract of salai guggal (AESG) was studied on cellular and humoral immune responses in mice and leucocyte migration in rats. Oral administration of AESG strongly inhibited the antibody production and cellular responses to sheep red blood cells in mice. It inhibited the infiltration of polymorphonuclear leucocytes and reduced the volume of pleural exudate in carrageenan induced pleurisy in rats. It showed no cytotoxic effect.

AGENTS AND ACTIONS SUPPLEMENTS
(REFERENCE 23 OF 123)
88046368
Braquet P Guinot P Touvay C
The role of PAF-acether in anaphylaxis demonstrated with the use of the antagonist BN 52021.
Agents Actions Suppl 1987;21:97-117
[No Abstract Available]

ALLERGY
(REFERENCE 24 OF 123)
83098321
Anfosso F Alcaraz G Vervloet D Charpin J
Variations in T cell subsets during hyposensitization of grass-sensitive patients with formaldehyde modified extracts: allergoids.
Allergy 1982 Nov;37(8):613-5

In atopic patients with clinical symptoms of hay fever, changes in T gamma and T mu cells were evaluated during desensitization. A significant increase in T mu and overall in T gamma cells was noted. These results suggested that T cell defect could be restored by desensitization treatment.

AMERICAN JOURNAL OF CHINESE MEDICINE
(REFERENCE 25 OF 123)
86183700
Sein GM
B.C.L. and immune response in mice.
Am J Chin Med 1986;14(1-2):33-6

The effects of Korean herbal medicine (B.C.L.) on some parameters of immunological response were studied in mice. B.C.L. pretreatment given either intraperitoneally or subcutaneously in a dose of 0.75 mg/mouse did not significantly inhibit lymphocyte transformation induced by concanavalin A. However, B.C.L. pretreatment in a dose of 2.25 mg/mouse was found to reduce significantly both the plaque-forming cells to sheep red blood cells immunization as well as total spleen cell population. Thus, B.C.L. pretreatment with a higher dose (2.25 mg/mouse) can selectively depress the humoral immune response. It is unclear, however, whether this action is mediated by the parent compound or its metabolites.

ANNALES ACADEMIAE MEDICAE STETINENSIS
(REFERENCE 26 OF 123)
84021873
Kucharska E
[Effect of biostymine on various immunological processes]
Ann Acad Med Stetin 1980;26:369-86 (Published in Polish)
[No Abstract Available]

ANTIBIOTIKI I KHIMIOTERAPIIA
(REFERENCE 27 OF 123)
90379787
Smirnov VV Mishenkova EL Grinevich IuA Petrenko GT Martynenko SV
[Immunomodulating mechanism of the antitumor effect of asterin]
Antibiot Khimioter 1990 Jun;35(6):31-4 (Published in Russian)

It was shown that asterin therapy performed on a model of spontaneous metastasis markedly changed the content of the thymus serum factor in mice and normalized its level. The inducing mechanism of the drug's antitumor action was realized both at the stage of the metastatic postinvasion phase and during its terminal period which was probably due to an increase in the influence of the thymus on the immune system and evident from an increase in the therapeutic action of the drug.

(REFERENCE 28 OF 123)
90247936
Mishenkova EL
[Study of the immunomodulating properties of antibiotics derived from higher plants]
Antibiot Khimioter 1990 Feb;35(2):33-7 (Published in Russian)

Investigations on screening of immunomodulating substances performed at the Antibiotic Department of the Institute of Microbiology and Virology of the Academy of Sciences of the Ukrainian SSR were analyzed. The analysis and detailed study of a screened antibiotic performed by the author showed that it was promising to use higher plants as organisms producing immunomodulators. A methodical approach was developed and recommended and graphs for screening immunomodulating agents of various origin were proposed.

ARCHIVES OF DERMATOLOGICAL RESEARCH
(REFERENCE 29 OF 123)
85224381
Baadsgaard O Geisler C Plesner T Thestrup-Pedersen K
Lymphocyte subsets in patients with compositae oleoresin dermatitis and increased UVA sensitivity during treatment with azathioprine.
Arch Dermatol Res 1985;277(4):304-6

Four patients with severe contact dermatitis resulting from compositae oleoresin were found to have increased sensitivity to ultraviolet light. All showed a clear reduction of Leu-3a-positive lymphocytes (T helper/inducer cells) and cells expressing the 1a phenotype in their blood. The numbers of T suppressor/cytotoxic (Leu 2a) lymphocytes, monocytes and B lymphocytes were within the normal range. Treatment with azathioprine (150 mg daily) improved the eczema. The number of Leu-3a-positive lymphocytes normalized during therapy, but the number of 1a-positive cells did not.

ARCHIVUM IMMUNOLOGIAE ET THERAPIAE EXPERIMENTALIS
(REFERENCE 30 OF 123)
88182698
Prusek W Jankowski A Radomska G Wieczorek E Podwysocka M
Immunostimulation in recurrent respiratory tract infections therapy in children.
Arch Immunol Ther Exp (Warsz) 1987;35(3):289-302

Selected immunologic parameters and effectivity of immunotherapy were evaluated in 117 children (12 months to 10 years old) suffering from recurrent respiratory tract infections. All the children displayed a profound depression of T lymphocytes number, which resembles the situation seen in AIDS patients. An increase of serum IgM concentration was also noted. Immunotherapy included treatment with the following preparations: TFX and Levamisol which stimulate T cell functions, Broncho-Vaxom which stimulates specific antibody production and a complex herb preparation PADMA showing undefined general stimulatory activity. Separate group of children was subjected to climatotherapy in Czerniawa Sanatorium and received no immunostimulants. All methods of treatment employed had beneficial effect. The highest percentage of positive results was obtained in children receiving TFX and Levamisol. In all groups under study, an elevation of T cells percentage was observed. This was especially evident in Levamisol treated patients. There was no correlation, however, between T cells number and clinical improvement.

ARCHIVES ROUMAINES DE PATHOLOGIE EXPERIMENTALE ET DE MICROBIOLOGIE
(REFERENCE 31 OF 123)
88339566
Olinescu A Hristescu S Poliopol M Agache F Kerek F
The effects of Boicil on some immunocompetent cells. II. In vitro and of the mouse cellular and humoral immune response.
Arch Roum Pathol Exp Microbiol 1987 Apr-Jun;46(2):147-58
[No Abstract Available]

ARZNEIMITTEL-FORSCHUNG
(REFERENCE 32 OF 123)
91254389
Schumacher A Friedberg KD
[The effect of Echinacea angustifolia on non-specific cellular immunity in the mouse]
Untersuchungen zur Wirkung von Echinacea angustifolia auf die unspezifische zellulare Immunantwort der Maus.
Arzneimittelforschung 1991 Feb;41(2):141-7 (Published in German)

Echinacea belongs to the most usable plants in medical treatment since many years. It is applicable in the fields of homeopathy and allopathy, however, there are many different ways of treatment. Two species are listed in the European Pharmacopoeia: Echinacea angustifolia and Echinacea purpurea. They differ in morphology and their chemical composition. There have been chemical and biological analyses of Echinacea for about 80 years. After exact investigations of these reports, the following results were found: Most chemical analyses were done with Echinacea angustifolia, especially the older ones, whereas biological activity was tested with Echinacea purpurea. In almost all of these experiments, proprietaries were preferred to use in contrast to any plant extracts. Most of the reports which declared the stimulating biological activity of Echinacea could not resist any critical opinion. So the frequency of medical application of this drug is mainly due to delivered practical knowledge. The experiments described in this study were practised with a water-soluble plant extract of Echinacea angustifolia. Echinacosid, one of its low-molecular weight compounds, is found in preparations of this plant. Their influence on the unspecified cellular immunity of the mouse after intraperitoneal, intravenous or peroral application was investigated. Under various conditions no effects on the immune system could be found using the carbon clearance test.

BIOCHEMICAL AND BIOPHYSICAL RESEARCH COMMUNICATIONS
(REFERENCE 33 OF 123)
90121239
Yamada H Nagai T Takemoto N Endoh H Kiyohara H Kawamura H Otsuka Y
Plantagoside, a novel alpha-mannosidase inhibitor isolated from the seeds of Plantago asiatica, suppresses immune response.
Biochem Biophys Res Commun 1989 Dec 29;165(3):1292-8

A hot-water extract from the seed of Plantago asiatica showed a potent inhibitory activity against jack bean alpha-mannosidase, and a flavanone glucoside, plantagoside, was isolated as the inhibitor. Plantagoside was a specific inhibitor for jack bean alpha-mannosidase (IC50 at 5 microM) and appeared to be a non-competitive inhibitor of the enzyme. Whereas, negligible or weak inhibitory activities were observed for beta-mannosidase, beta-glucosidase, and sialidase tested. Plantagoside also inhibited alpha-mannosidase activities in mouse liver lysosomal and microsomal fractions, and the enzyme inhibitory activity in microsomal fraction was enhanced in the presence of glucosidase inhibitor, castanospermine. Plantagoside suppressed antibody response to sheep red blood cells and concanavalin A induced lymphocyte proliferation which was measured by [3H] thymidine incorporation.

BIOMEDICINE
(REFERENCE 34 OF 123)
78211567
Shohat B Kirson I Lavie D
Immunosuppressive activity of two plant steroidal lactones withaferin A and withanolide E.
Biomedicine 1978 Jan-Feb;28(1):18-24

Withaferin A and withanolide E, two steroidal lactones of plant origin, were demonstrated to have specific immunosuppressive effects on human B and T lymphocytes as well as on mice thymocytes. E rosettes and EAC rosette formation by normal human T and B lymphocytes were inhibited by the two compounds at very low concentrations. The formation of mouse red blood rosettes by chronic lymphatic leukemic cells were only inhibited by withaferin A. The functional activity of normal human T lymphocytes as assessed by a local xenogeneic graft versus host reaction was also affected by these two plant steroidal lactones. These experiments demonstrate a specific action of the compound on antigen recognition as well as proliferative capacity of T lymphocytes and B lymphocytes.

CANCER IMMUNOLOGY, IMMUNOTHERAPY
(REFERENCE 35 OF 123)
92346623
Chai JG Bando T Kobashi S Oka M Nagasawa H Nakai S Maeda K Himeno K Sato M Ohkubo S
An extract of seeds from Aeginetia indica L., a parasitic plant, induces potent antigen-specific antitumor immunity in Meth A-bearing BALB/c mice.
Cancer Immunol Immunother 1992;35(3):181-5

The antitumor activity of an extract of seeds from Aeginetia indica L., a parasitic plant, was investigated. BALB/c mice, inoculated i.p. 1 x 10(5) syngeneic Meth A tumor cells, were administered 2.5 mg/kg A. indica extract i.p. every 2 days from day

0. The untreated mice died of an ascitic form of tumor growth within 21 days, whereas all the treated mice completely recovered from tumor challenge without any side effects. The extract did not exert direct cytotoxic activity against Meth A in vitro. Mice that survived after the first challenge as a result of A. indica treatment overcame the rechallenge with homologous Meth A without additional administration of the extract. On the other hand, those mice could not survive after rechallenge with Meth 1 tumor cells, which were also established in BALB/c mice but were different in antigenicity from Meth A, suggesting the development of antigen-specific concomitant immunity in the A. indica-cured mice. In the induction phase of antitumor resistance in this system, CD4+ T cells appeared to be the main contributors, since in vivo administration of anti-CD4 mAb completely abolished such resistance. In contrast, anti-CD8 mAb administration did not influence the effect of A. indica. The importance of CD4+ T cells in antitumor immunity was again clarified by Winn assay; that is, spleen and lymph node cells depleted of CD4+ T cells in vitro prior to assay abolished antitumor activity on co-grafted Meth A tumor cells in vivo.

CANCER INVESTIGATION
(REFERENCE 36 OF 123)
93007283
Lersch C Zeuner M Bauer A Siemens M Hart R Drescher M Fink U Dancygier H Classen M
Nonspecific immunostimulation with low doses of cyclophosphamide (LDCY), thymostimulin, and Echinacea purpurea extracts (echinacin) in patients with far advanced colorectal cancers: preliminary results.
Cancer Invest 1992;10(5):343-8

Outpatients (n = 15) with metastasizing far advanced colorectal cancers received immunotherapy consisting of low-dose cyclophosphamide (LDCY) 300 mg/m2 every 28 days i.v., thymostimulin 30 mg/m2, days 3-10 after low-dose cyclophosphamide i.m. once daily, then twice a week, and echinacin 60 mg/m2 together with thymostimulin i.m. All patients had had previous surgery and/or chemotherapy and had progressive disease upon entering the study. Two months after onset of therapy a partial tumor regression was documented in one and a stable disease in 6 other patients by abdominal ultrasonography, decrease of the tumor markers carcinoembryonic antigen (CEA), CA 19-9, CA 15-3, and/or chest roentgenography, which may also be attributed to the natural course of disease. Mean survival time was 4 months, 2 patients survived for more than 8 months. Immunotherapy was well tolerated by all patients without side effects.

CESKOSLOVENSKA FARMACIE
(REFERENCE 37 OF 123)
90367149
Fuska J Proksa B
[Metabolites with immunoregulatory effects isolated from higher plants]
Cesk Farm 1990 Jun;39(4):181-7 (Published in Slovak)
[No Abstract Available]

CHINESE MEDICAL JOURNAL
(REFERENCE 38 OF 123)
91347737
Wu S Hua ZJ Xiao YL Wang Y Zhang J Zhang HY Du WY
Effect of ginsenopolypeptide on the 3H-TdR integration of human blood lymphocyte.
Chin Med J (Engl) 1991 May;104(5):399-401

This paper reports the study of the effect of ginsenopolypeptide on 3H-TdR integration in normal human blood lymphocytes in vitro with micro-blood culture method of 3H-TdR integration. The results showed that the effect of ginsenopolypeptide on 3H-TdR integration in normal human peripheral blood lymphocytes which can be activated by phytoagglutinin was enhanced at low dosage and inhibited at high dosage, and its stimulating spike was 10(-6) micrograms/ml (P less than 0.01).

CHUNG HSI I CHIEH HO TSA CHIH CHINESE JOURNAL OF MODERN DEVELOPMENTS

(REFERENCE 39 OF 123)
92127656
Wang DZ Wang ZQ Zhang ZF
[Treatment of endometriosis with removing blood stasis and purgation method]
Chung Hsi I Chieh Ho Tsa Chih 1991 Sep;11(9):524-6, 515 (Published in Chinese)

According to the method of differentiation of symptom complexes of traditional Chinese medicine (TCM), endometriosis is a disease of blood stasis and mass in the lower portion of abdomen. 76 cases were treated by TCM prescription named endometriotic pill No 1 with rhubarb as the main ingredient. The chief functions of the rhubarb were removing blood stasis, disintegrating mass and purgation. The total effective rate was 80.26%. Among them, the effective rate of dysmenorrhea was 88.89%, that of pelvic pain was 66.72%, that of intercourse pain 72.12%, and diminishing in size of mass or nodule 22.15%; 3 cases of 22 infertility got pregnant (13.63%). The results revealed that the endometriotic pill No 1 yielded distinct improvement in the treatment of endometriosis, including clinical symptoms and signs, laboratory assay of blood rheology, serum Ig, subgroup of T lymphocyte (OKT system) and PG.

(REFERENCE 40 OF 123)
92127647
Ma QH Ju YL Zhang ZL
[Immunological study of inefficiency schizophrenics with deficiency syndrome treated with xin shen ling]
Chung Hsi I Chieh Ho Tsa Chih 1991 Apr;11(4):215-7, 197 (Published in Chinese)

This paper reports 30 cases of chronic schizophrenics with deficiency syndrome who had chronically taken many sorts of neuroleptic medications and other therapies which were ineffective. The 7 immunological functioning markers were detected: phytohemagglutinin (PHA) intradermic test; circulating immune complex (CIC); T, B lymphocytes, null (N), double (D) cell; and large granular lymphocyte (LGL) and to be compared with a control group of 30 healthy individuals. The result showed that 6 immunological markers (PHA, CIC and T, B, N and D cell) were significantly different as compared with the control group (P less than 0.01). In order to regulate proportion and function to immune cell, the 30 patients were given to take immunomodulating herbs (xin shen ling, XSL) during 6 weeks, while their 7 immunological markers were detected before treatment (BT) and after treatment (AT). The results showed that 5 immunological markers (PHA, CIC, T, N, and D cell) of BT were significantly different as compared with that of AT (P less than 0.01). However, the 5 immunological markers (PHA, CIC, and T, N and D cell) of AT were not significantly different as compared with that of the control group (P less than 0.05). The brief psychosis rating scale (BPRS) and nurses observation scale for inpatient evaluation (NOSIE) were used as evaluating changes of clinical symptoms BT and AT. The results showed that BPRS and NOSIE of BT were significantly different as compared with that of AT (P less than 0.05). The clinical efficacia rate was 67%. We have followed up the results for near 3 years which had a relapse of 5 cases of 20 cases to be discharged. It seemed that XSL may be one of the preventive relapse agents for these patients.

(REFERENCE 41 OF 123)
91004420
Duan S
[Adjustable action of pi-shen recipe on immune function in mice with L1210 ascites]
Chung Hsi I Chieh Ho Tsa Chih 1990 Jul;10(7):426-8, 390 (Published in Chinese)

Proliferation of Con A stimulated splenic lymphocyte was examined by incorporation of 3H-thymidine. Fluorescence polarization of DPH labelled splenic lymphocyte and bone marrow cells was measured. Proliferation of Con A stimulated splenic lymphocyte in DBA inbred healthy mice was higher than that of L1210 mice but fluorescence polarization of DPH labelled splenic lymphocyte in same healthy mice was lower than that of L1210 mice. i.e. membranous lipid lymphocyte fluidity of lymphocyte in the healthy mice was smaller than that of L1210 mice. 9 days after administration of Pi-Shen recipe by stomach tube proliferation of Con A-lymphocyte in the healthy mice has been increased. The recipe adjusted splenic lymphocyte membrane lipid fluidity of L1210 mice to level of those in healthy mice. Effects of Pi-Shen recipe on lipid fluidity of bone marrow cell membrane of L1210 mice were almost similar to that in splenic lymphocytes. These studies suggest that the mechanism or adjustable role of Pi-Shen recipe on T-lymphocyte function related to lymphocyte membrane lipid fluidity.

(REFERENCE 42 OF 123)
91004412
Zhang J
[Cell-mediated immunity in chronic pyelonephritis]
Chung Hsi I Chieh Ho Tsa Chih 1990 Jul;10(7):402-3, 388 (Published in Chinese)

The authors used monoclonal antibody (CD3, CD4, CD8) and indirect immunofluorescence technique to study peripheral blood lymphocyte surface markers in patients with chronic pyelonephritis (CPN) and in normal controls. In CPN patients, a significant decrease in CD3, a lower percentage of CD4 and significant higher percentage of CD8 leading to a decrease in the CD4/CD8 ratio were noted. No differences could be observed between Spleen-Kidney Yang deficiency and Kidney Yin deficiency. The overall picture shown by the CPN patients was compatible to a cell-mediated immune response defection. The CPN patients were then treated with Zi-Ling capsule (ZLC)/transfer factor (TF) and various antibiotics for three months, during which period the authors found a significant increase in CD3, CD4, but no significant change in CD8. Symptoms such as lumbago, fatigue, frequency of urination were improved. A significant decrease in CD4 after cessation of treatment with ZLC and TF was observed. These observations suggested that both ZLC and TF could also improve the immune function, however, they mainly affect CD4 but not CD8 cells, and the effect lasted for only a short period. In conclusion, ZLC/TF and antibiotics administered together would serve as a useful therapeutic measure to be recommended for patients with CPN.

(REFERENCE 43 OF 123)
85025149
Li QL
[Effect of "si jun zi tang" on nucleic acid contents of the thymus gland and T lymphocytes in the peripheral circulation]
Chung Hsi I Chieh Ho Tsa Chih 1984 Jun;4(6):366-7 (Published in Chinese)
[No Abstract Available]

(REFERENCE 44 OF 123)
83285594
Zhou JH
[Progress in pharmacological research of classical Chinese prescriptions in compliance with the principles of traditional Chinese medicine (II)]
Chung Hsi I Chieh Ho Tsa Chih 1983 Mar;3(2):118-20 (Published in Chinese)
[No Abstract Available]

(REFERENCE 45 OF 123)
83155900
Tian LQ
[Massive infusion with Chinese herbal preparations—a preliminary clinical and experimental study of "fluid-replacing" and "yin-restoring" injections]
Chung Hsi I Chieh Ho Tsa Chih 1982 Jul;2(3):153-5 (Published in Chinese)
[No Abstract Available]

(REFERENCE 46 OF 123)
83155887
Yu H
[Traditional Chinese medicine. Chinese medicinal herbs and immunology]
Chung Hsi I Chieh Ho Tsa Chih 1982 Jan;2(1):48-51 (Published in Chinese)
[No Abstract Available]

(REFERENCE 47 OF 123)
90124800
Li CY
[Immunologic changes in active pulmonary tuberculosis treated with a fuzheng guben pill]
Chung Hsi I Chieh Ho Tsa Chih 1989 Nov;9(11):663-5, 645 (Published in Chinese)

This paper reports the changes of immunity in treatment of active pulmonary tuberculosis with Fuzheng Guben Pill (FGP). The chemotherapy group consisted of 11 cases of active pulmonary tuberculosis & was cured by streptomycin (SM) & isonicotinylhydrazide (INH). The FGP group consisted of 14 cases of active pulmonary tuberculosis and was cured by SM and INH in combination with FGP. After 60 days of treatment, the subtype T-cell mediated immunity in the FGP group was recovered to normal level. (OKT3: 46.07 +/- 6.92 to 54.8 +/- 8.74; OKT4: 36.14 +/- 4.79 to 41.00 +/- 4.13, etc). The chemotherapy group had no obvious immunological change after medication. It was shown that FGP had an immunological modulation in active pulmonary tuberculosis patients.

(REFERENCE 48 OF 123)
90090792
Cai ZD
[Recent advances in studies on tonics in Chinese herbal medicine in China]
Chung Hsi I Chieh Ho Tsa Chih 1989 Aug;9(8):508-11 (Published in Chinese)
[No Abstract Available]

(REFERENCE 49 OF 123)
90090783
Sun JS
[Prevention and treatment of recurrent urinary tract infection with yishenkang granule]
Chung Hsi I Chieh Ho Tsa Chih 1989 Aug;9(8):469-71, 45 (Published in Chinese)

In this study, 35 female adult patients who were married and suffered from recurrent urinary tract infection in remission stage with the type of the deficiency of Kidney-Qi were admitted as the objects for this study. Before and after treatment, the T lymphocyte subtype of peripheral blood (OKT3, OKT4, OKT8), serum immunoglobulins (IgG, IgA, IgM, IgD), urinary sIg (sIgA) were performed by the ways of monoclonal antibody technique and radio-immunity analysis. The results proved that disturbances of cell mediated immunity, humoral immunity and local immune function were involved in the pathogenesis of the disease. These changes might be one of the susceptible factors that caused the repeated attacks of the disease, and the internal pathological basis of Kidney-Qi deficiency type. After taking Yishenkang granule according to the principle of benefiting Qi and invigorating the Kidney, the patients had been restored fairly from the disease on the low levels of the immune function, and strengthened on anti-infectious ability. From these, the attacks of the disease had been controlled effectively. The curative rate had reached 68.6%.

(REFERENCE 50 OF 123)
89376716
Chu DT Sun Y Lin JR
[Immune restoration of local xenogeneic graft-versus-host reaction in cancer patients in vitro and reversal of cyclophosphamide-induced immune suppression in the rat in vivo by fractionated Astragalus membranaceus]
Chung Hsi I Chieh Ho Tsa Chih 1989 Jun;9(6):351-4, 326 (Published in Chinese)

Through the process of fractionation, purification by gel filtration chromatography and thereafter the screening with an in vitro local xenogeneic graft-versus-host reaction (XGVHR) model, a fraction was identified as a potent immunorestorative agent and was designated "Fraction 3" (F3). Using the XGVHR in vitro as a model assay for T cell function again, F3 was studied on mononuclear cells (MNC) from 13 cancer patients and exhibited significant immunorestorative activity, with an increase in local XGVHR (compared to untreated cells) of 151.34 +/- 46.02 mm3 vs 57.80 +/- 16.44 mm3, P less than 0.001. The in vitro augmented immune reactions induced by F3 in cancer patients also significantly exceeded the local XGVHR observed in the untreated MNC derived from 9 normal donor controls (94.15 +/- 9.16 mm3, P less than 0.005). In a newly developed in vivo XGVHR animal model, pretreatment of rats with F3 resulted in a significant abrogation of the local XGVHR with a reversal of the immunosuppressive effect of cyclophosphamide from 99.42 +/- 9.2 mm3 (positive control) to 39.78 +/- 8.3 mm3 (P less than 0.001). This reversal was complete as the volume of the abrogated local XGVHR was comparable to that of the negative control (no cyclophosphamide-priming, saline injection only) 34.79 +/- 5.69 mm3 (P greater than 0.1). These results suggest that F3 retained the immunopotentiating activity of the original crude extract and form the rational basis for the use of Astragalus in immunotherapy.

(REFERENCE 51 OF 123)
89336872
He W Zhang DS
[Effects of kuo guan powder on immunologic functions in patients with ben-xu biaoshi syndrome in ischemic heart disease]
Chung Hsi I Chieh Ho Tsa Chih 1989 Apr;9(4):213-5, 196-7 (Published in Chinese)

Ischemic heart disease (IHD) is correlated with the Immunodisturbances. In this study, the immunological effects of Kuo Guan No 1, a powder for aiding Qi and activating the blood, in 17 cases of Qi Yang Xu Xue Yu (QYXXY) syndrome, Kuo Guan No 2, powder for nourishing the Yin and activating the blood, in 14 cases of Yin- Xu Xue-Yu (YXXY) syndrome had been observed in one month treatment. After treatment with both powder of Kuo Guan No 1 and Kuo Guan No 2, the increased levels of IgG, CIC, IC-IgG and IC-C3 in serum and the numbers of B cells in peripheral blood lymphocyte (PBL) of the patients with Ben-Xu Biao-Shi (BXBS) syndrome of IHD angina were markedly decreased and showed no significant difference while compared with the normal controls (P greater than 0.05); the numbers of OKT+3, OKT+4 and OKT+8 cells in PBL, which were lower before treatment in both groups, were obviously increased and showed no marked difference with the controls (P greater than 0.05); the higher ratio of T4/T8 was lowered in group of YXXY syndrome, and showed no difference while compared with the controls (P greater than 0.05), but the ratio in QYXXY syndrome group was lower than that in the controls (P less than 0.05). After the treatment with Kuo Guan No 1, the increased level of C3 in serum in QYXXY group was lowered down to that of the controls (P greater than 0.05). The results indicated that it is reasonable to consider that "Kuo Guan" powder is an immunoregulative preparation for patients with BXBS syndrome of IHD angina.

(REFERENCE 52 OF 123)
89288492
Li CG
[Histopathologic observation on the therapeutic effect of Tripterygium wilfordii in treating experimental allergic encephalomyelitis]
Chung Hsi I Chieh Ho Tsa Chih 1989 Feb;9(2):98-9, 70 (Published in Chinese)

The Tripterygium wilfordii (TW) was used to treat experimental allergic encephalomyelitis (EAE) in guinea pigs. The morphological change was observed by using light microscope. Lymphocytic histochemical staining was performed on the spinal cord from EAE in guinea pigs. The results were: The incidence of inflammatory reaction, neuraxial swelling, break and neuronal necrosis in the treatment group was lower than that in the control group (P less than 0.01-0.005); the variation of incidence of neurofibrillar demyelinating in the treatment group was smaller than that in the control group (P less than 0.025). The result of ANAE and ALP staining for lymphocytes in the spinal cord from EAE was T-cell. It showed TW could inhibit the allergic action and decrease tissular injury.

(REFERENCE 53 OF 123)
89275343
Zhang TZ Li W Yao PF
[Effect of Chinese herbal drugs on T-cell subsets and immune function in chronic senile bronchitis]
Chung Hsi I Chieh Ho Tsa Chih 1988 Nov;8(11):658-9, 644 (Published in Chinese)
[No Abstract Available]

(REFERENCE 54 OF 123)
89249558
Zhao J
[Advances in experimental research on the effects of anticarcinogenic, tonic herbal medicines on immune function]
Chung Hsi I Chieh Ho Tsa Chih 1988 Dec;8(12):754-6 (Published in Chinese)
[No Abstract Available]

(REFERENCE 55 OF 123)
88210747
Wang J Zhang DS
[Effect of shenqiwan on immunological function in the nephrotic syndrome of chronic glomerulonephritis patients]
Chung Hsi I Chieh Ho Tsa Chih 1987 Dec;7(12):731-3, 709 (Published in Chinese)
[No Abstract Available]

(REFERENCE 56 OF 123)
88080681
Dong DC Zhou LF Chen JX
[Changes in proteinuria, renal function and immunity after treatment with injections of a solution of Astragalus membranaceus]
Chung Hsi I Chieh Ho Tsa Chih 1987 Jul;7(7):403-4, 388 (Published in Chinese)
[No Abstract Available]

(REFERENCE 57 OF 123)
86298752
Hu GR
[T cell function in aged persons treated with a kidney-reinforcing principle]
Chung Hsi I Chieh Ho Tsa Chih 1986 May;6(5):264-7, 258 (Published in Chinese)
[No Abstract Available]

CHUNG-HUA CHENG HSING SHAO SHANG WAI KO TSA CHIH
(REFERENCE 58 OF 123)
90029852
Pang SF
[The effect of vitamin A and Astragalus on the splenic T lymphocyte-CFU of burned mice]
Chung Hua Cheng Hsing Shao Shang Wai Ko Tsa Chih 1989 Jun;5(2):122-4, 159 (Published in Chinese)

In present study the effects of vitamin A and Astragalus on the splenic TL-CFU of mice were studied by means of T-lymphocytes colony formation in semi-solid culture in vitro and incorporation of 3H-TdR. Marked reduction of the responsive reaction of TL-CFU and T-lymphocyte transformation were found. The TL-CFU of the experimentally burned mice untreated with vitamin A (i.e. group 1) were significantly inhibited (p less than 0.005) in comparison with the unburned control group (i.e. group 4). And the TL-CFU of the experimentally burned mice treated with vitamin A (i.e. group 3) increased significantly (p less than 0.005) in comparison with group 1. Incorporation of 3H-TdR showed that vitamin A might accelerate the proliferation of the TL-CFU of the burned mice. It means that vitamin A might be regarded as an effective agent for the reversal of the inhibition of cell-mediated immunity in post-burned state, whether Astragalus plays a role in regulating immune inhibition needs further investigation.

CHUNG-HUA CHUNG LIU TSA CHIH [CHINESE JOURNAL OF ONCOLOGY]
(REFERENCE 59 OF 123)
90126245
Wang DC
[Influence of Astragalus membranaceus (AM) polysaccharide FB on immunologic function of human periphery blood lymphocyte]
Chung Hua Chung Liu Tsa Chih 1989 May;11(3):180-3 (Published in Chinese)

Chemotherapy and/or radiotherapy are believed to further lower the already low cellular immunologic response of cancer patients giving poorer prognosis. A number of Chinese medicinal herbs known as Fuzheng therapy (FZT), in which AM is an active one, are being used to enhance the natural host defence function in cancer patients. Among some fractions of AM polysaccharide extracts, FB was the strongest. In vitro restorative effects of FB in 18 normal healthy individuals and in 9 previously untreated advanced cancer patients are reported. Local graft versus host (GVH) reaction and blastogenic response of lymphocytes in vitro (BRL) were used as test index for T-cell function. GVH reaction nodules with a volume greater than or equal to 50 mm3 were considered as positive GVH reaction. FB 100 micrograms/ml induced a restored reaction in 18 normal donors with an increase in local GVH reaction from 69.6 +/- 20.8 mm3 to 148.9 +/- 40.8 mm3 (P less than 0.001) and in 9 cancer patients with an increase in local GVH reaction from 29.3 +/- 9.5 mm3 to 137.2/ - 35.8 mm3 (P less than 0.001). The local GVH reaction of the 9 cancer patients went from negative to positive. FB on BRL was detected. 10 micrograms/ml of FB augmented the spontaneous 3H-TdR incorporation in the lymphocyte of 18 normal subjects from 310.2 to 910.9 counts per minute (cpm) and of 9 patients from 248.5 to 642.2 cpm, but the effects were not strong. The effect of single mitogen was not remarkable. (ABSTRACT TRUNCATED AT 250 WORDS)

CHUNG-HUA I HSUEH TSA CHIH [CHINESE MEDICAL JOURNAL]
(REFERENCE 60 OF 123)
92248481
Cheng Q
[Effect of cordyceps sinensis on cellular immunity in rats with chronic renal insufficiency]
Chung Hua I Hsueh Tsa Chih 1992 Jan;72(1):27-9, 63 (Published in Chinese)

Animal model of chronic renal failure (CRF) was induced in wistar rats by 5/6 nephrectomy. Half of the rats were treated with Cordyceps sinensis (CS) in form of decoction. It was found that CS has mitogenic effect on spleen lymphocytes, and is capable of increasing the production of IL-2 from splenocytes of the CRF rats. IL-2 absorbency of the splenocytes was promoted by CS. CS also exhibited such therapeutic effects on CRF animals as to decrease the level of BUN and serum creatinine and to increase the level of hemoglobin. These results indicate that CS has a regulative effect on cellular immunity in CRF rats.

CHUNG-HUA KOU CHIANG I HSUEH TSA CHIH
(REFERENCE 61 OF 123)
89250910
Zhao RF
[Juvenile periodontitis patients taking gu chi gao]
Chung Hua Kou Chiang Hsueh Tsa Chih 1988 Nov;23(6):368-70, 385 (Published in Chinese)
[No Abstract Available]

CHUNG-HUA YU FANG I HSUEH TSA CHIH [CHINESE JOURNAL OF PREVENTIVE MEDICINE]
(REFERENCE 62 OF 123)
92298813
Yan YS
[Effect of Chinese tea extract on the immune function of mice bearing tumor and their antitumor activity]
Chung Hua Yu Fang I Hsueh Tsa Chih 1992 Jan;26(1):5-7 (Published in Chinese)

The dynamic changes of cellular immune function and antitumor effect of GTE (green tea extract) in the BALB/c mice bearing EAC, HAC and S-180 tumor were investigated. Results showed that intraperitoneal injection GTE daily dose of 80 mg/kg stimulates the proliferation of T-Lymphocyte S-180 tumor bearing mice, the 125-IudR incorporation value (cpm) of control group was 932 and that of GTE treated group increased to 2988. The Natural Killer cell's activity (cpm) of treated group was raised from 10.7% of control group to 41%. Daily dose 50 mg/kg inhibited the EAC, HAC and the life span of GTE mice bearing EAC ascites tumor prolonged 128%. The GTE were effective on growth activity against mouse Ehrlich tumor at a dose of 500 mg/kg by oral administration (P less than 0.05), the inhibition ratio being about 32%. The authors suggested the mechanism of antitumor effects of GTE possibly included both cellular immune function and the inhibition of tumor growth.

(REFERENCE 63 OF 123)
92146157
Cao ZL
[The effect of Bulbus allii on precancerous lesions of the esophagus due to N-methyl-N-amylnitrosamine in rats]
Chung Hua Yu Fang I Hsueh Tsa Chih 1991 Jul;25(4):208-10 (Published in Chinese)

In so much as precancerous lesions of the esophagus are a stage that must pass in the course of formation of carcinoma of the esophagus, inhibiting its occurrence is an important measure in the prevention of esophageal. The test was carried out in 84 Wistar rats of both sexes randomly divided into 2 groups, one group fed with 50% aqueous extract of Bulbus allii and the other as control. After 105th day of experiment, results showed that Bulbus allii inhibited significantly precancerous lesions of the esophagus due to N-methyl-N-amyl-nitrosamine (P less than 0.05) increases of the splenic index (P less than 0.001) in rate and the percentage of peripheral T-lymphocyte (P less than 0.01) in rats. The results suggested that Bulbus allii had a preventive action against carcinoma of the esophagus, which could be attributed to increasing the immunity.

CHUNG-KUO CHUNG HSI I CHIEH HO TSA CHIH
(REFERENCE 64 OF 123)
93005451
Yu YP
[Correlation between syndrome types of traditional Chinese medicine and peripheral T lymphocyte subsets in Graves' disease]
Chung Kuo Chung Hsi I Chieh Ho Tsa Chih 1992 May;12(5):274-6, 260 (Published in Chinese)

This paper reports the determined results of OKT3, OKT4, OKT8, ERFC, smIg and CIC, TMCA, TGA in 31 cases of Graves' disease and in 20 normal controls. The results showed that the OKT3, OKT4, OKT8, and ERFC were significantly lower than those in the normal controls, whereas the smIg was higher than that in normal controls. The difference between the two groups was very significant, even though the ratio of OKT4/OKT8 showed no significance of both. Typology of Graves' disease according to the theory of TCM, all 31 cases were divided into two types: (1) 14 cases of depression of Liver-energy and asthenia of Spleen; (2) 17 cases of deficiency of Yin leads to hyperactivity of Fire. The OKT8 and the ratio of OKT4/OKT8 in the latter respectively were lower and higher than those of the former. The difference between the two types was significant (P less than 0.01, P less than 0.05) whereas the positive rates of the CIC, TMCA, TGA also were higher in the deficiency of Yin leads to hyperactivity of Fire than those in the depression of Liver-energy and asthenia of Spleen. After treatment with combined TCM-WM on 31 cases of Graves' disease, it was found that the OKT4, OKT8, ERFC were significantly elevated, and the smIg was more decreased than those without treatment. It was also found that smIg markedly decreased in two types, OKT8, ratio of OKT4/OKT8 in the latter, and ERFC in both types all returned to normal. Remainder indexes had no obvious change before and after treatment. (ABSTRACT TRUNCATED AT 250 WORDS)

CHUNG-KUO CHUNG YAO TSA CHIH [CHINA JOURNAL OF CHINESE MATERIA]
(REFERENCE 65 OF 123)
93039609
Zhang H Liang H Zhang Z
[Effect of mieyanling oral liquid on the immune responses in normal and cyclophosphamide treated mice]
Chung Kuo Chung Yao Tsa Chih 1992 May;17(5):303-6, backcover (Published in Chinese)

It has been proved that Mieyanling in Vivo & in Vitro can augment the lymphocyte transformation rate induced by PHA, Con-A or LPS in mice. The suppressed immune function caused by cyclophosphamide can also be significantly relieved by Mieyanling Oral Liquid.

CHUNG-KUO I HSUEH KO HSUEH YUAN HSUEH PAO [ACTA ACADEMIAE MEDICINAE]
(REFERENCE 66 OF 123)
84026761
Zheng JR Xu LF Ma L Wang DH Gao JW
[Studies on pharmacological actions of total glycosides in Tripterygium wilfordii]
Chung Kuo I Hsueh Ko Hsueh Yuan Hsueh Pao 1983 Feb;5(1):1-8 (Published in Chinese)
[No Abstract Available]

(REFERENCE 67 OF 123)
82070569
Yao CZ Li F Liu YL Zhang ZD Wang JW Cai BJ Liu YY Cheng JH Zhao SL
[Influence of Chinese herb Lysimachia christinae Hance on immune responses in mice. I. Immunosuppressive effect (author's transl)]
Chung Kuo I Hsueh Ko Hsueh Yuan Hsueh Pao 1981 Jun;3(2):123-6 (Published in Chinese)
[No Abstract Available]

CHUNG YAO TUNG PAO [BULLETIN OF CHINESE MATERIA MEDICA]
(REFERENCE 68 OF 123)
85025122
Chen XS
[On the quality control of Chinese herbal drugs with "heat clearing and detoxicating" properties—selection of bioassay parameters according to the therapeutic principle of traditional Chinese medicine]
Chung Yao Tung Pao 1984 May;9(3):98-102 (Published in Chinese)
[No Abstract Available]

(REFERENCE 69 OF 123)
84082377
Chen YP
[Studies on immunological actions of Cordyceps sinensis. I. Effect on cellular immunity]
Chung Yao Tung Pao 1983 Sep;8(5):33-5 (Published in Chinese)
[No Abstract Available]

(REFERENCE 70 OF 123)
83025340
Yang GH
[Research on protective effects of Chinese tonic herbs against microwave radiation]
Chung Yao Tung Pao 1982 May;7(3):32-4 (Published in Chinese)
[No Abstract Available]

(REFERENCE 71 OF 123)
89304242
Cao ZL Zhu M Liu HX Xiao ZM
[Effects of radix Rehmanniae and processed radix Rehmanniae on some immune functions in mice]
Chung Yao Tung Pao 1988 Oct;13(10):22-4, 62-3 (Published in Chinese)
[No Abstract Available]

DISS ABSTR INT [B]
(REFERENCE 72 OF 123)
92082257C
Tadi PP
ANTICARCINOGENIC, ANTITUMOR, AND ANTIFUNGAL PROPERTIES OF ALLIUM SATIVUM
Diss Abstr Int [B] 1992

In this study the antimutagenic/anticarcinogenic, immune enhancing, antitumor and antifungal effects of a crude extract and organosulfur compounds of garlic were determined. Diallyl sulfide (DAS) and ajoene, each at 100 ug/ml, and garlic extract (GE, 12.5 mg/ml) inhibited rat liver 9000 x g supernatant (S-9)-dependent mutagenesis in Salmonella typhimurium TA100 induced by either aflatoxin B1 (AFB1) or benzo(a)pyrene (B[a]P). The garlic compounds were shown to inhibit the binding of [3H]AFB1 to calf thymus DNA and the formation of specific AFB1-DNA adducts. These effects on mutagenesis and DNA binding correlated with an inhibition of the metabolism of [3H]AFB1. Ajoene and DAS did not affect glutathione-S-transferase, an enzyme important to the conjugation of compounds to glutathione. GE was tested for its effects on immune function in a murine model by injecting C3H/He mice with Candida albicans. GE appeared to control Candida albicans as exhibited in blood and kidney cultures. Peritoneal exudate cells obtained for chemiluminescent assays from garlic-treated mice exhibited an increased oxidative burst. The cytotoxic effects of diallyl disulfide (DADS, 5-200 ug/ml), DAS (200 ug/ml), dimethyl disulfide (DMDS, 5-400 ug/ml) and allyl methyl sulfide (AMS, 5-400 ug/ml), were determined with in vitro cultures of MBT-2, R3327, HL-60 and K562 tumor cells. DADS exhibited toxicity against all the tumor cell lines tested. DMDS was cytotoxic to K562 tumor cells and AMS was cytotoxic to MBT-2 cells. The effects of DADS, DAS, DMDS and AMS on the in vitro growth of C albicans were investigated. Inhibitory concentrations mg/ml of DAS, DMDS, AMS and DADS were in the range of 0.625-1.250, 5-20, 10-20 and 156-625 ug/ml, respectively. The results of this study suggest that garlic compounds inhibited rat liver S-9-mediated AFB1 metabolite binding to calf thymus DNA, AFB1-DNA adduct formation and AFB1-induced mutagenesis in S typhimurium TA100 by inhibition of microsomal mixed-function oxidase activity. Garlic compounds exhibited antifungal activity and enhanced phagocytic activity. In addition, garlic compounds were cytotoxic to several tumor cell lines. (Full text available from University Microfilms International, Ann Arbor, MI, as Order No. AAD92-02458.)

DOKLADY AKADEMII NAUK SSSR

(REFERENCE 73 OF 123)
83157179
Pigarevskii PV Mokhnach IV
[Immunomorphological changes in mouse lymphoid tissue as affected by Aconitum soongaricum Stapf., levamisole and sodium nucleinate]
Dokl Akad Nauk SSSR 1983;268(3):754-6 (Published in Russian)
[No Abstract Available]

EXPERIENTIA

(REFERENCE 74 OF 123)
86247999
Ribereau-Gayon G Jung ML Baudino S Salle G Beck JP
Effects of mistletoe (Viscum album L.) extracts on cultured tumor cells.
Experientia 1986 Jun 15;42(6):594-9

Bacterially fermented mistletoe preparations (BFMP) were tested on rat hepatoma tissue culture (HTC) cells & human leukemia Molt 4 cells. A dose-dependent inhibition of the growth rate of the cells was observed. For both cell lines, cytostatic concentrations, expressed in weight of fresh plant, were 0.5 mg/ml culture medium for oak BFMP and 1 mg/ml for apple tree BFMP. However, the action of the two preparations was markedly different on each cell line. Non-viable HTC cells were not stained by trypan blue while non-viable Molt 4 cells were fully colored by this reagent. A lysis of cellular membranes of HTC cells was observed by electron microscopy. Furthermore, oak BFMP inhibited the growth of virus transformed 3T3-SV40 cells more than that of non-transformed 3T3 cells. In contrast to BFMP, non-fermented extracts and a purified mistletoe lectin showed a greater inhibition of the growth of Molt 4 cells than of HTC cells. Samples withdrawn at different times during fermentation gradually lost their inhibitory effect on the growth of Molt 4 cells while their action on HTC cells increased up to the 4th day of fermentation. These results are discussed in relation to the cytotoxic substances of mistletoe already characterized.

FEBS LETTERS

(REFERENCE 75 OF 123)
91032105
Lee-Huang S Huang PL Nara PL Chen HC Kung HF Huang P Huang HI Huang PL
MAP 30: a new inhibitor of HIV-1 infection and replication.
FEBS Lett 1990 Oct 15;272(1-2):12-8

A new inhibitor of human immunodeficiency virus (HIV) has been isolated and purified to homogeneity from the seeds and fruits of the Momordica charantia. This compound, MAP 30 (Momordica Anti-HIV Protein), is a basic protein of about 30 kDa. It exhibits dose-dependent inhibition of cell-free HIV-1 infection and replication as measured by: (i) quantitative focal syncytium formation on CEM-ss monolayers; (ii) viral core protein p24 expression; and (iii) viral-associated reverse transcriptase (RT) activity in HIV-1 infected H9 cells. The doses required for 50% inhibition (ID50) in these assays were 0.83, 0.22 and 0.33 nM, respectively. No cytotoxic or cytostatic effects were found under the assay conditions. These data suggest that MAP 30 may be a useful therapeutic agent in the treatment of HIV-1 infections. The sequence of the N-terminal 44 amino acids of MAP 30 has been determined.

FOLIA HAEMATOLOGICA. INTERNATIONALES MAGAZIN FÜR KLINISCHE UND

(REFERENCE 76 OF 123)
68006592
Reissmann G
[Nonspecific stimulus therapy and the properdin system]
Folia Haematol Int Mag Klin Morphol Blutforsch 1966;85(2):125-31 (Published in German)
[No Abstract Available]

FORTSCHRITTE DER MEDIZIN

(REFERENCE 77 OF 123)
79214729
Mayr A Raettig H Stickl H Alexander M
[Paraimmunity, paraimmunization, paraimmunity inducers. 2. Paraimmunity inducers, own studies, discussion]
Fortschr Med 1979 Jul 19;97(27):1205-10 (Published in German)
[No Abstract Available]

GAN TO KAGAKU RYOHO [JAPANESE JOURNAL OF CANCER AND CHEMO-THERAPY]

(REFERENCE 78 OF 123)
89272038
Okamoto T Motohasi H Takemiya S Sugimasa Y Sairenji M Kobayasi S
[Clinical effects of Juzen-daiho-to on immunologic and fatty metabolic states in post-operative patients with gastrointestinal cancer]
Gan To Kagaku Ryoho 1989 Apr;16(4 Pt 2-2):1533-7 (Published in Japanese)

Juzen-daiho-to is one of the Chinese traditional medicines which is usually applied with patients suffering from anemia or chronic exhaustive disease. Twenty-three patients after gastrectomy & 16 patients after colectomy were studied for NK cell activity, blastogenesis by PHA, several T-lymphocyte subsets, serum triglyceride and serum lipo-protein before drug administration at one, three, six, nine months and one year after the start of drug administration respectively. A remarkable elevation in NK cell activity was noted 3 and 6 months after the drug administration. Statistical analysis shows a significant converse correlation between NK cell activity and lipo-protein value in the group given Juzen-daiho-to.

(REFERENCE 79 OF 123)
87074931
Xian MS
[Relation between cancer immunity and combination therapy by Chinese traditional medicine and Western medicine and its prognosis]
Gan To Kagaku Ryoho 1986 Dec;13(12):3334-42 (Published in Japanese)
[No Abstract Available]

HAWAII MEDICAL JOURNAL

(REFERENCE 80 OF 123)
90337747
Chien YK Liu YH Massey DG
Interleukin-3 and anti-aging medication: a review.
Hawaii Med J 1990 May;49(5):160-1, 165
[No Abstract Available]

IMMUNOPHARMACOLOGY AND IMMUNOTOXICOLOGY

(REFERENCE 81 OF 123)
91225383
Yonekura K Kawakita T Mitsuyama M Miura O Yumioka E Suzuki A Nomoto K
Induction of colony-stimulating factor(s) after administration of a trad. Chinese medicine, xiao-chai-hu-tang (Japanese name: shosaiko-to).
Immunopharmacol Immunotoxicol 1990;12(4):647-67

Colony stimulating factor (CSF)-rich serum was obtained from mice injected intraperitoneally (ip) with shosaiko-to, a traditional Chinese herbal medicine. Transfer of the CSF-rich serum into naive mice augmented the resistance against Listeria monocytogenes. A dose-dependent induction of CSF was observed in mice given shosaiko-to via intravenous route as well as via intraperitoneal route. Since the serum CSF induction was observed in both lipopolysaccharide (LPS)-responder C3H/He mice and LPS-non-responder C3H/HeJ mice, the effect of shosaiko-to seemed to be independent of possibly contaminating LPS. The level of serum CSF induced by shosaiko-to in athymic nude mice was similar to that in control euthymic mice, and the induction of CSF was completely blocked by the previous administration of carrageenan, a selective macrophage-blocker. In mice treated ip with shosaiko-to CSF activity was detected in the peritoneal cavity, the site of injection, and the time course was similar to that of serum CSF induction. In a bone marrow culture system, the composition of colonies formed by shosaiko-to-induced CSF was similar to that formed by standard GM-CSF. The CSF activity was scarcely affected by treatment of the sera with anti-M-CSF antibody. These results suggest that shosaiko-to augments the host defense by inducing mainly GM-CSF, and that CSF is produced by cells of macrophage lineage. In addition, it was shown that CSF could be induced even after oral administration of herbal medicines.

(REFERENCE 82 OF 123)
89067354
Kawakita T Yamada A Mitsuyama M Kumazawa Y Nomoto K
Protective effect of a trad.Chinese medicine, xiao-chai-hu-tang (Japanese name: shosaiko-to), on Listeria monocytogenes infection in mice.
Immunopharmacol Immunotoxicol 1988;10(3):345-64

Lethal effect of Listeria monocytogenes (L. monocytogenes) in mice was prevented by an intraperitoneal (ip) injection of a traditional Chinese herbal medicine, xiao-chai-hu-tang (Japanese name: shosaiko-to), 4 days before ip bacterial infection. The numbers of bacteria in the peritoneal cavity and liver were smaller in shosaiko-to treated mice from one day after the infection. Macrophage accumulation in the peritoneal cavity after ip inoculation of L. monocytogenes was observed in both untreated and shosaiko-to treated mice. Although rates of such increases were almost the same between both groups, the absolute number of macrophages was larger in shosaiko-to treated than in untreated mice because of a higher level of the macrophage number at 4 days after ip injection of shosaiko-to. In untreated mice, bactericidal activity of peritoneal macrophages decreased from 1 day to 3 days after ip injection of killed L. monocytogenes. Such an activity was maintained at the same level from 1 to 3 days in shosaiko-to treated mice. Augmented accumulation of macrophages and maintenance of their bactericidal activity may be main mechanisms of the augmented resistance in shosaiko-to treated mice. Augmented resistance against bacterial growth in the thigh muscle in ip shosaiko-to treated mice may be caused by such mechanisms. The effect of shosaiko-to observed at an early stage of infection may be T-cell independent, since such an effect was observed in athymic nude mice and delayed footpad reaction could not be detected at such a timing in euthymic normal mice.

INDIAN JOURNAL OF PHYSIOLOGY AND PHARMACOLOGY
(REFERENCE 83 OF 123)
84134357
Vyas DS Acharya RP Dadhich AP Godhwani JL Purohit VS
Effect of Allium cepa (onion) on immune response in rabbit [letter]
Indian J Physiol Pharmacol 1983 Jul-Sep;27(3):259-60
[No Abstract Available]

JOURNAL OF MEDICINAL CHEMISTRY
(REFERENCE 84 OF 123)
92284470
Gustafson KR Cardellina JH 2d McMahon JB Gulakowski RJ Ishitoya J Szallasi Z
Lewin NE Blumberg PM Weislow OS Beutler JA et al
A nonpromoting phorbol from the Samoan medicinal plant Homalanthus nutans in-
hibits cell killing by HIV-1.
J Med Chem 1992 May 29;35(11):1978-86

Extracts of Homalanthus nutans, a plant used in Samoan herbal medicine, exhibited
potent activity in an in vitro, tetrazolium-based assay which detects the inhibition of
the cytopathic effects of human immunodeficiency virus (HIV-1). The active constituent was identified as prostratin, a relatively polar 12-deoxyphorbol ester.
Noncytotoxic concentrations of prostratin from greater than or equal to 0.1 to greater
than 25 microM protected T-lymphoblastoid CEM-SS and C-8166 cells from the killing effects of HIV-1. Cytoprotective concentrations of prostratin greater than or equal
to 1 microM essentially stopped virus reproduction in these cell lines, as well as in
the human monocytic cell line U937 and in freshly isolated human monocyte/mac-
rophage cultures. Prostratin bound to and activated protein kinase C in vitro in CEM-
SS cells and elicited other biochemical effects typical of phorbol esters in C3H10T1/
2 cells; however, the compound does not appear to be a tumor promoter. In skin of
CD-1 mice, high doses of prostratin induced ornithine decarboxylase only to 25-30%
of the levels induced by typical phorbol esters at doses 1/30 or less than that used for
prostratin, produced kinetics of edema formation characteristic of the nonpromoting
12-deoxyphorbol 13-phenylacetate, and failed to induce the acute or chronic
hyperplasias typically caused by tumor-promoting phorbols at doses of 1/100 or less
than that used for prostratin.

JOURNAL OF PHARMACOBIODYNAMICS
(REFERENCE 85 OF 123)
86226957
Iwama H Amagaya S Ogihara Y
Studies of the combined use of steroid and Shosaiko-to, one of the Kampohozai
(Chinese traditional medicine), on pituitary adrenocortical axis function and immune
responses.
J Pharmacobiodyn 1986 Feb;9(2):189-96

The combined effects of Shosaiko-to, one of the Kampohozai (Chinese traditional
medicine), and prednisolone were examined for suppressive actions on pituitary
adrenocortical axis function and immune response induced by prednisolone using
rats and mice. The administration of Shosaiko-to, 1.2 g/kg p.o., for 45 d showed a
tendency to increase adrenal weight. By the combined use of Shosaiko-to, 0.12 and
1.2 g/kg p.o., and prednisolone, 0.016 g/kg p.o., for 45 d, the decrease of adrenal
weight induced by the treatment with prednisolone was restored. The administration
of Shosaiko-to, 1.2 g/kg p.o., elevated the blood corticosterone level. In the case of
combined use, Shosaiko-to, 0.12 and 1.2 g/kg p.o., inhibited the decrease of blood
corticosterone level induced by the treatment with prednisolone, 0.004 g/kg p.o.,

and Shosaiko-to, 1.2 g/kg p.o., inhibited the decrease of blood corticosterone level induced by the treatment with prednisolone, 0.016 g/kg p.o. On the other hand, the administration of Shosaiko-to, 1.2 g/kg p.o., for 7 d reduced the number of hemolytic plaque forming cells (HPFC) in spleen cells. But Shosaiko-to, 1.2 g/kg p.o., administered for 7 d inhibited the decrease of the number of HPFC induced by the treatment with prednisolone, 0.01 and 0.03 g/kg s.c., for 3 d. Furthermore, Shosaiko-to, 1.2 g/kg p.o., restored the number of rosette forming cells (RFC) which decreased by prednisolone, 0.03 g/kg s.c. The decrease of 7S HA titer of the serum by the treatment with prednisolone, 0.01 g/kg s.c., was also inhibited by the combination with Shosaiko-to, 1.2 g/kg p.o.

(REFERENCE 86 OF 123)
86036748
Kumazawa Y Nakatsuru Y Fujisawa H Nishimura C Mizunoe K Otsuka Y Nomoto K
Lymphocyte activation by a polysaccharide fraction separated from hot water extracts of Angelica acutiloba Kitagawa.
J Pharmacobiodyn 1985 Jun;8(6):417-24

The action of a polysaccharide fraction obtained from hot water extracts of Angelica acutiloba Kitagawa, termed as Angelica immunostimulating polysaccharide (AIP) fraction, on murine lymphocytes participating in antibody responses was investigated. When AIP fraction was injected concomitantly into mice immunized with antigens, immunoglobulin M (IgM) and IgG antibody responses against sheep erythrocytes (SRBC) increased significantly, but IgM response against T-independent antigens such as trinitrophenylated lipopolysaccharide (TNP-LPS) and TNP-Ficoll did not augment. Murine B lymphocytes were polyclonally activated in vitro and in vivo by AIP fraction to differentiate into antibody-forming cells as functionally matured cells. The differentiation of B lymphocytes to an intermediate stage capable of responding to helper T lymphocytes was also stimulated by the administration of AIP fraction into CDF1 and C3H/HeJ mice. A concomitant injection of AIP fraction with SRBC for carrier priming resulted in the increment of anti-TNP IgM antibody response in cultures reconstituted with unprimed B and SRBC-primed T lymphocytes, indicating that AIP fraction can stimulate T lymphocytes.

JOURNAL OF TONGJI MEDICAL UNIVERSITY
(REFERENCE 87 OF 123)
93085799
Zhang GM Hao TL Yang YZ Feng ZH Jiang ZY Zhou B Zhang H
Effect of "re du qing" on the activation, proliferation and membrane fluidity of lymphocytes.
J Tongji Med Univ 1992;12(3):150-3

Effects of Chinese Medicinal Preparation "Re Du Qing" (RDQ) on the activation, proliferation and membrane fluidity of T lymphocytes from human peripheral blood were studied by means of 3H-TdR incorporation and DPH fluorescence polarization. The results showed that "RDQ" can: 1) significantly inhibit the activation of T lymphocytes; 2) restrain the proliferation of activated T lymphoblasts in the presence of exogenous interleukin-2 (IL-2); and 3) increase the membrane fluidity of T lymphocytes and antagonize the decreased fluidity of lymphocyte membrane mediated by Con A or PHA. The functional abnormalities of T lymphocytes in some autoimmune diseases such as arthritis and the usefulness of RDQ in the treatment of these diseases were also discussed.

JOURNAL OF TRADITIONAL CHINESE MEDICINE

(REFERENCE 88 OF 123)
90065675
Zhang JQ
Clinical and experimental studies on yang-deficiency.
J Tradit Chin Med 1982 Sep;2(3):237-42
[No Abstract Available]

(REFERENCE 89 OF 123)
85035108
Yang GZ Geng PL
Effects of Yang-promoting drugs on immunological functions of Yang-deficient animal model induced by prednisolone.
J Tradit Chin Med 1984 Jun;4(2):153-6
[No Abstract Available]

(REFERENCE 90 OF 123)
84293936
Jiang TL Yan SC Wang SF Wu GL Feng GW Li LF Li XM Shen JH
Effect of "liuwei dihuang decoction" on prevention and treatment of tumor.
J Tradit Chin Med 1984 Mar;4(1):59-68
[No Abstract Available]

(REFERENCE 91 OF 123)
83243214
Chen WB Li TQ Yan LQ Li ZY Liu MY
Boosting effects of drugs benefiting vital energy & activating blood and transfer factor on the immunity of patients with chronic cor pulmonale.
J Tradit Chin Med 1983 Mar;3(1):63-6
[No Abstract Available]

JAPANESE JOURNAL OF PHARMACOLOGY

(REFERENCE 92 OF 123)
89069153
Mori H Xu QA Sakamoto O Uesugi Y Ono Y Koda A Nishioka I
Immunological mechanisms of antitumor activity of some kinds of Chinese herbs: Meth A-induced delayed type hypersensitivity.
Jpn J Pharmacol 1988 Sep;48(1):37-46

In the present paper, we confirmed that a delayed type hypersensitivity response can be elicited against Meth A tumor (Meth A-DTH) in BALB/c mice bearing the primary tumor. This response was augmented by lipopolysaccharide. We examined the effects of 4 kinds of Chinese herbs including A. capillaris, S. doederleinii, A. macrocephala and S. subprostrata on the Meth A-DTH, and the results were compared with that of the herbs on picryl chloride-induced delayed type hypersensitivity (PC-DTH). All of the herbs examined augmented the Meth A-DTH 10 days after the primary tumor transplantation, and S. doederleinii, A. macrocephala and S. subprostrata prevented the decay of the response on the 20th day, but A. capillaris did not. On the other hand, none of the herbs affected the PC-DTH. When both DTH responses were caused simultaneously in the same mouse, Meth A-DTH decayed 20 days after the transplantation but PC-DTH did not. In this case, the effects of these 4 herbs on Meth A-DTH and PC-DTH were essentially the same as those seen in the case of separate experiments. The previous and present results suggest that A. capillaris shows antitumor activity mainly through a direct cytotoxicity, although this herb might have certain components to enhance Meth A-DTH, and the other herbs display the activity through the enhancement of T cell-mediated tumor immunity, particularly tumor specific DTH.

KLINICHESKAIA MEDITSINA
(REFERENCE 93 OF 123)
89260141
Simvolokov SI Nikitin AV Iakovleva LG
[Clinico-immunologic effectiveness of chlorophyllypt in the treatment of acute destructive pneumonia]
Klin Med (Mosk) 1989 Feb;67(2):108-12 (Published in Russian)
An attempt has been made to replace antibiotics by chlorophyllypt (0.25 percent solution in physiological sodium chloride solution administered by intravenous drip). The clinical, laboratory and X-ray parameters in 22 patients treated by this drug normalized in earlier terms than those in 19 patients who received the traditional antibiotic therapy. Chlorophyllypt was found to have the immunocorrective effect manifested by the normalization of the T-lymphocyte number and its theophylline-resistant subpopulation. No such effect was achieved when broad-action antibiotics were used.

MEDICAL HYPOTHESES
(REFERENCE 94 OF 123)
79220988
Horrobin DF
Multiple sclerosis: the rational basis for treatment with colchicine and evening primrose oil.
Med Hypotheses 1979 Mar;5(3):365-78

Multiple sclerosis (MS) is a disease with no known treatment. In view of this and of its distressing nature patients are attracted by any new concepts. As a reaction to this neurologists are sometimes excessively sceptical and fail to consider new approaches seriously. Recent attempts have been made to treat multiple sclerosis with polyunsaturated fatty acids and with colchicine. This approach is not arbitrary and is firmly grounded in fundamental basic scientific concepts. In patients with multiple sclerosis there is evidence of both an abnormality in essential fatty acid metabolism and an abnormality in lymphocyte function. It is now apparent that the fatty acid abnormality may cause the lymphocyte abnormality and that both may be improved by dietary manipulation. There is also evidence that the demyelination may be associated with recurrent inflammatory episodes and with entry of calcium into the cytoplasm. In vitro colchicine has been shown to have actions compatible with regulation of cytoplasmic calcium and in two diseases characterized by intermittent inflammatory episodes (Behcets syndrome and familial Mediterranean fever) it has been found to prevent or to reduce the severity of such episodes. Preliminary results suggest that combined therapy with evening primrose oil and colchicine may be of considerable value.

MICROBIOLOGY AND IMMUNOLOGY
(REFERENCE 96 OF 123)
80032214
Nakashima S Umeda Y Kanada T
Effect of polysaccharides from Ganoderma applanatum on immune response. I. Enhancing effect on induction of delayed hypersensitivity in mice.
Microbiol Immunol 1979;23(6):501-13
[No Abstract Available]

MIKROBIOLOGICHESKII ZHURNAL

(REFERENCE 97 OF 123)
80120037
Beloklitskaia GF Diachenko IuV
[Experimental effect of chlorophyllypt on immunity indices]
Mikrobiol Zh 1979 Jul-Aug;41(4):404-9 (Published in Russian)
[No Abstract Available]

MOLECULAR BIOTHERAPY

(REFERENCE 98 OF 123)
92000401
Peng SY Norman J Curtin G Corrier D McDaniel HR Busbee D
Decreased mortality of Norman murine sarcoma in mice treated with the immunomodulator, Acemannan.
Mol Biother 1991 Jun;3(2):79-87

An extract from the parenchyma of Aloe barbadensis Miller shown to contain long chain polydispersed beta (1,4)-linked mannan polymers with random O-acetyl groups (acemannan, Carrisyn) was found to initiate the phagocyte production of monokines that supported antibody dependent cellular cytotoxicity and stimulated blastogenesis in thymocytes. Acemannan, in both enriched and highly purified forms, was administered intraperitoneally to female CFW mice into which murine sarcoma cells had been subcutaneously implanted. The rapidly growing, highly malignant and invasive sarcoma grew in 100% of implanted control animals, resulting in mortality in 20 to 46 days, dependent on the number of cells implanted. Approximately 40% of animals treated with acemannan at the time of tumor cell implantation (1.5 x 10(6) cells) survived. Tumors in acemannan-treated animals exhibited vascular congestion, edema, polymorphonuclear leukocyte infiltration, and central necrosing foci with hemorrhage and peripheral fibrosis. The data indicate that in vivo treatment of peritoneal macrophages stimulates the macrophage production of monokines, including interleukin-1 and tumor necrosis factor. The data further indicate that sarcomas in animals treated i.p. with acemannan at the time of tumor cell implantation were infiltrated by immune system cells, became necrotic, and regressed. The combined data suggest that acemannan-stimulated synthesis of monokines resulted in the initiation of immune attack, necrosis, and regression of implanted sarcomas in mice.

(REFERENCE 99 OF 123)
92000394
Lau BH Yamasaki T Gridley DS
Garlic compounds modulate macrophage and T-lymphocyte functions.
Mol Biother 1991 Jun;3(2):103-7

Organosulfur compounds of garlic have been shown to inhibit growth of animal tumors and to modulate the activity of diverse chemical carcinogens. There is also evidence that garlic may modulate antitumor immunity. In this study, we determined the effects of an aqueous garlic extract and a protein fraction isolated from the extract on the chemiluminescent oxidative burst of the murine J774 macrophage cell line and thioglycollate-elicited peritoneal macrophages obtained from BALB/c mice. T-lymphocyte activity was determined using mouse splenocytes incubated with phytohemagglutinin, labeled with [3H]-thymidine and assayed for lymphoproliferation. Significant dose-related augmentation of oxidative burst was observed with garlic extract and the protein fraction. The protein fraction also enhanced the T-lymphocyte blastogenesis. The data suggest that garlic compounds may serve as biological response modifiers by augmenting macrophage and T-lymphocyte functions.

NÄHRUNG

(REFERENCE 100 OF 123)
86203554
Aboul-Enein AM
Inhibition of tumor growth with possible immunity by Egyptian garlic extracts.
Nährung 1986;30(2):161-9

Garlic bulbs (Allium sativum) were extracted with distilled water or ethanol. The extracts were then incubated with Ehrlich ascites carcinoma cells at 37 degrees C for 1 h. These pretreated cells were injected into swiss albino mice which survived over 12 weeks. To the contrary, tumor cells which were pretreated with garlic extracts, produced ascites tumor in all mice that died 2 or 4 weeks after intraperitoneal injection. When mice were treated twice at intervals of 7 days with freshly prepared tumor cells exposed to watery or ethanolic extracts of fresh garlic, they acquired resistance against a challenge with Ehrlich ascites tumor cells. Administration of garlic extracts to mice for at least 2 weeks before tumor transplantation, caused a slight delay of 10-20 days in tumor growth and animal death. Generally, the ethanolic extract of garlic gave more pronounced effect as tumor inhibitor as well as immunity induction than watery extract. No change in serum electrophoretic pattern was detected in mice, whether the tumor cells injected were incubated or not with garlic extract. In animals treated with unincubated tumor cells, albumin and globulin percentages as well as albumin:globulin ratios (A/G) were decreased as compared to normal mice. A/G ratio was also decreased in immunized mice, pretreated with garlic extract, due to the increase of gamma globulin and unchanging of albumin.

NIPPON EISEIGAKU ZASSHI [JAPANESE JOURNAL OF HYGIENE]

(REFERENCE 101 OF 123)
74045984
Nakata T
[Tumor transplantation immunity induced with tumor cells treated with allicin contained in fresh garlic extract (author's transl)]
Nippon Eiseigaku Zasshi 1973 Jun;28(2):261-9 (Published in Japanese)
[No Abstract Available]

NIPPON JINZO GAKKAI SHI

(REFERENCE 102 OF 123)
90065208
Nagata M Kawaguchi H Komatsu Y Hattori M Itoh K
[The effects of sairei-to on nephrotoxic serum nephritis in rats—possible effects on intraglomerular cell mediated immunity]
Nippon Jinzo Gakkai Shi 1989 Jul;31(7):713-21 (Published in Japanese)

Sairei-to, one of the herb drugs, has been demonstrated to have several effects. Clinically, evidence has been accumulated showing that sairei-to has been able to reduce the frequency of relapse in minimal change nephrotic syndrome. It has also been found that sairei-to has improved proteinuria in minimal change nephrotic syndrome as well as chronic glomerulonephritis in man. Although the mechanism of such effects is still unclear, it is supposed that it is the immune modulating actions that have been reported. In this study, we quantitated the number of intrarenal Ia positive cells and T cells in nephrotoxic nephritis in rats in order to clarify the intrarenal immune actions of sairei-to on immune mediated glomerulonephritis. Four groups of rats with nephrotoxic nephritis were experimented on. The first group was the controlled group, which had no treatment whatsoever. The second group was administered MPSL (solumedrol 20 mg/kg, alternate day). The fourth group with both sairei-to and MPSL. The level of proteinuria in three groups treated was almost the same, that is, less than that of controlled group. On light microscopy, sairei-to suppressed glomerular inflammation such as endocapillary proliferative lesions and mesangial expansion, which were shown in controlled group. The histological improvement was almost that found in rats treated with MPSL and both. Sairei-to suppressed infiltrations of intraglomerular Ia positive cells (P less than 0.01) and T cells (P less than 0.01) on the 7th day and 14th day as well. Remarkable suppression of T cells infiltration was noted in rats treated with MPSL along with sairei-to on the 14th day (P less than 0.01). (ABSTRACT TRUNCATED AT 250 WORDS)

NIPPON SAIKINGAKU ZASSHI [JAPANESE JOURNAL OF BACTERIOLOGY]
(REFERENCE 103 OF 123)
76123320
Shimura K Shiomi T
[Tumor immunity induced by Ehrlich tumor (study of antineoplastic polysaccharides. 13)]
Nippon Saikingaku Zasshi 1975 Jan;30(1):225 (Published in Japanese)
[No Abstract Available]

NIPPON YAKURIGAKU ZASSHI [FOLIA PHARMACOLOGICA JAPONICA]
(REFERENCE 104 OF 123)
80158120
Yanagihara Y Koda A
[Immunopharmacological study of buckwheat hypersensitivity III. Effect of dialysate-conjugated T cell mitogen on IgE formation]
Nippon Yakurigaku Zasshi 1979 Oct;75(7):755-63 (Published in Japanese)

It has already been reported that dialysate (BWD) separated from the aqueous extract of buckwheat is a haptenic substance capable of neutralizing specific IgE antibody both on mast cells and on B cells in some species. The present work represents a study carried out to determine the effect of BWD conjugated with T cell mitogen such as phytohemagglutinin-P (PHA) and concanavalin A (Con A) on IgE formation in mice. Anti-buckwheat IgE formation was little affected by the pretreatment of these conjugates given i.v. 3 days before the immunization, but was effectively suppressed by the pretreatment of BWD-PHA or BWD-Con A given i.p. together with incomplete Freund's adjuvant 2 weeks before the immunization. BWD-PHA induced a more potent suppression of IgE formation as compared with BWD-Con A, Con A or PHA. The transfer of T cells obtained from spleen cells primed with BWD-PHA, which responded with buckwheat and exerted a slight helper function for adoptive anti-DNP IgE formation to DNP-buckwheat, suppressed anti-buckwheat IgE formation in recipients with no effect on the anti-KLH IgE response. Our findings suggest that suppressor T cells specific to buckwheat are induced in spleen cells of mice treated with BWD-PHA.

(REFERENCE 105 OF 123)
80158117
Yanagihara Y Koda A
[Immunopharmacological study of buckwheat hypersensitivity (II). Effect of dialysate on antibody formation (author's transl)]
Nippon Yakurigaku Zasshi 1979 Oct;75(7):721-30 (Published in Japanese)

It was reported that dialysate (BWD) separated from the aqueous extract of buckwheat was a haptenic substance capable of neutralizing IgE antibody on mast cells and that the activity was specific to non-dialysate (BWND)-induced hypersensitivity reaction. The effect of BWD on antibody formation was investigated in the present paper. In rats, anti-buckwheat IgE formation was slightly depressed by the administration of BWD, but both anti-DNP IgE and IgG formations in rats immunized with DNP-BWND were unaffected. In mice, anti-buckwheat IgE formation was suppressed by BWD administration. A good correlation was noted between a decrease of surface IgE population on B cells and that of IgE titer in serum. However, the helper function of T cells for adoptive anti-DNP IgE formation was little affected by BWD treatment. Lymphocyte transformation to BWND and other non-specific mitogens using spleen cells obtained from sensitized mice was inhibited in a dose-dependent fashion by the addition of BWD. However, lymphocyte transformation using spleen cells pretreated with BWD was not affected by other non-specific mitogens except for BWND and pokeweed mitogen.

PLANTA MEDICA
(REFERENCE 106 OF 123)
92131941
Wang JZ Mao XJ Ito H Shimura K
Immunomodulatory activity of polysaccharide from Acanthopanax obovatus roots.
Planta Med 1991 Aug;57(4):335-6

The effects of the Acanthopanax obovatus polysaccharide (AOPS) as well as its combination with cyclophosphamide (CY) or prednisolone on immune responses were investigated in mice. AOPS (250 mg/kg i.p. x 5) increased the spleen weight and the number of spleen cells, and augmented the phagocytosis of peritoneal macrophages both in normal mice and in immunosuppressed mice. In a haemagglutinin assay AOPS increased the production of specific antibodies and antagonized the suppressive effect of CY. AOPS not only enhanced the degree of in vitro spleen cell-mediated red blood cells (SRBC) hemolysis (quantitative hemolysis of SRBC) but also restored the suppressive effect of CY completely. From these results, AOPS was shown to have an enhancing and a modulating activity on immune responses.

(REFERENCE 107 OF 123)
83144788
Bloksma N Schmiermann P de Reuver M van Dijk H Willers J
Stimulation of humoral and cellular immunity by Viscum preparations.
Planta Med 1982 Dec;46(4):221-7
[No Abstract Available]

(REFERENCE 108 OF 123)
86094768
Beuscher N Kopanski L
[Stimulation of immunity by the contents of Baptisia tinctoria]
Stimulation der Immunantwort durch Inhaltsstoffe aus Baptisia tinctoria.
Planta Med 1985 Oct(5):381-4 (Published in German)
[No Abstract Available]

PRESSE MEDICALE
(REFERENCE 109 OF 123)
85088404
Homberg JC
[Autoimmunity induced by drugs. Immunological characteristics and etiopathogenic hypotheses]
Presse Med 1984 Dec 15;13(45):2755-60 (Published in French)

Drug-induced autoimmune diseases have two immunological peculiarities. Firstly, some autoantibodies are present, which are virtually never seen in spontaneous human diseases and may be regarded as specific. This applies to antimitochondria antibody type 3 (anti M3) in the lupus-like syndrome caused by Venocuran, to antimitochondria antibody type 6 (anti M6) in iproniazide-induced hepatitis, to anti-insulin antibody found after treatment with methimazole, and to anti liver/kidney microsome antibody type 2 (anti LKM2) associated with hepatitis induced by tielinic acid. Secondly, a search for other autoantibodies shows that the immune disorder is much more limited than in spontaneous autoimmune diseases. Thus, contrary to myasthenia and idiopathic autoimmune haemolytic anaemia, we never found autoantibodies specifically directed against the thyroid, the stomach or the adrenal gland during treatment with D-penicillamine and alpha-methyldopa. Only some hypotheses may account for these peculiarities. Cross-reaction between drug and autoantigen may occur, but the fact that the antigen-antibody reaction is not inhibited by the drug or its metabolites does not support this explanation. Much more attractive is the "T-cell bypass" theory, according to which autoreacting suppressor T-cells are circumvented by helper T-cells stimulated by the drug-modified autoantigen. In this case, the autoimmune reaction would indicate to which body substance the drug is bound, thus making it immunostimulant, and not a structural similarity between the drug and the autoantigen.

PROBLEMY TUBERKULEZA
(REFERENCE 110 OF 123)
90245813
Nersesian ON Bogatyreva EV
[Effect of chemotherapy combined with the use of tissue preparations on nonspecific immunity in patients with pulmonary tuberculosis]
Probl Tuberk 1990(1):28-31 (Published in Russian)

General and local nonspecific immunity was studied in 143 new cases of pulmonary tuberculosis (71 and 72 persons, respectively). The results showed that combination of chemotherapy using desensitizing agents and tissue preparations according to V. P. Filatov (a suspension of placenta tissue and aloe) had an immunomodulating effect. The efficacy of the combined chemotherapy amounted to 87 percent with an account of the general immunity status.

TANPAKUSHITSU KAKUSAN KOSO [PROTEIN, NUCLEIC ACID, ENZYME]
(REFERENCE 111 OF 123)
77014110
Maeda YY Ishimura K Chihara G
[Antitumor polysaccharides and host defense against cancer: A new way for cancer immunochemotherapy (author's transl)]
Tanpakushitsu Kakusan Koso 1976;21(6):425-35 (Published in Japanese)
[No Abstract Available]

THERAPIE DER GEGENWART
(REFERENCE 112 OF 123)
82085218
Schimmel KC Werner GT
[Non-specific increase of the body's own immunity by Echinacin administration]
Ther Ggw 1981 Nov;120(11):1065-76 (Published in German)
[No Abstract Available]

UGESKRIFT FOR LAEGER
(REFERENCE 113 OF 123)
92056102
Pedersen A Klausen B Hougen HP Ryder L Winther K
[Immunomodulating effect of LongoVital in patients with recurrent aphthous stomatitis. 2]
Ugeskr Laeger 1991 Sep 9;153(37):2561-4 (Published in Danish)

LongoVital (LV) (DK. reg. no. 5178/75) is a herbal-based tablet enriched with recommended doses of vitamins. Peripheral lymphocyte subsets: T-helper/CD4 (OKT4+) and T-suppressor/cytotoxic/CD8 (OKT8+) were studied quantitatively in 31 otherwise healthy patients with minor recurrent aphthous ulceration (RAU) during six months' daily LV intake in a double-blind, randomized, crossover 1-year study. Fourteen had had LV during the first six months (GrA) and 17 LV during the latter six months (GrB). OKT4+ percentages increased significantly during the LV period in both groups (p less than 0.05). OKT8+ percentages increased in both groups, however, only significantly in GrA (P less than 0.05). It is concluded that LV acts as an immunostimulator in patients with RAU and that the increase in T-lymphocyte subsets may account for the previously reported benefit of LV in RAU prevention.

VETERINARIIA
(REFERENCE 114 OF 123)
76272616
Grigorian GS Manasian AV Manukian VA Petrosian SA
[Effect of an Eleutherococcus extract on the body of animals]
Veterinariia 1976 Apr(4):100-1 (Published in Russian)
[No Abstract Available]

VOENNO-MEDITSINSKII ZHURNAL
(REFERENCE 115 OF 123)
88128593
Novikov VS Bortnovskii VN Mastriukov AA Lotovin AP Arzumanov AA
[Efficacy of the use of biologically active substances to increase the body resistance in sailors]
Voen Med Zh 1987 Oct(10):50-1 (Published in Russian)
[No Abstract Available]

VOPROSY ONKOLOGII
(REFERENCE 116 OF 123)
86291257
Kupin VI Polevaia EB
[Stimulation of the immunological reactivity of cancer patients by Eleutherococcus extract]
Vopr Onkol 1986;32(7):21-6 (Published in Russian)

In vitro treatment of lymphocytes with eleutherococcal preparation produced an immune-boosting effect both in cancer patients and healthy controls. The results of a randomized study pointed to eleutherococcus' capability of stimulating general nonspecific resistance and immunologic vigor in the course of cytostatic and radiation treatment for breast cancer. Since eleutherococcus is free of toxicity and allergenicity in prolonged treatment, it is indicated in patients receiving intensive antitumor therapy. Drug concentration should be tailored individually.

VRACHEBNOE DELO
(REFERENCE 117 OF 123)
84198011
Smirnov VV Mishenkova EL
[Various aspects of the immunobiological action of preparation K]
Vrach Delo 1984 Feb(2):108-11 (Published in Russian)
[No Abstract Available]

(REFERENCE 118 OF 123)
82177803
Gruzina EA Shvedov LM Barba EI Lakiza VV Perminov IA
[Effect of tissue therapy on body nonspecific reactivity in diabetes mellitus]
Vrach Delo 1982 Jan(1):68-70 (Published in Russian)
[No Abstract Available]

(REFERENCE 119 OF 123)
89333091
Mel'nik VP
[Immune reactivity of patients with pulmonary tuberculosis suffering from chronic alcoholism]
Vrach Delo 1989 Apr(4):82-5 (Published in Russian)

The immunological reactivity was studied in 152 patients with pulmonary tuberculosis of whom 112 suffered also of alcoholism. All patients with association of the two diseases showed inhibition of the functional activity and reduction of the number of T-lymphocytes while those without alcoholism showed these changes in 80%. Use of T-activin and electrophoresis of chlorophyllypt allowed to restore the moderately reduced reactivity in most patients. In markedly reduced inhibition of cellular immunity T-activin proved more effective.

WISCONSIN MEDICAL JOURNAL
(REFERENCE 120 OF 123)
74085680
Hofmann JW Heim LR Boulanger WJ DeCosse JJ
The effect of surgery on cellular immunity.
Wis Med J 1973 Dec;72(12):249-53
[No Abstract Available]

WORLD HEALTH ORGANIZATION TECHNICAL REPORT SERIES
(REFERENCE 121 OF 123)
70067695
Cell-mediated immune responses. Report of a WHO scientific group.
World Health Organ Tech Rep Ser 1969;423:1-61
[No Abstract Available]

YAKUGAKU ZASSHI [JOURNAL OF THE PHARMACEUTICAL SOCIETY OF JAPAN]
(REFERENCE 122 OF 123)
88300474
Chihara G
[Current status and possible future of antitumor drugs. With special reference to pharmacology of Oriental medicine]
Yakugaku Zasshi 1988 Mar;108(3):171-86 (Published in Japanese)
[No Abstract Available]

ZHURNAL MIKROBIOLOGII, EPIDEMIOLOGII I IMMUNOBIOLOGII
(REFERENCE 123 OF 123)
86237979
Zakharova NS Remova TN Shepeleva IB Bazhanova IG Britsina MV
[Action of plant extracts on the natural immunity indices of animals]
Zh Mikrobiol Epidemiol Immunobiol 1986 Apr(4):71-5 (Published in Russian)

The influence of extracts from oak bark, St. John's-wort leaves and pine buds on natural immunity characteristics of mice has been studied. The injection of these extracts into mice has been found to enhance their resistance to infection with Staphylococcus aureus and Bordetella pertussis virulent cultures, to decrease the enzymatic activity of 5'-nucleotidase in the peritoneal exudate macrophages of mice and to increase the level of lysozyme in their blood. The action of these extracts has proved to depend on their dosage and the time of observation.

List you want to Display: I (PLANTS, MEDICINAL+DRUGS, CHINESE HERBAL +HIV)

88037725
Tyms AS Berrie EM Ryder TA Nash RJ Hegarty MP Taylor DL Mobberley MA Davis JM Bell EA Jeffries DJ et al
Castanospermine and other plant alkaloid inhibitors of glucosidase activity block the growth of HIV [letter]
Lancet (1987 Oct 31) 2(8566):1025-6

92142533
Yao XJ Wainberg MA Parniak MA
Mechanism of inhibition of HIV-1 infection in vitro by purified extract of Prunella vulgaris.
Virology (1992 Mar) 187(1):56-62
[ABSTRACT ONLINE]

91319727
Lee-Huang S Huang PL Kung HF Li BQ Huang PL Huang P Huang HI Chen HC
TAP 29: an anti-human immunodeficiency virus protein from Trichosanthes kirilowii that is nontoxic to intact cells.
Proc Natl Acad Sci U S A
[ABSTRACT ONLINE]

89165274
Ngan F Chang RS Tabba HD Smith KM
Isolation, purification and partial characterization of an active anti-HIV compound from the Chinese medicinal herb viola yedoensis.
Antiviral Res (1988 Nov) 10(1-3):107-16

88292932
Chang RS Yeung HW
Inhibition of growth of human immunodeficiency virus in vitro by crude extracts of Chinese medicinal herbs.

Antiviral Res (1988 Apr) 9(3):163-75
Twenty-seven medicinal herbs reputed in ancient Chinese folklore to have anti-infective properties were extracted by boiling underreflux. The extracts were tested for inhibitory activity against the human immunodeficiency virus in the H9 cell line at concentrations nontoxic to growth of the H9 cells. Using a significant reduction (greater than 3 S. D. below the mean) in the percentage of cells positive for specific viral antigens in three successive assays as indicative of activity against the virus, 11 of the 27 extracts were found to be active. One of the extracts (Viola yedoensis) was studied in greater depth. At a subtoxic concentration, this extract shut off completely the growth of HIV in virtually all experiments. It did not inactivate HIV extracellularly, did not induce interferon and did not inhibit the growth of herpes simplex, polio or vesicular stomatitis viruses in human fibroblast culture. Chinese medicinal herbs appeared to be a rich source of potentially useful materials for the treatment of human immunodeficiency virus infection.

93037375
Balzarini J Neyts J Schols D Hosoya M Van Damme E Peumans W De Clercq E
The mannose-specific plant lectins from Cymbidium hybrid and Epipactis helleborine and the (N-acetylglucosamine) n-specific plant lectin from Urtica dioica are potent and selective inhibitors of human immunodeficiency virus and cytomegalovirus replication in vitro.
Antiviral Res (1992 Jun) 18(2):191-207
[ABSTRACT ONLINE]

93012797
Ng TB Chan WY Yeung HW
Proteins with abortifacient, ribosome inactivating, immunomodulatory, antitumor and anti-AIDS activities from Cucurbitaceae plants.
Gen Pharmacol (1992 Jul) 23(4):579-90
[ABSTRACT ONLINE]

91103217
Gau JP Lin CK Lee SS Wang SR
The lack of antiplatelet effect of crude extracts from ganoderma lucidum on HIV-positive hemophiliacs.
Am J Chin Med (1990) 18(3-4):175-9
[ABSTRACT ONLINE]

91207055
Buimovici-Klein E Mohan V Lange M Fenamore E Inada Y Cooper LZ
Inhibition of HIV replication in lymphocyte cultures of virus-positive subjects in the presence of shosaiko-to, an oriental plant extract.
Antiviral Res (1990 Oct-Nov) 14(4-5):279-86
[ABSTRACT ONLINE]

89308985
Sanders PL
Acupuncture and herbal treatment of HIV infection.
Holist Nurs Pract (1989 Aug) 3(4):38-44
[ABSTRACT ONLINE]

92256931
Zhang X Tang X Chen H
Inhibition of HIV replication by baicalin and S. baicalensis extracts in H9 cell culture.
Chin Med Sci J (1991 Dec) 6(4):230-2
[ABSTRACT ONLINE]

89312735
Duke JA
Castanospermum and anti-AIDS activity.
J Ethnopharmacol (1989 Apr) 25(2):227-8
[NO ABSTRACT ONLINE]

92247333
Zhu Y
[Research on the development of Chinese materia medica and natural drug for AIDS]
Chung Kuo Chung Yao Tsa Chih (1991 Dec) 16(12):707-10, 761
[NO ABSTRACT ONLINE]

90227785
In vitro screening of traditional medicines for anti-HIV activity: memorandum from a WHO meeting.
Bull World Health Organ (1989) 67(6):613-8
[ABSTRACT ONLINE]

91243215
Tang X
[Inhibition of human immunodeficiency virus reverse transcriptase in vitro by extracts of Chinese medicinal herbs]
Chung Kuo I Hsueh Ko Hsueh Yuan Hsueh Pao (1990 Dec) 12(6):391-5
[ABSTRACT ONLINE]

91292606
Tang XS
[Research methodology of anti-AIDS agents]
Chung Hsi I Chieh Ho Tsa Chih (1991 Mar) 11(3):173-6
[NO ABSTRACT ONLINE]

91207058
Kreis W Kaplan MH Freeman J Sun DK Sarin PS
Inhibition of HIV replication by Hyssop officinalis extracts.
Antiviral Res (1990 Dec) 14(6):323-37
[ABSTRACT ONLINE]

91199729
Balick MJ
Ethnobotany and the identification of therapeutic agents from the rainforest.
Ciba Found Symp (1990) 154:22-31; discussion 32-9
[ABSTRACT ONLINE]

91032105
Lee-Huang S Huang PL Nara PL Chen HC Kung HF Huang P Huang HI Huang PL
MAP 30: a new inhibitor of HIV-1 infection and replication.
FEBS Lett (1990 Oct 15) 272(1-2):12-8
[ABSTRACT ONLINE]

92284470
Gustafson KR Cardellina JH 2d McMahon JB Gulakowski RJ Ishitoya J Szallasi Z Lewin
NE Blumberg PM et al
A nonpromoting phorbol from the Samoan medicinal plant Homalanthus nutans in-
hibits cell killing by HIV-1
J Med Chem (1992 May 29) 35(11):1978-86
[ABSTRACT ONLINE]

92325696
Beutler JA Cardellina JH 2d McMahon JB Boyd MR Cragg GM
Anti-HIV and cytotoxic alkaloids from Buchenavia capitata.
J Nat Prod (1992 Feb) 55(2):207-13
[ABSTRACT ONLINE]

92277084
Chen K Shi Q Kashiwada Y Zhang DC Hu CQ Jin JQ Nozaki H Kilkuskie RE
Tramontano E Cheng YC et al
Anti-aids agents, 6. Salaspermic acid, an anti-HIV principle from Tripterygium wilfordii,
and the structure-activity correlation with its related compounds.
J Nat Prod (1992 Mar) 55(3):340-6
[ABSTRACT ONLINE]

91350800
Vlietinck AJ Vanden Berghe DA
Can ethnopharmacology contribute to the development of antiviral drugs?
J Ethnopharmacol (1991 Apr) 32(1-3):141-53
[ABSTRACT ONLINE]

92061397
Kassler WJ Blanc P Greenblatt R
The use of medicinal herbs by human immunodeficiency virus-infected patients.
Arch Intern Med 1991 Nov;151(11):2281-8

The use of herbs has been advocated as an alternative treatment strategy for human
immunodeficiency virus-related illness. To describe the use of medicinal herbs among
acquired immunodeficiency syndrome clinic patients and to investigate possible toxic
effects, we interviewed 114 randomly selected patients attending a university-based
acquired immunodeficiency syndrome clinic and performed a structured review of
the literature to identify potential adverse effects of herbal use. Twenty-five partici-

pants (22%) reported using one or more herbal products in the past 3 months. Of those taking herbs, six (24%) were unable to identify the herb that they had used. The mean number of herbal tablets taken was 4.5 tablets per day, and 12 patients (48%) reported taking herbs for longer than 90 days. The median cost to patients for their herbs was $18 per month. Of those taking herbs, five (20%) stated that their primary medical provider was unaware of their herb use, and four (16%) were involved in clinical drug trials while using herbs. Several patients reported taking herbs in doses at which potential adverse effects were identified in our literature review. These adverse effects include dermatitis, nausea, vomiting, diarrhea, thrombocytopenia, coagulopathies, altered mental states, hepatotoxicity, and electrolyte disturbances. Seven patients (28%) reported experiencing symptoms that could have been caused by one or more of the herbal products that they were taking. Physicians and clinical investigators need to inquire about patients' use of herbs. Patient care and clinical trials could be distorted because pharmacologic effects of herbs can resemble commonly occurring symptoms in human immunodeficiency virus disorders as well as side effects of prescribed or investigational medications.

90067309
Davis D
New remedies: check the facts [letter; comment]
Nursing 1989 Dec;19(12):6
[No Abstract Available]

92054528
Treating AIDS with worts [news] [published erratum appears in Science 1992 Oct 30;258(5083):following 725]
Science 1991 Oct 25;254(5031):522
[No Abstract Available]

91207055
Buimovici-Klein E Mohan V Lange M Fenamore E Inada Y Cooper LZ
Inhibition of HIV replication in lymphocyte cultures of virus-positive subjects in the presence of shosaiko-to, an oriental plant extract.
Antiviral Res 1990 Oct-Nov;14(4-5):279-86

An oriental remedy, Shosaiko-to (SST) consisting of a mixture of aqueous extracts from seven different plants and whose most active component is the chemically defined compound baicalein was tested for its ability to inhibit the production of the human immunodeficiency virus (HIV). The testing was done with cultures of human lymphocytes obtained from HIV-positive asymptomatic subjects and patients with ARC or AIDS. The replication of the virus was monitored by quantitative assay of the reverse transcriptase (RT) activity and of the synthesis of antigen p24. The lymphocyte cultures (LC) were maintained in the absence and in the presence of 25, 50 or 100 micrograms/ml of SST, and monitored for up to 5 weeks. The results showed that in LC from asymptomatic subjects RT activity and synthesis of p24 was completely inhibited by low concentrations of SST. High concentrations of SST inhibited virus replication in 80% of LC from ARC patients, but were completely ineffective in LC from AIDS patients. It was observed that the RT activity was more sensitive to inhibition by SST than the synthesis of p24, and that the antiviral effect was dependent on the virus load of the LC.

90227785

In vitro screening of traditional medicines for anti-HIV activity: memorandum from a WHO meeting.
Bull World Health Organ 1989;67(6):613-8

Many plant products are being used by patients with acquired immunodeficiency syndrome (AIDS) in some countries without any scientific proof that they possess anti-HIV (human immunodeficiency virus) activity. Traditional healers are now offering their remedies for scientific evaluation, and a few studies provide information on the inhibitory activity against HIV of plants such as Viola yedoensis, Arctium lappa, Epimedium grandiflorum, Glycyrrhiza uralensis and Castanospermum australe. Natural products can be selected for biological screening based on ethnomedical use, random collection or a chemotaxonomic approach (i.e., screening of species of the same botanical family for similar compounds), but the follow-up and selection of plants based on literature leads would seem to be the most cost-effective way of identifying plants with anti-HIV activity. No single in vitro screening methodology for anti-HIV activity is ideal and confirmatory assays in multiple systems are needed to examine completely the potential use of a compound. To promote further research in traditional medicine and AIDS, appropriate institutions will be identified where the different activities for the scientific evaluation of plants and their extracts for possible treatment of AIDS can be carried out.

91292607
Zhang X
[Treating AIDS by integrated traditional and Western medical method]
Chung Hsi I Chieh Ho Tsa Chih 1991 Mar;11(3):177-8 (Published in Chinese)
[No Abstract Available]

91292606
Tang XS
[Research methodology of anti-AIDS agents]
Chung Hsi I Chieh Ho Tsa Chih 1991 Mar;11(3):173-6 (Published in Chinese)
[No Abstract Available]

88311312
Yu J Chen KJ
[Clinical study of AIDS treated with traditional Chinese medicine]
Chung Hsi I Chieh Ho Tsa Chih 1988 Feb;8(2):71-3, 67-8 (Published in Chinese)
[No Abstract Available]

92247333
Zhu Y
[Research on the development of Chinese materia medica and natural drug for AIDS]
Chung Kuo Chung Yao Tsa Chih 1991 Dec;16(12):707-10, 761 (Published in Chinese)
[No Abstract Available]

91032105
Lee-Huang S Huang PL Nara PL Chen HC Kung HF Huang P Huang HI Huang PL
MAP 30: a new inhibitor of HIV-1 infection and replication.
FEBS Lett 1990 Oct 15;272(1-2):12-8

A new inhibitor of human immunodeficiency virus (HIV) has been isolated and purified to homogeneity from the seeds and fruits of the Momordica charantia. This compound, MAP 30 (Momordica Anti-HIV Protein), is a basic protein of about 30 kDa. It exhibits dose-dependent inhibition of cell-free HIV-1 infection and replication as measured by: (i) quantitative focal syncytium formation on CEM-ss monolayers; (ii) viral core protein p24 expression; and (iii) viral-associated reverse transcriptase (RT) activity in HIV-1 infected H9 cells. The doses required for 50% inhibition (ID50) in these assays were 0.83, 0.22 and 0.33 nM, respectively. No cytotoxic or cytostatic effects were found under the assay conditions. These data suggest that MAP 30 may be a useful therapeutic agent in the treatment of HIV-1 infections. The sequence of the N-terminal 44 amino acids of MAP 30 has been determined.

89308985
Sanders PL
Acupuncture and herbal treatment of HIV infection.
Holist Nurs Pract 1989 Aug;3(4):38-44
The validity of TCM remains controversial in the Western culture. Nonetheless, the value of these adjunctive and complementary therapies in treatment of HIV will continue to gain attention as clients experience its benefit. Nurses have the opportunity to validate and educate clients in their search for useful therapies. For nurses counseling and administering care to HIV-infected clients, knowledge of TCM can be useful. TCM offers another view of illness, health, and treatment that can improve the quality of life for our clients.

92284680
Wu B
Recent development of studies on traditional Chinese medicine in prophylaxis and treatment of AIDS.
J Tradit Chin Med 1992 Mar;12(1):10-20
[No Abstract Available]

92177808
Lu W
Treatment of AIDS by traditional Chinese medicine and materia medica.
J Tradit Chin Med 1991 Dec;11(4):249-52
[No Abstract Available]

91318796
Su C
Trial treatment of AIDS by TCM—a clinical report of 30 cases.
J Tradit Chin Med 1991 Jun;11(2):91-8
[No Abstract Available]

92284640
Recht C Mittmann S
[Alternative nursing possibilities for patients with AIDS]
Alternative Pflegemöglichkeiten bei Aidskranken.
Krankenpfl Soins Infirm 1992 Apr;85(4):60-4 (Published in German)
[No Abstract Available]

93060806
Mittmann S Recht C
[Alternative care for patients with AIDS]
Soins alternatifs pour les patients atteints du sida.
Krankenpfl Soins Infirm 1992 Aug;85(8):25-9 (Published in French)
[No Abstract Available]

89313509
Sergio W
Mulberry roots and seeds may be effective in the treatment of AIDS.
Med Hypotheses 1989 May;29(1):75-6
A natural substance, 1-deoxynojirimycin, found in mulberry roots and seeds may be effective in the treatment of AIDS infection.

89159067
Gandolfi A
[Race against time in the fight against AIDS and cancer: research on rare plants]
Minerva Stomatol 1988 Nov;37(11):IX (Published in Italian)
[No Abstract Available]

89314683
Getting to the root of AIDS [news]
Occup Health Saf 1989 Jun:16
[No Abstract Available]

Adjuvants, Immunologic and Plants, Medicinal

Atal CK Sharma ML Kaul A Khajuria A
Immuomodulating agents of plant origin. I: Preliminary screening.
J Ethnopharmacol (1986 Nov) 18(2):133-41

The immunobiological activity was investigated of certain medicinal plants widely used in the Ayurvedic and Unani systems of medicine for treatment of chronic infections and immunological disorders. The effect of an ethanolic extract of each drug was studied on delayed type hypersensitivity, humoral responses to sheep red blood cells, skin allograft rejection, and phagocytic activity of the reticuloendothelial system in mice. Picrorhiza kurroa was found to be a potent immunostimulant, stimulating both cell-mediated and humoral immunity. Tylophora indica, Aconitum heterophyllum and Holarrhena antidysenterica appeared to stimulate phagocytic function while inhibiting the humoral component of the immune system. Tinospora cordifolia and Ocimum gratissimum appeared to improve the phagocytic function without affecting the humoral or cell-mediated immune system. Hemidesmus indicus suppressed both the cell-mediated and humoral components of the immune system.

Beusher N Stolze H
[Plant immunostimulants (letter)]
Dtsch Med Wochenschr (1990 Feb 23) 115(8):317-8

Beuscher N Kopanski L
[Stimulation of immunity by the contents of Baptisia tinctoria]
Planta Med (1985 Oct) (5):381-4

Beuscher N Scheit KH Bodinet C Kopanski L
[Immunologically active glycoproteins of Baptisia tinctoria]
Planta Med (1989 Aug) 55(4):358-63

Chromatographically purified fractions of aqueous-ethanolic extracts from Baptisia tinctoria roots contained a strong lymphocyte DNA synthesis-stimulating activity. Electrophoretic analysis of these fractions revealed four distinct protein bands with molecular masses of P1=58 kD; P4=31 kD; P5=26 kD; and P6=14 kD. They contained carbohydrate as determined by periodic acid Schiff staining. An estimation of the approximate amount of sugar was done by using human transferrin as a reference; this method revealed the following values: P1=27%; P4=12%; P5=14%; and P6=8%. The mixture of proteins and every single band were immunoreactive with a polyclonal antiserum against Baptisia proteins determined in immune and dot blots, respectively. Electrophoretically purified proteins were characterized by tryptic cleavage and determination of their amino acid content. They contained several common amino acids, predominantly aspartic acid, glutamic acid, threonin and alanine. The content of glucosamine and/or galactosamine was less than 0.2 Mol-percent. The four proteins revealed pI values between 5.3 and 4.7. Protein P4 was immunochemically related to phytohemagglutinin but, in contrast to PHA-P, it exhibited no hemagglutinating activity and no leucagglutinating activity like PHA-L.

Brossat JY Ledeaut JY Ralamboranto L Rakotovao LH Solar S Gueguen A Coulanges P
[Immunostimulating properties of an extract isolated from Aloe vahombe.2. Protection in mice by fraction against infections by Listeria monocytogenes, Yersinia pestis, Candida albicans and Plasmodium berghei]
Étude des propriétés immunostimulantes d'un extrait isolé à partir d'Aloe vahombe.
Arch Inst Pasteur Madagascar (1981) 48(1):11-34

A partially purified extract of leaves of Aloe vahombe, a plant endemic in the south of Madagascar, administered intravenously to mice, protects them against infection of bacteria (Listeria monocytogenes, Yersinia pestis), parasites (Plasmodium berghei) and fungus (Candida albicans). The protective fraction must be administered two days before inoculation of the pathogenic agent. These results significantly confirm those we obtained in an earlier study on mice infection by Klebsiella pneumoniae. Currently we are testing the protective action of the purified extract on the experimental development of sarcomas, and we are in the process of analyzing the mode of action of this nonspecific immunostimulant.

Chubarev VN
[The immunotropic action of preparations made from medicinal plants]
Immunotropnoe deistvie preparatov iz lekarstvennykh rastenii.
Med Sestra (1990 Nov) 49(11):47-51

Chubarev VN Rubtsova ER Filatova IV Krendal' FP Davydova ON
[Immunotropic effect of a tincture of the tissue culture biomass of ginseng cells and of an Eleutherococcus extract in mice]
Immunotropnoe vliianie nastoiki iz biomassy kul'tury tkani kletok zhen'shenia i ekstrakta eleuterokokka u myshei.
Farmakol Toksikol (1989 Mar-Apr) 52(2):55-9

The tincture from biomass of ginseng tissue culture was shown to exert the immunomodulatory effect on humoral immunity and to increase the thymus and spleen weight. It is of interest to note that the biomass preparation did not change the immunity of intact animals but exerted a strong immunomodulatory action on mice previously treated with cyclophosphane. Similar results have been obtained also for another adaptogen—Eleutherococcus.

Cyong J Otsuka Y
A pharmacological study of the anti-inflammatory activity of Chinese herbs. A review.
Acupunct Electrother Res (1982) 7(2-3):173-202

A considerable number of Chinese medical herbs have been found to be anti-inflammatory upon screening for the inhibition of acute inflammation and allergic reaction, and for the suppression of adjuvant arthritis. Most of this research has been published exclusively in Japanese, and consequently is little known internationally. In this review, we will introduce the most recent conclusions drawn from current pharmacological research on the anti-inflammatory action of various Chinese medicinal herbs being undertaken in Japan. Due to the limitations of space, we mention only herbs showing anti-inflammatory activity in vivo when administered intra-orally, and having low toxicity. We will also introduce some popular Chinese medical prescriptions used in the treatment of arthritis, hepatitis and nephritis and attempt to explain their anti-inflammatory action resulting from the synergistic action of the herbs contained in these prescriptions. All references cited in this review were either written originally in English or have an English abstract.

Dalsgaard K
Saponin adjuvants. 3. Isolation of a substance from Quillaja saponaria Molina with adjuvant activity in foot-and-mouth disease vaccines.
Arch Gesmate Virusforsch (1974) 44(3):243-54

Grigorescu E Stanescu U
[Immunotherapeutic quality of medicinal plants]
Rev Med Chir Soc Med Nat Iasi (1987 Apr-Jun) 91(2):319-24

Hou YD
[Study on the biologically active constituents of Astragalus membranaceus]
Chung Hsi I Chieh Ho Tsa Chih (1984 Jul) 4(7):42-4

Iwama H Amagaya S Ogihara Y
**Effects of five kampohozais on the mitogenic activity of lipopolysaccaride, con-
canavalin A, phorbol myristate acetate and phytohemagglutinin in vivo.**
J Ethnopharamacol (1986 Nov) 18(2):193-204

Mitogenic activity of lipopolysaccaride (LPS), concanavalin (Con A), phorbol myristate
acetate (PMA) and phytohemagglutinin (PHA) was investigated using spleen cells prepared from C57BL/6 orally pretreated with one of five kampohozai extracts (Shosaiko-
to, Daisaiko-to, Hochuekki-to, Juzen-daiho-to and Tokishakuyakusan). Shosaiko-to
and Daisaiko-to elevated the mitogenic activity of LPS and reduced those of Con A.
The mitogenic activities of PMA and PHA were elevated by low doses of Shosaiko-to
and Daisaiko-to and suppressed by high doses. Juzen-daiho-to and Tokishakuyakusan
showed no effect on the mitogenic activity of LPS and Con A, but increased those of
PMA and PHA. Hochuekki-to increased the mitogenic activity of LPS, Con A, PMA
and PHA. In the absence of mitogens, these five kampohozais showed no mitogenic
activity. These results indicate that the kampohozais used in this experiment appear
to possess the immunomodulating or immunostimulating activities that might be expected from clinical experiences in Japan and China.

Kimura M Kobayashi S Luo B Kimura I
**Selective inhibition by magnosalin and magnoshinin, compounds from "shin-i"
(Flos magnoliae), of adjuvant-induced angiogenesis and granuloma formation in
the mouse pouch.**
Int Arch Allergy Appl Immunol (1990) 93(4):365-70

Inhibitory effects of magnosalin and magnoshinin, compounds from the crude drug
"Shin-i" (Flos magnoliae), of angiogenesis and pouch granuloma formation induced
by an adjuvant containing croton oil were investigated. Magnosalin inhibited
angiogenesis 2.4-fold (intra-pouch) and 9.7-fold (intraperitoneal) more strongly than
granuloma formation. The inhibition of angiogenesis by magnosalin was 5-fold (intra-
pouch) and 21-fold (intraperitoneal) weaker than that by hydrocortisone. In contrast,
intraperitoneal magnoshinin inhibited granuloma formation 2.5-fold more strongly
than angiogenesis. The regression coefficients of anti-angiogenesis vs. the inhibition
of granuloma formation were 1.79 for magnosalin, 1.11 for hydrocortisone, and 0.61
for magnoshinin. These results show that the anti-chronic inflammatory effect of "Shin-
i" was caused by selective inhibition of angiogenesis by magnosalin and of granuloma
formation by magnoshinin.

Kiyohara H Yamada H
**Carbohydrate chains for expression of complement activating activity in pectic
polysaccarides from the root of Angelica acutiloba kitagawa.**
Kitasato Arch Exp Med (1991 Dec) 64(4):167-77

Kolesnikova AG
[Bactericidal and immunocorrective properties of plant extracts]
Zh Mikrobiol Epidemiol Immunobiol (1986 Mar) (3):75-8

Extracts from oak cork, St. John's wort leaves and flowers and pine buds possess more pronouced bactericidal properties with respect to staphylococci, shigellae, Escherichia coli than decoctions from these medicinal plants. Such extracts may be included into complexes for the treatment of otorhinolaryngological diseases, enterocolitis in children and bacterial eczema. As a medicinal form, extracts prepared from medicinal plants are more convenient for storage and permit more exact dosage.

Kucharska E
[Effect of biostymine on various immunological processes]
Wplyw biostyminy na niektore procesy immunologiczne.
Ann Acad Med Stetin (1980) 26:369-86

Kumazawa Y Mizunoe K Otsuka Y
Immunostimulating polysaccharide separated from hot water extract of Angelica acutiloba kitagawa (Yamato tohki).
Immunology (1982 Sep) 47(1):75-83

Separation of immunostimulating polysaccharide (AIP) from Angelica and its biological activities were investigated. AIP was separated as an acetone-insoluble and non-dialysable fraction from hot water extract obtained by heating the root of Angelica acutiloba in water at 95-98 degrees for 30 minutes. It is a water-soluble heteropolymer(s) consisting of uronic acid, hexose and peptide. The anti-tumor activity of AIP was observed in terms of prolongation of the survival period of mice bearing Ehrlich ascites cells. The uptake of tritiated thymidine into murine and human spleen cells could be stimulated by AIP in a dose-dependent manner. Murine B cells were activated polyclonally by AIP and differentiated to antibody-forming cells even in the absence of either helper T cells or macrophages. The possibility that the biological activity of AIP might be due to contamination by bacterial lipopolysaccharides (LPS) or lipid A-associated protein (LAP) was ruled out for the following reasons: (i) polyclonal B-cell activation by AIP was shown in spleen cell cultures of C3H/HeJ mice, a low responder strain to LPS; (ii) the activity of AIP disappeared completely after a mild periodate oxidation whereas that of LPS containing LAP was not lost by similar treatment. In addition, the primary antibody response to sheep-erythrocytes was markedly augmented by an intraperitoneal injection of AIP. This result shows that AIP is a potent adjuvant.

Kupin VI Polevaia EB
[Stimulation of the immunological reactivity of cancer patients by Eleutherococcus extract]
Vopr Onkol (1986) 32(7):21-6

In vitro treatment of lymphocytes with eleutherococcal preparation produced an immune-boosting effect both in cancer patients and healthy controls. The results of a randomized study pointed to eleutherococcus' capability of stimulating general nonspecific resistance and immunologic vigor in the course of cytostatic and radiation treatment for breast cancer. Since eleutherococcus is free of toxicity and allergenicity in prolonged treatment, it is indicated in patients receiving intensive antitumor therapy. Drug concentration should be tailored individually.

Labadie RP van der Nat JM Simons JM Kroes BH Kosasi S van den Berb AJ t'Hart LA van der Sluis WG et al
An ethnopharmacognostic approach to the search for immunomodulators of plant origin.
Planta Med (1989 Aug) 55(4):339-48

The search for immunomodulating plant constituents through basic field inquiries into the literature and practices of traditional Indian medicine is treated. The strategy of data collecting proceeds through aspects of an ethnobotanical, an ethnopharmaceutical, an ethnopharmacological, and an ethnomedical nature. In the experimental immunopharmacognostic phase, immunomodulatory compounds are isolated and purified through action-guided fractionation procedures. The results described here refer to activities found on human complement activation and on PMN leucocytes activation. The immunomodulating plant compounds included in this reports were isolated from Azadirachta indica bark, Woodfordia fructicosa flowers, Picrorhiza kurroa roots, and Jatropha multifida latex.

Michel P Pignon T Ralamboranto L Randrianandraina S Ratovonarivo A Coulanges P
[Prospective study of the immunomodulator properties of i.m. administered "ALVA" extract in patients with solid tumors under a course of chemical immunosuppressive therapy]
Étude prospective des propriétés immunomodulatrices de l'extrait "ALVA" utilisé en "I.M." chez des patients atteints de tumeurs solides et en cours de therapie immunosuppressive chimique.
Arch Inst Pasteur Madagascar (1989) 56(1):253-9

Mishenkova EL
[Study of the immunomodulating properties of antibiotics derived from higher plants]
Issledovanie immunomoduliruiuschchikh svoistv antibiotikov iz vysshikh rastenii.
Antibiot Khimioter 1990 Feb;35(2):33-7

Investigations on screening of immunomodulating substances performed at the Antibiotic Department of the Institute of Microbiology and Virology of the Academy of Sciences of the Ukrainian SSR were analyzed. The analysis and detailed study of a screened antibiotic performed by the author showed that it was promising to use higher plants as organisms producing immunomodulators. A methodical approach was developed and recommended and graphs for screening immunomodulating agents of various origin were proposed.

Nersesian ON Bogatyreva EV
[Effect of chemotherapy combined with the use of tissue preparations on nonspecific immunity in patients with pulmonary tuberculosis]
Probl Tuberk 1990(1):28-31

General and local nonspecific immunity was studied in 143 new cases of pulmonary tuberculosis (71 and 72 persons, respectively). The results showed that combination of chemotherapy using desensitizing agents and tissue preparations according to V. P. Filatov (a suspension of placenta tissue and aloe) had an immunomodulating effect. The efficacy of the combined chemotherapy amounted to 87 percent with an account of the general immunity status.

Oakovlev AI Konoplia AI Laskova IL Kedrovskaia NN
[The mechanisms of the immunostimulating action of plant heteropolysaccharides]
Izuchenie mekhanizmov immunostimuliruiushchego deistviia nekotorykh rastitel'nykh geteropolisakharidov.
Farmakol Toksikol (1988 Sep-Oct) 51(5):68-72

In experiments on Wistar rats it was found that oral administration of heteropolysaccharide preparations isolated from medicinal plants of Asteraceae, Tiliaceae and Polygonaceae families induces the appearance in the blood serum and supernatant fluid of cells of the spleen and thymus of humoral immunostimulating substances. Similar factors appear in the supernatant fluid of cells of the spleen and thymus after their treatment with sera of the rats receiving polysaccharides. The administration of the preparations significantly changes the appearance of the immunostimulating factors in animals with the toxic liver damage as well as under intensive physical exercise.

Osterlind K Hansen HH Hansen M Dombernowsky P
[Herbal medicine compared with a placebo in adjuvant treatment of patients after radical operation for squamous cell carcinoma of the lung]
Naturmedicin versus placebo i den adjuverende behandling af patienter med radikalt opereret planocellulaer lungecancer.
Ugeskr Laeger (1985 Jan 14) 147(3):156-60 (Published in Danish)

Pigarevskii PV Mokhnach IV
[Immunomorphological changes in mouse lymphoid tissue as affected by Aconitum soongaricum Stapf., levamisole and sodium nucleinate]
Immunomorfologicheskie izmeneniia v limfoidnoi tkani myshei pod vliianiem akonita dzhungarskogo, levamizola i nukleinata natriia.
Dokl Akad Nauk SSSR 1983;268(3):754-6

Prusek W Jankowski A Radomska G Wieczorek E Podwysocka M
Immunostimulation in recurrent respiratory tract infections therapy in children.
Arch Immunol Ther Exp (Warsz) 1987;35(3):289-302

Selected immunologic parameters and effectivity of immunotherapy were evaluated in 117 children (12-month-10-years old) suffering from recurrent respiratory tract infections. All the children displayed a profound depression of T lymphocytes number, which resembles the situation seen in AIDS patients. An increase of serum IgM concentration was also noted. Immunotherapy included treatment with the following preparations: TFX and Levamisol which stimulate T cell functions, Broncho-Vaxom which stimulates specific antibody production and a complex herb preparation PADMA showing undefined general stimulatory activity. Separate group of children was subjected to climatotherapy in Czerniawa Sanatorium and received no immunostimulants. All methods of treatment employed had beneficial effect. The highest percentage of positive results was obtained in children receiving TFX and Levamisol. In all groups under study, an elevation of T cells percentage was observed. This was especially evident in Levamisol treated patients. There was no correlation, however, between T cells number and clinical improvement.

Sergeev AV Revazova ES Denisova SI Kalatskaia OV Rytenko AN
[Immunomodulating and antitumor activity of polysaccharides of plant origin]
Immunomoduliruiushchaia i protivoopukholevaia aktivnost' polisakharidov rastitel'nogo proiskhozhdeniia.
Biull Eksp Biol Med (1985 Dec) 100(12):741-3

The effect of the polysaccharides tagetan, palustran, and zymosan injections to BALB/c mice on the formation of cytotoxic T-lymphocytes in allogenic mixed culture has been studied. Lymphocytes from a 5-day-old mixed culture were characterized by the greatest cytotoxic activity, with splenocytes serving as reacting cells in mice injected 12-50 mg/kg of tagetan, 20 mg/kg of zymosan and 10-100 mg/kg of palustran, 7, 3, and 5 days, respectively, before the beginning of allogeneic stimulation in vitro. To determine correlation between immunostimulating and antitumor activity 25 mg/kg of tagetan every 14 days, 20 mg/kg of zymosan every 6 days, and 10 mg/kg of palustran every 6 days, were injected to BALB/c and BALB/c nu/nu mice prior to and following subcutaneous implantation of Crocker sarcoma cells. By the end of the first month of immunotherapy the tumor size in mice on tagetan or zymosan was 2-2.5 times smaller than in control animals. Tumor growth inhibition with palustran was about 30%. Polysaccharide administration to BALB/c nu/nu mice was not accompanied by tumor growth inhibition. The data obtained suggest that inhibition of Crocker sarcoma growth in mice injected the above polysaccharides is mediated by stimulation of antitumor T-cell activity.

Schonhofer PS Schulte-Sasse H
[Are botanical immunostimulants effective and harmless?]
Sind pflanzliche Immunstimulantien wirksam und unbedenklich?
Dtsch Med Wochenschr (1989 Nov 17) 114(46):1804-6

Simons JM t'Hart LA van Dijk H Fischer FC de Silva KT Labadie RP
Immunomodulatory compounds from Picrorhiza kurroa: isolation and characterization of two anti-complementary polymeric fractions from an aqueous root extract.
J Ethnopharmacol (1989 Sep) 26(2):169-82

Two aqueous root extracts of Picrorhiza kurroa, one prepared by extraction at 4 degrees C and the other by refluxing, were purified using the guidance of modulation of classical (CP) and alternative (AP) pathway complement activity. By means of methanol extraction and gel filtration chromatography, two polymeric fractions were isolated from the cold water extract. A methanol-soluble polymeric fraction (CS1) was highly active in inhibiting CP complement activity exclusively, whereas a methanol-insoluble polymeric fraction (CI1) exhibited an inhibitory effect on both CP and AP complement activity. Preliminary chemical analysis of the anti-complementary fractions revealed the presence of structures of carbohydrate and of peptide nature in CS1 and CI1. The modulation of CP complement activity by CS1 was studied in more detail. Its inhibitory effect was proven to be based on complement consumption rather than on chelation of $Ca2+$ and/or $Mg2+$ or on stabilization of the target cells in the complement-assay. The purification of the aqueous extract prepared by refluxing resulted in the isolation of a polymeric fraction with the same qualitites as CS1. However, a fraction with properties similar to CI1 could not be isolated from this extract.

Solar S Zeller H Rasolofonirina N Coulanges P Ralamboranto L Andriatsimahavandy AA Rakotovao LH Le Deaut JY
[Immunostimulant properties of an extract isolated and partially purified from Aloe vahombe]
Mise en evidence et étude des propriétés immunostimulantes d'un extrait isolé et partiellement purifié à partir d'Aloe vahombe.
Arch Inst Pasteur Madagascar (1980) 47(1):9-39

When the mice are given a hypodermic infection of unrefined Vahombe extract (the Aloe called Vahombe is a liliaceous plant growing in the South of Madagascar), they are protected against the infection caused by the Klebsiella, a pneumonia vector to man, giving rise to an experimental septicaemia in the mouse. Neither bactericide nor bacteriostatic activity has been detected yet about Aloe extract. The anti-infectious activity is proportional to the dose of extract injected, the protecting power is the greatest when the mice have been treated with Aloe, two or three days previously to the infection due to Klebsiella pneumoniae. We have determined the LD50 (Lethal dose 50) for the check batches (non-treated mice) and for the batches of protected mice. We were able to show that the previous injection developed the resistance to infection, multiplied from thirtyfold to a hundredfold. We have tackled the purification of the substance—made soluble after lyophilization of the crude extract—by means of filtration with Sephadex G50. It would be the first time, for all we know, that a substance was endowed with organism. At present we are proceeding with the purification of the active principle and contemplating trying the protective power upon virus infections as well as upon cancerous or parasitic ones.

Standring R Lavender EA Wheeler AW Spackman VM Moran DM
Induction of T-helper cell activity by fragments of rye grass pollen extract produced by digestion with chymotrypsin.
Int Arch Allergy Appl Immunol (1988) 87(4):337-41

Stanescu U Grigorescu E
[Immunotherapeutic properties of medicinal plants. II. Plant immunomodulator macromolecules]
Calitatea imunoterapeutica a plantelor medicinale (II).Macromolecule vegetale imunomodulatoare.
Rev Med Chir Soc Med Nat Iasi (1987 Oct-Dec) 91(4):731-9

Sun YH
[Cordyceps sinensis and cultured mycelia]
Chung Yao Tung Pao (1985 Dec) 10(12):3-5

Sun Y Hersh EM Talpaz M Lee SL Wong W Loo TL Mavligit GM
Immune restoration and/or augmentation of local graft versus host reaction by traditional Chinese medicinal herbs.
Cancer (1983 Jul 1) 52(1):70-3
The in vitro restorative effect of aqueous extracts from two traditional Chinese medicinal herbs were studied in 19 cancer patients and in 15 normal healthy donors. Using the local graft versus host (GVH) reaction as a test assay for T-cell function, the extract from astragalus membranaceus (10 microgram/ml) induced a restored reaction in nine of ten patients with an increase in local GVH reaction from 18.2 plus/minus 15.8 mm3 to 112.9 plus/minus 94.2 mm3 (P less than 0.01). The extract from ligustrum lucidum likewise effected an immune restoration in nine of 13 cancer patients with an increase in local GVH reaction from 32.3 plus/minus 36.1 mm3 to 118 plus/minus 104.9 mm3 (P less than 0.01). This degree of immune restoration appears to be complete as it equals the local GVH reaction observed among untreated mononuclear cells from normal healthy donors (82.8 plus/minus 41.1 mm3, P greater than 0.1). These results suggest that both extracts of the traditional Chinese medicinal herbs contain potent immune stimulants which may provide the rational basis for their therapeutic use as biological response modifiers.

Thabrew MI de Silva KT Labadie RP de Bie PA van der Berg B
Immunomodulatory activity of three Sri-Lankan medicinal plants used in hepatic disorders.
J Ethnopharmacol (1991 May-Jun) 33(1-2):63-6

The effects of aqueous extracts of Osbeckia octandra whole plant, Melothria maderaspatana whole plant and Phyllanthus debilis leaves on the human immune system were investigated. The extracts showed strong anticomplement effects on both the classical and alternate pathways of the human complement system in vitro. The effects were dose-dependent and most pronounced in the classical complement pathway assay. The extract also exhibited a direct dose-dependent inhibition with luminol-induced chemiluminescence of human polymorphonuclear leukocytes upon stimulation with zymosan.

Thatte UM Dahanukar SA
Comparative study of immunomodulating activity of Indian medicinal plants, lithium carbonate and glucan.
Methods Find Exp Clin Pharmacol (1988 Oct) 10(10):639-44

The protective effects of Asparagus racemosus (AR) and Tinospora cordifolia (TC) against myelosuppression induced by single doses of cyclophosphamide (CP) have been previously reported. Presented here are the results of a comparative study between AR, TC, glucan and lithium carbonate against the myelosuppressive effects of single and multiple doses of cyclophosphamide in mice. Cyclophosphamide was administered as a single dose 200 mg/kg subcutaneously to one group of mice, while a second group received 3 doses of 30 mg/kg intraperitoneally. Both groups received AR, TC and lithium orally for 15 days before CP. Glucan was administered intravenously in 3 doses, before cyclophosphamide in the first group and together with cyclophosphamide in the second group. In both groups peripheral and differential WBC counts were done before and after drug treatment and serially after cyclophosphamide injection. All four drugs produced leucocytosis with neutrophilia. When compared to the control group, all 4 drugs prevented, to varying degrees, leucopenia produced by cyclophosphamide. We conclude, therefore, that both indigenous plants, AR and TC, are potent immunostimulants, with effects comparable to lithium and glucan. They need further evaluation in patients receiving cytotoxic drugs.

t'Hart LA van den Berg AJ Kuis J van Dijk H Labadie RP
An anti-complementary polysaccharide with immunological adjuvant activity from the leaf parenchyma gel Aloe vera.
Planta Med (1989 Dec) 55(6):509-12

The aim of the study is to develop new substances with immunomodulatory activity. To this end, extracts from plants used in traditional medicine are used as starting material. This study deals with the mucilagenous leaf-gel of Aloe vera which is well reputed for its therapeutical effect on inflammatory-based disorders. The purification of an aqueous gel-extract guided by inhibition of complement activity in HPS is described. Using anion-exchange and gel permeation chromatography, a highly active polysaccharide fraction was isolated that is present in the various chain lengths. The polysaccharides consist of several monosaccharides of which mannose is dominant. The inhibition is based on alternative pathway activation, resulting in consumption of C3. With respect to their biological activity the polysaccharides inhibit the opsonization of zymosan in HPS and display adjuvant activity on specific antibody production and the induction of delayed type hypersensitivity in mice.

t'Hart LA van Enckevort PH van Dijk H Zaat R de Silva KT Labadie RP
Two functionally and chemically distinct immunomodulatory compounds in the gel of Aloe vera.
J Ethnopharmacol (1988 May-Jun) 23(1):61-71

An aqueous extract of Aloe vera gel was analyzed guided by modulatory activity with regard to the in vitro activation of human complement and of human polymorphonuclear leucocytes (PMN). Upon ultrafiltration a high (h-Mr) and a low (l-Mr) molecular mass fraction were obtained. Pre-incubation of human pooled serum with the h-Mr fraction resulted in a depletion of classical and alternative pathway complement activity. In contrast, only the l-Mr fraction could inhibit the production of free oxygen radicals by activated PMNs. The latter activity cannot be attributed to nonspecific effects like toxicity, interference with stimulant binding or scavenger activity.

Vasil'eva V   Tatskaia VN   Reznik SR
[Experience with using plant and microbial adjuvants for producing immune ascitic fluids in laboratory animals]
Sproba zastosuvannia roslynnoho i mikrobnoho ad'iuvantiv dlia oderzhannia imunnykh astsytnykh ridyn u laboratornykh tvaryn
Mikrobiol Zh (1974 May-Jun) 36(3):358-60

Wagner H
[Plant preparations for immunostimulation]
Phytopraparate zur Immunstimulierung.
Internist (Berl) (1988 Jul) 29(7):472-8

Wagner H   Kreutzkamp B   Jurcic K
[Contents and pharmacology of Okoubaka aubrevillei-Rinde]
Planta Med (1985 Oct) (5):404-7

Wang YP
[Progress of pharmacological research on angelica polysaccharide]
Chung Hsi I Chieh Ho Tsa Chih (1991 Jan) 11(1):61-3

Weng XC   Zhang P   Gong SS   Xiai SW
Effect of immuno-modulating agents on murine IL-2 production.
Immunol Invest (1987 Apr) 16(2):79-86

The effect of two Chinese traditional drugs, Dang Gui injection prepared from Angelica sinensis and C 21 Ester glucoside (GB) extracted from Cyanchus auriculatus on in vitro production of IL-2 has been studied. The IL-2 was produced by Con A stimulation of mouse spleen mononuclear cells. The IL-2 activity was assayed using Con A stimulated blast cells as the target. It was found that Dang Gui increased and GB decreased the production of IL-2. In the control experiments for immuno-modulating effect, prostaglandin E2 (PGE2) was found to suppress and indomethacin to increase IL-2 production. The stimulatory effect of Dang Gui was totally abrogated by PGE2.

Wu RT   Chiang HC   Fu WC   Chien KY   Chung YM   Horng LY
Formosanin-C, an immunomodulator with antitumor activity.
Int J Immunopharmacol (1990) 12(7):777-86

Paris formosana Hayata (Liliaceae) grown in the mountain areas of Taiwan, has been used as a folk remedy for a snake bite, and as an anti-inflammatory or anti-neoplastic agent. The effects of formosanin-C, a diosgenin saponin isolated from Paris formosana, on immune responses and transplantable murine tumor were studied. In culture systems, formosanin-C (0.03-0.16 microM) displayed significant enhancement of the blastogenic response of human peripheral blood cells to phytohemagglutinin. Formosanin-C also significantly increased the 3H-thymidine incorporation of Con A-stimulated lymphocytes at concentrations of 0.1 and 0.01 microM. The responsiveness of the granulocyte/macrophage colony-forming cells (GM-CFC) to mouse fibroblast cells L929 conditioned medium was altered in the presence of 0.01 and 0.001 microM of formosanin-C. In addition, formosanin-C given intraperitoneally activated natural killer cell activity at doses of 1-2.5 mg/kg. An intraperitoneal injection of 2.5 mg/kg of formosanin-C markedly induced interferon production, the peak blood level of which was observed 24 h after formosanin-C injection. Growth of subcutaneously transplanted MH-134 mouse hepatoma was retarded by intraperitoneal treatment with 1-2.5 mg/kg of formosanin-C. The activity of fluorouracil against MH-134 mouse hepatoma was potentiated by intraperitoneal treatment with formosanin-C.

These results suggest that formosanin-C might display antitumor activity in association with modification of the immune system.

Xu YM Lu PC
[Experimental studies on immunostimulatory effects of the Isatis indigotica polysaccharide]
Chung Hsi I Chieh Ho Tsa Chih (1991 Jun) 11(6):357-9, 325-6

Polysaccharides extracted from the root of Isatis indigotica (IIP, 50 mg/kg.d, ipx8d) significantly increased the weight of spleen and number of white blood cells and lymphocytes in peripheral blood in normal ICR mice, and antagonized the immunosuppressive actions of hydrocortisone. There were marked potentiating effects on delayed hypersensitivity reaction induced by 2, 4-dinitrochlorobenzene in normal NIH mice treated with IIP as well as in immunodepressed mice induced by cyclophosphamide. By administration of IIP, the percentage of ANAE+ lymphocytes stained with acid alpha-naphthyl acetate esterase method was significantly increased in peripheral blood of normal ICR mice, and the decreases in number of ANAE+ lymphocytes in mice induced by hydrocortisone were prevented to a certain extent. But IIP could not enhance Con A-induced lymphocyte proliferation of C57BL mouse spleen cells in vitro measured with MTT colorimetric assay. In addition, the plaque-forming cells in 5 x 10(6) splenocytes of NIH mice treated with IIP were higher than that of the control group (P less than 0.01). IIP could also elevate the clearance rate of intravenous charcoal particles in normal mice, i.e., stimulated the phagocytic activity of macrophages. The result indicates that IIP is capable of increasing humoral and cellular immune functions and enhancing the functions of reticuloendothelial system, and might be a good immunopotentiator.

Xu RS Zhu QZ Xie YY
Recent advances in studies on Chinese medicinal herbs with physiological activity.
J Ethnopharmacol (1985 Nov-Dec) 14(2-3):223-53

Medicinal plants with physiological activity studied in China during recent years are classified into three types: (1) drugs originating from traditional medicine and ancient prescriptions; (2) drugs originating from folk prescriptions or experienced prescriptions; (3) drugs originating from Chinese drugs with modified structures of the active principles and now in common use. The physiological activities are discussed in separate sections according to their therapeutic effects: nervous system; parasites; cardiovascular system; cancer; birth control; immunoactivity.

Younis GM Pavelescu M Stanescu U Grigorescu E
[Pharmacodynamic screening of the immunostimulant activity of products from the plant Solenostema argel (Del.) Hayne]
Rev Med Chir Soc Med Nat Iasi (1988 Jan-Mar) 92(1):59-60

Chapter 5

Glossary and Other Useful Information

Herb Names and Plant Taxonomy

The botanical name of a plant, often in Latin or Greek, can be a great source of information. However, this is often ignored by herbalists as binomials can be very intimidating! If their derivation and the reasoning behind their choice is grasped this intimidation changes into empowerment—or at least simple bewilderment.

The selection and use of botanical names occur in the field of taxonomy. Taxonomy is the arrangement of living organisms into categories based on natural similarities, such as structure, development, biochemical or physiological functions, and evolutionary history. This is done to identify relationships between different ancient and modern groups; to indicate the evolutionary pathways along which present-day organisms may have developed; and to provide a basis for comparing experimental data about different plants and animals. As many characteristics as possible are used, including the organism's anatomy, biochemistry, embryology, molecular biology, behavior, and distribution.

The system of classification was introduced by Carolus Linnaeus, a Swedish botanist, in 1753. The basic unit in the Linnaean classification of living forms is the species: a group of organisms both resembling each other more closely than the organisms of any other group and capable of mating with one another to produce fertile offspring. According to internationally accepted rules, a species is always identified by two technical Latin names, or a binomial. For example, the species of common Yarrow is known technically as *Achillea millefolia*. The first name always identifies the genus, which is a group of species more closely related to one another than to any other group. The second word, the specific epithet, identifies a particular species within a genus. Thus Yarrow belongs to the genus *Achillea*, but this genus also contains other species, such as *Achillea ptarmica*—the sneezewort.

Species are arranged into higher groupings that are progressively more inclusive. Species that are closely related are grouped together into a genus. Genera with similar characteristics and origins are grouped into families. Families, in turn, are grouped into orders, orders into classes, and classes into phyla in animals and into divisions in plants. Finally, related phyla or divisions are placed together into kingdoms. Sometimes it is desirable to make finer distinctions between two consecutive ranks. In that case an additional rank may be inserted between the original two, and the prefix sub- or super- is then added to one of the main ranks. Between an order and a family, for example, the order may contain several suborders, each suborder several superfamilies, and each superfamily several families.

Traditionally organisms have been classified into two kingdoms, plant and animal, but the most popular classification system now is the five-kingdom grouping. Here organisms are classified according to whether they are procaryotic—meaning single-celled, like bacteria, with neither internal membranes nor organelles—or eucaryotic, meaning composed of one or more cells containing membrane-bound nuclei and organelles; whether they are unicellular or multicellular; and whether they obtain food by photosynthesis, ingestion, or absorption of organic matter from their surroundings. The five kingdoms established according to these properties are:

1. **Monera**, including bacteria and blue-green algae; single-celled or colony-forming procaryotes; if colonial, no specialization or division of labor occurs among the cells. They are classified by the nature of their cell walls, type of motility, and mode of nutrition.

2. **Protista**, including protozoa and some single-celled algae; they, and all other living things except the Monera, have eucaryotic cell structure. Two major subgroups are the algae which photosynthesize, and protozoa which live by ingesting or absorbing organic matter.

3. **Fungi**, plant-like, many-celled organisms that live by absorbing nutrients from their surroundings. These organisms, classified by body structure and type of reproduction, include yeast, slime mold, mold, and mushrooms.

4. **Plantae** (plants); many-celled organisms that live by photosynthesis. They have leaves or leaflike structures specialized for photosynthesis; stems or stemlike structures that hold the leaves; and roots specialized for anchoring the plant in a growth medium and absorbing water. The plants fall into two groups: bryophytes (liverworts and mosses), which have no tissues for transporting water and minerals from roots; and the more numerous vascular plants, which include both ferns and seed plants.

5. **Animalia** (animals), comprising sponges; coelenterates, such as jellyfish; annelids, such as earthworms, leeches, and clamworms; mollusks, such as clams, snails, and squid; arthropods, such as insects, spiders, and lobsters; echinoderms, such as starfish and sea urchins; and vertebrates—the fish, amphibians, reptiles, birds, and mammals.

As an example of the application of the Linnaean system consider Peppermint, *Mentha piperita*.

Kingdom—Plant

Division—Angiospermae
The flowering plants which include more than 250,000 species of "herbs," shrubs and trees.

Class—Dicotyledoneae
Characterized by seeds having 2 cotyledons. Approximately 48 orders and 289 families.

Order—Tubiflorae
The Tubiflorae contain 26 families with many important medicinal species. Usually order names end in "-ales" (e.g., Papaverales, the order containing California poppy).

Family—Labiatae (Lamiaceae)
Approximately 200 genera and 3,000 species. Family names usually end in "-aceae."

Genus—*Mentha*
25 species with many hybrids. The genus name should be capitalized and either in italics or underlined.

Species—*Mentha piperita* Linnaeus (Peppermint)
The binomial is followed by the name of the botanist who first characterized the species.

Kinds of Names

The names used in taxonomy can be grouped into various types. A few examples are given here.

Mythological Names

A number of names are taken from mythology, such as Nymphaea, the water lily, from the Latin **Nympha**, goddess of waters, meadows and forest.

Geographical Names

These are often self-explanatory (e.g., sinensis = China, californica = California, alabamensis = Alabama).

Classical Names

Apparently every name of a plant used in classical Greek has been used in modern nomenclature, and these have been modified until they form a large number of the designations in common use. Consider Psyllium from the Greek **psylla**, flea; Greek name of *Plantago Psyllium*. The seeds of this species resemble fleas.

Personal Names

Derived from the name of the collector of the species on which the genus was based, like Lobelia after Matthias de l'Obel, Flemish botanist (1538-1616). Another example is the California Poppy, *Eschscholtzia californica*, named after the botanist Eschscholtz.

Historical Names

Derived from the name of a historical figure such as *Agrimonia eupatoria* named for Eupator, a surname of Mithridates, King of Pontus.

Descriptive Names

Names indicative of habitat, size, form, color, and resemblance may be found in almost endless variety. As examples consider:

- an anatomical feature—*Hypericum perforatum*, St. John's Wort, characterized by small perforations along the edge of the leaf.
- size is indicated in all gradations (e.g., Plantago major, Greater Plantain).
- white color—*Lamium album*, White Deadnettle.

- yellow color—*Xanthium canadense*, Burweed.
- disagreeable odors as suggested by such names as foetidus as in *Symplocarpus foetidus*, Skunk Cabbage.
- ecological characteristic—*Arnica montana*, Arnica from mountains.
- living in the water—*Hydrocotyle asiatica*, Gotu Cola.

Uses or Properties

As many of the botanical systemizers were also doctors, a number of names reflect this interest and knowledge of the therapeutic uses of the plants.

- *Leonurus cardiaca*, Motherwort that helps the heart.
- *Taraxacum officinalis*, Dandelion, once in the official pharmacopoeia.
- *Rhamnus catharticus*, Purging Buckthorn.
- *Fagopyrum esculentum*, Buckwheat that is good to eat.

Selected Examples of Binomial Meanings

abrax	**abraxas**, mystical word formed from Greek letters.
absinthium	Gr. name of a plant in Xenophon.
abund-	L. **abundo**, to overflow, to abound with plants, grow up with luxuriance.
Achillea	Gr. **Achilleus**, hero of Homer's "Iliad" who is said to have discovered the virtues of a certain plant.
Aconitum	Gr. **akoniton**, a kind of poisonous plant, monk's hood.
Acorus	Gr. the sweet flag found in Dioscorides.
aculeatus	thorny, prickly.
Aesculus	L. name for a kind of oak.
agnus-castus	L. pure, innocent.
Agrimonia	L. **agrestis**, pertaining to land, rural; Gr. monos, solitary.
Agropyron	Gr. **agros**, a field; Gr. **pyr**, wheat.
alba -idum, -bum	L. white.
Alchemilla	from the Arabic for alchemy.
Allium	L. garlic.
Aloe	Gr. name for the plant.
alternifolia	L. alternate leaves.
Althaea	Gr. **althaino**, to heal.
amara	L. bitter tasting.
Anemone	daughter of the wind, from Gr. **anemos**, the wind.
Anethum	Gr. **anethon**, anise, dill.
Angelica	Gr. **angelikos**, angelic, heavenly, divine.
Anisum	Gr. **anison**, anise, dill.
Apium	L. parsley.
arborescens	L. planted with trees.
archangelica	said to have been revealed by the Archangel Gabriel.
Arctium lappa	Gr. **arctos**, a bear because of roughness.
Arctostaphylos	Gr. bear and bunch of grapes.
Aristolochia	Gr. best, birth.
Artemisia	name, in Dioscorides, of a plant, called after Artemis (Diana).
arvense	L. **arvensis**, of or belonging to a field.
arvensis	growing on arable land.
Asclepias	Gr. **asklepias**, named for Asklepios, god of medicine and healing.
Asparagus	from the ancient Greek name for the plant.
Astragalus	Gr. **astragalos**, name of a kind of leguminous plant.
Atropa	Gr. **Atropos**, one of the three goddesses of fate, the unbending one.
aureus	L. gold.

Avena	L. **avena**, an old name for oats.
Ballota	Gr. **ballote**, a name for black horehound.
Baptisia	Gr. to dip under water, dye.
Barosma	Gr. **baros**, weight, heaviness.
basilicum	Gr. **basilikos**, royal, kingly.
belladonna	It. beautiful lady.
Bellis	L. **bellus**, neat, charming, handsome.
benedictus	L. **bene**, well, agreeable.
Berberis	L. **berberis**, the barberry.
Betonica	Vettonica, the name in Pliny of a medicinal plant growing in the region of Spain called Vectones or Vettones.
Betula	L. **betula**, the birch.
Borago	L. **burra**, a shaggy garment, referring to the rough foliage.
Brassica	L. **brassica**, cabbage.
bursa-pastoris	L. **bursa**, a pouch, purse made of skin; **pastor**, shepherd.
calamus	L. **calamus**, a reed.
Calendula	L. **Kalendae**, the first day of the month in the Roman calendar. Monthly blooming.
campestris	L. **campus**, a plain; relating to a plain, growing in a field.
Cannabis	L. **cannabis**, hemp.
Capsella	L. **capsa**, box, from the form of the fruits.
Capsicum	Gr. **kapto**, to bite.
cardamomum	from Gr. name for the plant.
Carum	Gr. **karon**, name of caraway in Dioscorides.
Cascara	Spanish **cascara**, bark.
Castanea	L. name from **castania,** N. Greece which was known for its trees.
cataria	L. **catarius**, of cats; old name of a plant attractive to cats.
Caulophylum	Gr. **kaulos**, the stem of a plant, a cabbage stalk.
Centaurea	called after Chiron the Centaur, who had wide knowledge of herbs.
Centella	Gr. **kenteo**, to prick.
Cephaëlis	Gr. **kephalotos**, with a head.
cerifera	L. **cera**, wax or L. **cereus**, a wax candle.
Cetraria	L. **cetra**, a sort of leather shield.
Chamaelirium	L. **chamaeleon**, ground-lion.
Chamomilla	Gr. **chamaimelon**, name, in Dioscorides, of a plant that smelt of apples.
Chelone	Gr. **chelone**, a tortoise.
Chionanthus	Gr. **chion**, snow, white as snow.
Chondus	Gr. **chone**, funnel, tube.
Chrysanthe-mum	Gr. **chrysos**, gold; **anthemon**, flower.

Cimicifuga	L. **cimicinus**, smelling like or of bugs.
cinerea	L. **cinereus**, ash-colored.
Cnicus	Gr. **knekos**, a thistle-like plant used for dyeing.
Commiphora	Gr. **kommi**, gum.
communis, e	L. **communis**, common, general.
Convallaria	L. **convolvere,** to entwine.
cordata	L. **cordis**, the heart.
Coriandrum	ancient name for coriander.
Crataegus	Gr. **krataigos**, name of a tree in Theophrastus.
crispus	L. **crispus**, curled, curly, with wavy margins.
Curcuma	Arabic **Kirkum**, turmeric.
Cypripedium	Gr. **Kypridios**, belonging to Aphrodite.
diffusa, us, um	L. loosely spreading, spread, scatter.
Digitalis	translation of German name **Fingerhut**, thimble.
dioica	Gr. **di**, two.
Dioscorea	named after the Greek herbalist Dioscorides.
distichon	Gr. **distichos**, in two rows.
Drosera	Gr. **droseros**, dewy, referring to the clear, dew-like drops on the leaf glands.
Dryopteris	Gr. **Dryope**, daughter of Dryops and a playmate of the woodnymphs.
Elattaria	L. **elatus**, elevating.
Ephedra	Gr. **ephedra**, sitting upon a seat.
Equisetum	L. **equus**, horse; L. **seta**, bristle, hair.
erythraea	Gr. **erythros**, red, reddish.
Eschscholzia	called after Johann Friedrich Eschscholtz (1793-1831).
Eucalyptus	Gr. **eu** (used before roots beginning with a consonant), good, well, true, nice; Gr. **kalyptos**, covered, hidden.
Eupatorium	called after Eupator, a surname of Mithridates, king of Pontus.
Euphorbia	called by King Juba II of Mauretania after his physician in ordinary, Euphorbus.
Euphrasia	Gr. **euphrasia**, delight, mirth.
felix-mas	L. **felix**, fruitful, productive; L. **mas**, a male.
ficaria	L. **ficus**, a fig tree.
foetidus	L. **foetidus**, stinking.
Fragaria	L. **fragum**, a strawberry plant.
fulva	L. **fulvus**, reddish yellow, tawny, gold colored.
Fumaria	L. **fumus**, smoke.
Galega	Gr. **galaktos**, milky.
Galium	name, in Dioscorides, of *G. verum*, used to curdle milk for making cheese.

Gaultheria	Gr. **gaulos**, a pail, a round-bottomed vessel.
Gelsemium	It. **gelsomino**, jessamine.
Gentiana	called after Gentius, an Illyrian king.
Geranium	Gr. **geranos**, a kind of bird called the crane, from the beak-like fruit.
Ginkgo	Jap. **gingko**, vernacular name of the maidenhair fern tree.
glaucus, a, um	Gr. **glaukos**, silvery, gleaming, covered with a bloom like a plum.
Glechoma	Gr. **glechon**, pennyroyal.
globulus	L. **globulus**, a globe, ball, round as a ball.
Glycyrrhiza	Gr. **glykys**, sweet, pleasant.
gracilis, e	L. **gracilis**, slender.
graveolens	L. **grave**, heavy.
Grindelia	called after David Hieronymus Grindel (1776-1836).
Guaiacum	West Indian name for lignum-vitae.
Hamamelis	Gr. **hama**, all together, at the same time.
Harpagophy-tum	Gr. **harpagos**, robbing, rapacious.
Hedera	L. **hedera**, ivy.
hederacea	L. **hederaceus**, of ivy, ivy-green.
hippocasta-num	Gr. **hippos**, horse, and Gr. **Kastanus**, chestnut, meaning chestnut unfit for food.
hirtus, a, um	L **hirtus**, hairy.
Hordeum	L. **hordeum**, barley.
horridus, a, um	L. **horridus**, bristly, prickly.
hortensis, e	L. **hortensis**, cultivated in gardens.
Humulus	Latinized form of a Teutonic word for hops.
Hydrastis	Gr. **hydor**, water + **drao**, to act; an agent, performer.
Hypericum	Gr. **Hyperikon**, the St. John's wort.
Hyssopus	Gr. **Hyssopos**, an aromatic plant.
idaeus	of Mt. Ida, a mountain in Crete.
inflata	L. **inflatus**, inflated.
Iris	Gr. **iris**, rainbow—name of a kind of lily.
Juglans	Jupiter's nut, L. **Jovis glans**.
Labiatae	meaning lipped, referring to the 2-lipped corolla, L. **labium**, lip.
Lactuca	Latin name for lettuce, **lac**, milk, from the white juice.
Lappa	L. **lappa**, a bur.
Lavandula	L. **lavo**, to wash.
Leonurus	L. **leo**, lion.

leuco-	Gr. **leukos**, white.
Ligusticum	name of a plant growing in Liguria.
Ligustrum	name, in Virgil, of a plant with white flowers.
Linum	L. **linum**, flax, thread, rope.
Lobelia	called after Matthias de l'Obel, Flemish botanist (1538-1616).
longus, a, um	L. **longus**, tall, long.
lucidus, a, um	L. **lucidus**, shining.
lupulus	L. **lupus**, a wolf.
luteum, us, a	L. **luteus**, golden-yellow.
Lycopus	Gr. **lykos**, a wolf.
macro-	Gr. **makros**, large.
maculatus, a, um	L. **macula**, spotted, speckled.
majalis	used in botany to signify flowering during May.
major	L. **major**, greater.
Malva	Gr. **malasso**, to soften.
marianum, us, a	said to refer to Mary. According to legends, the white marks on the leaves of *Silybum marianum* represent drops of milk spilt when feeding the infant Jesus during the flight to Egypt.
Marrubium	Gr. **maron**, a bitter herb.
Matricaria	L. **matrix**, womb.
media, um, us	L. **medius**, middle, intermediate.
Melaleuca	Gr. **melas**, **melaina**, or **malania**, black, blackness, clothed in black.
melano-	Gr. **melas**, black.
Melissa	Gr. **melissa**, honeybee, nymph who kept bees.
Mentha	Gr. **mentha**, mint.
Menyanthes	Gr. **menyo**, to disclose.
millefolium	L. **mille**, thousand, and **folium**, leaf.
minimum, us, a	L. least, smallest, very small.
minor, us	L. smaller.
mono-	Gr. **monos**, alone, single.
montana, us, um	L. growing in mountainous places.
multi-, multus, a, um	L. **multus**, many.
muralis, e	L. **murus**, a wall; of, growing on, walls.
muscosus, a, um	L. **muscus**, moss; moss-like.
Myrica	Gr. **myrike**, ancient name of the tamarisk. Gr. **myro**, to flow, since it grows on banks of running streams.
Myristica	Gr. **myristikos**, fit for anointing.

myrtillus	Gr. **Myrtilos**, son of Mercury, charioteer of Oenomaus.
napellus	L. **napus**, a kind of turnip.
Nasturtium	L. **nasus**, nose, and L. **tortus**, twisting away or torment.
neglectus, a, um	L. **neglectus**, neglected, overlooked.
Nepeta	L. **nepa**, a scorpion.
niger, gra, grum	L. **nigra**, black.
nitens	L. **nitens**, shining.
nivalis, e	L. **nivis**, growing in or near snow.
nobilis, e	L. **nobilis**, famous, noted, celebrated.
nodosa, a, um	L. **nodus**, knotty, referring to tubers or swollen nodes.
nudi-, nudus, a, um	L. **nudus**, naked.
Nymphaea	L. **nympha**, goddess of waters, meadows and forests.
occidentalis	L. **occidentalis**, western.
odorata	L. **odoratus**, sweet-smelling.
officinale, is	L. **officinalis**, kept at the druggist's shop, i.e. used medicinally.
Olea	L. **olea**, olive.
Oxalis	Gr. **oxys**, sharp, acid.
Paeonia	Gr. **Paion**, physician of the gods.
palmatum	L. **palmatus**, marked like the palm of the hand.
paluster, tris, tre	L. **palustre**, marsh; growing in swampy places.
Panax	Gr. **panacaea**, an herb which was supposed to heal all diseases.
Papaver	L. **papaver,** poppy.
Parthenium	Gr. **parthenos**, virgin.
Passiflora	L. **passio**, a passion, also a suffering.
pellucidus, a, um	L. **pellucidus**, transparent.
peltatum	L. **peltatus**, armed with a shield.
pendulus, a, um	L. **pendulus**, hanging down.
perennis	L. throughout the year, through the year.
perforatum	L. **perforatus**, perforated.
Petroselinum	Gr. **petros**, a rock; Gr. **selinon**, parsley.
Phytolacca	Gr. **phyton**, tree, plant.
Piscidia	L. **piscis**, fish; L. **caedere**, to kill.
Plantago	L. **planta**, sole of the foot.
Polygala	Gr. **polys**, many or much; Gr. **gala**, milk.

Populus	L. **populus**, the poplar tree, so-called from the number and continual motion of its leaves.
pratense	L. **pratensis**, pertaining to or growing in a meadow.
Primula	L. **primus**, the first.
Prunella	from the German, as the herb was used to treat croup.
Psyllium	Gr. **psylla**, flea; Greek name of *Plantago Psyllium*. The seeds of this species resemble fleas.
pubescens	L. **pubescens**, hairs of puberty; covered with soft hairs.
Pulmonaria	L. **pulmonarius**, beneficial to the lungs.
pulsatilla	L. **pulsata**, beaten, driven about, from the beating of the flowers by the wind.
purpurea, us, um	L. applied to various shades of red.
Quercus	L. **quercus**, an oak.
racemosa	L. **racemus**, the stalk of a cluster, a bunch of berries.
Ranunculus	L. **rana**, a frog.
recutita	L. **recutitus**, having a fresh or new skin.
repens	L. **repo**, creeping.
Rheum	Gr. **rha**, rhubarb
riparius, a, um	L. growing by rivers and streams.
Rosmarinus	L. **Ros**, dew; L. **Marinus**, of the sea.
rotundifolia	L. **rotundus**, round.
Rubus	L. **rubus**, blackberry.
Rumex	L. for sorrel.
rupester, tris, tre	L. **rupes**, rock; growing on rocks.
Ruscus	L. **ruscarius**, of or for butcher's broom.
Salix	L. **salix**, the willow.
Salvia	name of a plant in Pliny, perhaps from **salvus**, safe, sound, **salus**, health.
Sambucus	L. for the elder tree.
Sanguinaria	L. **sanguis**, blood.
sativa, us, um	L. sown, planted, cultivated, as opposed to agrestis and silvestris, which mean wild.
scoparius	L. **scopula**, thin branches, twigs, a broom.
Scrophularia	from scrophula, i.e., tubercular glands of the neck.
Scutellaria	L. **scutella**, salver, dish, referring to the pouch on the calyx.
semi-	half.
Senecio	from L. **senex**, old man, because of the conspicuous white pappus.
serrulata	L. saw shaped, serrated.

silvaticus, a , um	L. growing in woods, L. **silva**, woodland.
Silybum	L. **Silybum**, a kind of thistle with edible stems.
Smilax	Gr. **smilax**, the yew; also a bindweed.
Solidago	L. **solidare**, to put together or make firm.
somnifer, era, erum	L. **somnus**, sleep; sleep-bringing, soporific.
spicata	L. **spica**, a point.
squalidus, a, um	L. rough, unkempt, neglected, squalid.
Stachys	Gr. **stachys**, an ear of grain, spike.
Stellaria	L. **stella**, star.
sylvatica	L. **sylvaticus**, growing among trees.
Symphytum	Gr. **symphyton**, name of a kind of plant with healing properties, comfrey.
Symplocarpus	Gr. **symploke**, a twisting together.
Taraxacum	medieval Latin, ultimately from Arabic, bitter potherb.
thalictroides	Gr. **thaliktron**, meadow-rue.
tham-	Gr. **thamees**, crowded, copious.
Thuja	Gr. **thya**, an African tree with fragrant, durable wood.
Thymus	Gr. **thymos**, to perfume or to sacrifice.
Tilia	L. **tilia**, the linden tree.
tinctoria	L. **tinctorius**, of or belonging to dyeing, bloodthirsty.
tremulus, a, um	L. **tremo**, shivering, trembling, quake, quiver.
tricho-	Gr. hairy, hair-like.
Trifolium	L. **tria**, thrice, and **folium**, leaf.
Trigonella	Gr. **trigonos**, triangular, three-cornered.
Trillium	L. **trillium**, an herb with leaves in whorls of three.
tuberosa	L. **tuberosus**, full of humps.
Tussilago	L. **tussis**, cough.
ulmaria	medieval name for the goats-beard, a plant with elm-like leaves
Ulmus	L. **ulmus**, the elm.
Urtica	L. **urtica**, nettle; derived from **urere**, to burn.
uva-ursi	L. **uva**, grape, and L. **ursi**, bear.
Valeriana	medieval name, perhaps from L. **valeo**, be well or strong.
Verbena	L. **verbenae**, sacred boughs.
versicolor	changing color.
verus, a, um	L. **verus**, true, genuine.
Viburnum	L. **viburnum**, the wayfaring tree.
villosa, us	L. **villosus**, hairy, shaggy, rough.

Vinca	L. **vinca**, the periwinkle.
Viola	L. **viola**, the violet.
virgaurea	L. **virga**, rod, and L. **aureus**, golden.
virosa	L. **virosus**, muddy, covered with slime, poison, fetid.
Viscum	L. **viscum**, bird-lime, made from the berries of mistletoe.
Vitex	L. **vitex**, the chaste tree.
vulgare, is	L. general, common, usual.
xanth(o)-	Gr. **xanthos**, yellow.
Zingiber	Gr. **zingiber**, ginger.

Herbs Listed by Latin Binomial

Abelmoschus moschatus	Muskseed
Abies balsamea	Balsam Fir
Abrus precatorius	Jequirity
Abutilon indicum	Atbala
Acacia arabica	Acacia Bark
Acacia catechu	Black Catechu
Acacia decurrens	Acacia Bark
Acacia senegal	Acacia Gum
Acer rubrum	Red Maple
Achillea millefolium	Yarrow
Achillea ptarmica	Sneezewort
Aconitum napellus	Aconite
Acorus calamus	Sweet Flag
Adhatoda vasica	Malabar Nut
Adiantum capillus-veneris	Maidenhair Fern
Adonis vernalis	False Hellebore
Aegopodium podagraria	Ground Elder
Aesculus hippocastanum	Horse Chestnut
Aethusa cynapium	Fool's Parsley
Aframomum melegueta	Grains of Paradise
Agathosma betulina	Buchu
Agrimonia eupatoria	Agrimony
Agropyron repens	Couch Grass
Ailanthus altissima	Tree of Heaven
Ajuga chamaepitys	Ground Pine
Ajuga reptans	Bugle
Alchemilla arvensis	Lady's Mantle
Aletris farinosa	True Unicorn Root
Alkanna tinctoria	Alkannet
Allium cepa	Onion
Allium sativum	Garlic
Alnus glutinosa	Alder
Aloe spp.	Aloe
Aloysia triphylla	Lemon Verbena
Alpinia officinarum	Galangal
Alstonia scholaris	Alstonia Bark
Althaea officinalis	Marshmallow
Amaranthus hypochondriacus	Amaranth
Anacardium occidentale	Cashew
Anacylus pyrethrum	Pellitory
Anagallis arvensis	Scarlet Pimpernel
Anchusa tinctoria	Alkanet root
Andira araroba	Cabbage Tree
Andrapogon muricatus	Vetiverian
Anemone pulsatilla	Pasque Flower
Anethum graveolens	Dill
Angelica archangelica	Angelica
Antennaria dioica	Life Everlasting
Anthemis cotula	Mayweed
Anthemis nobilis	Chamomile
Anthoxanthum odoratum	Sweet Vernal Grass

Apium graveolens	Celery Seed
Apocynum androsaemifolium	Bitter Root
Apocynum cannabinum	Canadian Hemp
Arachis hypogaea	Peanut
Aralia nudicaulis	False sarsaparilla
Aralia racemosa	American Spikenard
Aralis spinosa	Angelica tree
Aranthe elongata	Matico
Arctium lappa	Burdock
Arctostaphylos uva-ursi	Bearberry
Aristolochia spp.	Birthwort
Aristolochia serpentaria	Virginia snakeroot
Armoracia rusticana	Horseradish
Arnica montana	Arnica
Artemisia abrotanum	Southernwood
Artemisia absinthium	Wormwood
Artemisia dracunculus	Tarragon
Artemisia vulgaris	Mugwort
Arum maculatum	Cuckoopint
Arum triphyllum	Arum root
Asarum canadense	Wild Ginger
Asclepias incarnata	Swamp Milkweed
Asclepias syriaca	Milkweed
Asclepias tuberosa	Pleurisy root
Asparagus officinalis	Asparagus
Asparagus racemosus	Shatavari
Aspidosperma quebracho	Quebracho
Astragalus gummifer	Tragacanth
Astragalus membranaceus	Astragalus
Atropa belladonna	Belladonna
Avena sativa	Oats
Azadirachta indica	Azedarach
Azadiracta indica	Neem
Ballota nigra	Black Horehound
Bambusa arundinacea	Bamboo Manna
Baptisia tinctoria	Wild Indigo
Bellis perennis	Daisy
Berberis aquifolium	Mountain Grape
Berberis aristata	Berberis
Berberis vulgaris	Barberry
Betula lenta	Sweet birch
Betula spp.	Birch
Bidens tripartita	Burr Marigold
Bixa orellana	Annatto
Boerhaavia diffusa	Punarnava
Boletus ignarius	Agaric of oak
Borago officinalis	Borage
Boswellia thurifera	Frankincense
Brassica alba	White Mustard
Brassica nigra	Black Mustard
Brayers anthelmentica	Kooso
Brunfelsia hopeana	Manaca
Bryonia alba	White Bryony
Buxus sempervirens	Box

Caesalpinia bonducella	Nikkar Nuts
Caffea arabica	Coffee
Calamintha ascendens	Calamint
Calendula officinalis	Calendula
Calvatia species	Puff Ball
Camellia sinensis	Tea
Camphora officinalis	Camphor
Canella winterana	Canella
Cannabis sativa	Indian Hemp
Capsella bursa-pastoris	Shepherd's Purse
Capsicum minimum	Cayenne
Carica papaya	Papaya
Carthamus tinctorius	Safflower
Carum carvi	Caraway
Cascara sagrada	Cascara
Casparia febrifuga	Angostura
Cassava ssp.	Tapioca
Cassia angustifolia	Senna
Cassia fistula	Purging cassia
Cassia marilandica	American senna
Cassia senna	Senna
Castanea pumila	Dwarf chestnut
Castanea sativa	Chestnut
Caulophylum thalictroides	Blue Cohosh
Ceanothus americanus	Red Root
Celastrus scandens	Bittersweet, American
Centaurea cyanus	Cornflower
Centaurea nigra	Knapweed
Centaurium erythraea	Centaury
Centella asiatica	Hydrocotyle
Cephaëlis ipecacuanha	Ipecacuanha
Ceratonia siliqua	Carob
Cetraria islandica	Iceland moss
Chameamelum nobilis	Chamomile
Chamaelirium luteum	False Unicorn Root
Chelidonium majus	Greater Celandine
Chelone glabra	Balmony
Chenopodium ambrosioides	Wormseed
Chimaphila umbellata	Wintergreen
Chionanthus virginicus	Fringetree
Chondodendron tomentosum	Pareira-brava
Chondus crispus	Irish Moss
Chrysanthemum indicum	Chrysanthemum
Chrysanthemum cinerariaefolium	Pyrethrum
Chrysanthemum leucanthemum	Ox-Eye Daisy
Cichorium intybus	Chicory
Cimicifuga racemosa	Black Cohosh
Cinchona spp.	Cinchona
Cinnamomum aromaticum	Cassia
Cinnamomum camphora	Camphor
Cinnamomum verum	Cinnamon
Citrullus colocynthis	Colocynth
Citrus aurantifolia	Lime
Citrus aurantium	Orange

Citrus limon	Lemon
Cladonia pyxidata	Cupmoss
Claviceps purpurea	Ergot
Cnicus benedictus	Blessed thistle
Cochlearia officinalis	Scurvy Grass
Cola vera	Kola Nut
Colchicum autumnale	Colchicum
Coleus forskohlii	Coleus
Collinsonia canadensis	Stone Root
Commiphora mol-mol	Myrrh
Commiphora mukul	Guggulu
Conium maculatum	Hemlock
Convallaria majalis	Lily of the Valley
Convolvulus scammonia	Scammony
Copaifera langsdorffi	Copaiba
Copernicia cerifera	Carnauba
Coptis groenlandica	Gold Thread
Coptis trifolia	Gold Thread
Corallorhiza odontorhiza	Coral Root
Coriandrum sativum	Coriander
Cornus circinata	Round-leaved dogwood
Cornus florida	Common dogwood
Cornus sericea	Osier, Red, American
Crataegus monogyna	Hawthorn
Crataegus oxyacantha	Hawthorn
Crithmum maritimum	Samphire
Crocus sativus	Saffron
Croton eluteria	Cascarilla
Croton tiglium	Croton
Cucurbita pepo	Pumpkin
Cuminum cyminum	Cumin
Curcuma longa	Turmeric
Curcuma zedoaria	Zedoary
Cuscuta epithymum	Dodder
Cyclopia genistoides	Rooibosch
Cydonia oblonga	Quince
Cymbopogon citratus	Lemon Grass
Cynoglossum officinale	Houndstongue
Cyperus esculentus	Nutgrass
Cypripedium calceolus	Lady's Slipper
Daemonorops draco	Dragon's Blood
Daphne mezereum	Mezereon
Datura stramonium	Thorn apple
Daucus carrota	Wild Carrot
Delphinium consolida	Larkspur
Delphinium staphisagria	Stavesacre
Dicentra canadensis	Turkey Corn
Digitalis spp.	Foxglove
Dioscorea villosa	Wild Yam
Diospyros virginiana	Persimmon
Dipteryx odorata	Tonka Beans
Dorema ammoniacum	Ammoniacum
Dorstenia contrajerva	Contrajerva
Drimys winteri	Winter's Bark

Drosera rotundifolia	Sundew
Dryopteris felix-mas	Male Fern
Ecballium elaterium	Wild cucumber
Echinacea spp.	Echinacea
Eclipta alba	Bhringaraj
Elattaria cardamomum	Cardamom
Embelia ribes	Embelia
Emblica officinalis	Amla
Ephedra sinica	Ma Huang
Equisetum arvense	Horsetail
Erigeron canadense	Fleabane
Eriodictyon californicum	Yerba Santa
Eryngium aquaticum	Button snakeroot
Eryngium maritimum	Eryngo
Erythronium americanum	Adder's Tongue, American
Erythroxylum coca	Coca
Eschscholzia californica	Californian Poppy
Eucalyptus spp.	Eucalyptus
Eugenia caryophyllata	Cloves
Euonymus atropurpurea	Wahoo
Eupatorium cannabinum	Hemp Agrimony
Eupatorium perfoliatum	Boneset
Eupatorium purpureum	Gravel Root
Euphorbia corollata	Large flowering spurge
Euphorbia hirta	Euphorbia
Euphorbia ipecacuanha	American Ipecac
Euphorbia pilulifera	Pill Bearing Spurge
Euphorbia resinifera	Euphorbium
Euphrasia spp.	Eyebright
Euryale ferox	Chinese foxnuts
Exogonium purga	Jalap
Fabiana imbricata	Pichi
Fagopyrum esculentum	Buckwheat
Fagus sylvatica	Beech
Ferula assa-foetida	Asafetida
Ferula gummosa	Galbanum
Ferula rubicaulis	Galbanum
Ferula sumbul	Sumbul
Ficus carica	Fig
Filipendula ulmaria	Meadowsweet
Foeniculum vulgare	Fennel
Fragaria vesca	Strawberry
Frasera carolinensis	Columbo, American
Fraxinus excelsior	Ash
Fraxinus ornus	Manna
Fucus vesiculosus	Bladderwrack
Fumaria officinalis	Fumitory
Galega officinalis	Goat's Rue
Galipea officinalis	Angostura
Galium aparine	Cleavers
Galium odoratum	Woodruff
Galium verum	Lady's Bedstraw
Garcinia hanburyi	Gamboge
Garrya fremontii	Feverbrush

Gaultheria procumbens	Wintergreen
Gelidium amansii	Agar
Gelsemium sempervirens	Yellow Jasmin
Gentiana spp.	Gentian
Geranium maculatum	Cranesbill
Gerum rivale	Water avens
Gillenia stipulata	Indian Physic
Ginkgo biloba	Ginkgo
Glechoma hederacea	Ground Ivy
Glycine max	Soybean
Glycyrrhiza glabra	Liquorice
Gnaphalium uliginosum	Cudweed
Gossypium herbaceum	Cotton Root
Gratiola officinalis	Hedge Hyssop
Grindelia camporum	Gumweed
Grindelia squarrosa	Grindelia
Guaiacum officinale	Guaiacum
Guarea rusbyi	Cocillana
Haematoxylon campechianum	Logwood
Hagenia abyssinica	Kousso
Hamamelis virginiana	Witch Hazel
Harpagophytum procumbens	Devil's Claw
Hedeoma pulegioides	American pennyroyal
Hedera helix	Ivy
Helianthemum canadense	Frostwort
Helianthus annuus	Sunflower
Helichrysum stoechas	Eternal Flower
Helleborus foetidus	Fetid hellebore
Helleborus niger	Black Hellebore
Hepatica nobilis	American Liverwort
Heracleum lanatum	Masterwort
Herniaria glabra	Rupturewort
Heuchera americana	Alum root
Hevea ssp.	Rubber
Hieracium pilosella	Mouse Ear
Hordeum vulgare	Barley
Humulus lupulus	Hops
Hydrocarpus spp.	Chaulmoogra
Hydrangea arborescens	Hydrangea
Hydrastis canadensis	Golden Seal
Hydrocotyle asiatica	Gotu Kola
Hyoscyamus niger	Henbane
Hypericum perforatum	St. John's Wort
Hyssopus officinalis	Hyssop
Ilex aquifolium	Holly
Ilex paraguariensis	Paraguay Tea
Ilicium verum	Star Anise
Impatiens biflora	Jewel Weed
Inula helenium	Elecampane
Ipomemea digitata	Vidari Kanda
Ipomoea orizabensis	Mexican Scammony Root
Ipomoea purga	Jalap
Ipomoea turpethum	Turpeth
Iris caroliniana	Blue Flag

Iris florentina	Orris
Iris foetidissima	Gladwin
Iris germanica	Orris
Iris pallida	Orris
Iris pseudacorus	Yellow Flag
Iris versicolor	Blue Flag
Isonandra gutta	Gutta-percha
Jasminum grandiflorum	Jasmine
Jateorhiza palmata	Calumba
Juglans cinerea	Walnut
Juglans regia	Walnut
Juniperus communis	Juniper
Juniperus oxycedrus	Cade oil
Juniperus sabina	Savin
Juniperus virginiana	Red cedar
Kalmia latifolia	Mountain Laurel
Kickxia elatine	Fluellen
Krameria triandra	Rhatany
Lachnanthes tinctoria	Lachnanthes
Lactuca virosa	Wild Lettuce
Lamium album	Archangel
Larix decidua	Larch
Larix laricina	Tamarac
Larrea divaricata	Chaparral
Laurus nobilis	Laurel
Lavandula officinalis	Lavender
Lawsonia inermis	Henna
Ledum groenlandicum	Labrador Tea
Leonurus cardiaca	Motherwort
Leptandra virginicum	Black Root
Ligusticum porteri	Osha
Ligustrum spp.	Privet
Lilium candidum	Meadow Lily
Linaria vulgaris	Yellow Toadflax
Linum catharticum	Mountain Flax
Linum usitatissimum	Flaxseed
Lippia dulas	Lippia
Liquidambar orientalis	Storax
Liriodendron tulipifera	Tulip tree
Liriosma ovata	Muira-Puama
Lobaria pulmonaria	Lungmoss
Lobelia inflata	Lobelia
Lomatium dissectum	Lomatium
Lonicera caprifolium	Honeysuckle
Lophophora williamsii	Mescal Buttons
Lycopodium clavatum	Clubmoss
Lycopodium complanatum	American Ground Pine
Lycopus europaeus	Bugleweed
Lycopus virginicus	Bugleweed
Lysimachia vulgaris	Loosestrife
Lythrum salicaria	Purple Loosestrife
Magnolia glauca	Magnolia
Mahonia repens	Oregon Grape
Mallotus philippinensis	Kamala

Malva sylvestris	Mallow
Maranta arundinacea	Arrowroot
Marrubium vulgare	Horehound
Marsdenia condurango	Condurango
Matricaria recutita	Chamomile
Medicago sativa	Lucern
Melaleuca alternifolia	Ti Tree
Melaleuca leucadendron	Cajaput
Melia azedarach	Pride of India
Melissa officinalis	Balm
Mentha aquatica	Wild Mint
Mentha longifolia	English Horsemint
Mentha piperita	Peppermint
Mentha pulegium	Pennyroyal
Mentha spicata	Spearmint
Menyanthes trifoliata	Bogbean
Metroxylon rumphii	Sago
Mitchella repens	Partridge Berry
Monarda punctata	Horsemint
Monsonia ovata	Monsonia
Morus nigra	Mulberry
Mucuna pruriens	Cowhage
Myrcia acris	Bay
Myrica cerifera	Bayberry
Myrica gale	Sweet Gale
Myristica fragrans	Nutmeg
Myroxylon balsamum	Tolu Balsam
Myroxylon pereirae	Peruvian Balsam
Myrrhis odorata	Sweet Cicely
Myrtus communis	Myrtle
Nectandra rodiaei	Bebeeru
Nepeta cataria	Catmint
Nicotiana tabacum	Tobacco
Nymphaea odorata	American White Pond Lily
Ocimum basilicum	Basil
Oenanthe aquatica	Water Fennel
Oenanthe crocata	Water Dropwort
Oenothera biennis	Evening Primrose
Olea europaea	Olive
Onosis spinosa	Rest Harrow
Ophioglossum vulgatum	Adder's Tongue, English
Origanum majorana	Marjoram
Origanum vulgare	Oregano
Oryza sativa	Rice
Ourouparia gambir	Pale catechu
Oxalis acetosella	Wood Sorrel
Paeonia officinalis	Peony
Panax quinquefolius	Ginseng, American
Panax ginseng	Ginseng
Papaver rhoeas	Red Poppy
Papaver somniferum	Opium Poppy
Parietaria officinalis	Pellitory of the Wall
Passiflora incarnata	Passion Flower
Paullinia cupana	Guarana

Pausinystalia yohimbe	Yohimbé
Peltigera canina	English Liverwort
Petasites hybridus	Butterburr
Petroselinum crispum	Parsley
Peucedanum ostruthium	Masterwort
Peumus boldus	Boldo
Phoenix dactylifera	Date
Physalis alkekengi	Winter Cherry
Physostigma venenosum	Calabar Bean
Phytolacca americana	Poke
Phytolacca decandra	Poke
Picrorhiza Kurroa	Kutki
Pilocarpus microphyllus	Jaborandi
Pilocarpus species	Jaborandi
Pilosella officinarum	Mouse Ear
Pimenta dioica	Allspice
Pimpinella anisum	Aniseed
Pimpinella saxifraga	Burnet Saxifrage
Pinus Montana	Dwarf pine
Pinus mugo	Pine Oils
Pinus strobus	White Pine
Pinus sylvestris	Pine Oils
Piper angustifolia	Matico
Piper betle	Betel
Piper cubeba	Cubeb
Piper longum	Indian Long Pepper
Piper methysticum	Kava Kava
Piper nigrum	Pepper
Piscidia erythrina	Jamaican Dogwood
Pistacia lentiscus	Mastic
Plantago major	Plantain
Plantago psyllium	Psyllium
Podophyllum peltatum	American Mandrake
Pogostemon cablin	Patchouli
Polemonium caeruleum	Jacob's Ladder
Polemonium reptans	Abscess Root
Polygala rubella	Bitter polygala
Polygala senega	Snakeroot
Polygonatum multiflorum	Solomon's Seal
Polygonum bistorta	Bistort
Polygonum hydropiper	Smartweed
Polygonum multiflorum	Fo-ti
Polymnia uvedalia	Bearsfoot
Polypodium vulgare	Polypody root
Polystrichum juniperum	Hair cap moss
Pomaderris elliptica	Kumarhou
Populus alba	Poplar
Populus candicans	Balm of Gilead
Populus gileadensis	Balm of Gilead
Populus nigra	Balm of Gilead
Populus tremuloides	White Poplar
Potentilla anserina	Silverweed
Potentilla reptans	Five-leaf-grass
Potentilla tormentilla	Tormentil

Primula veris	Cowslip
Primula vulgaris	Primrose
Prunella vulgaris	Self-heal
Prunus amygdalus	Almond
Prunus armeniaca	Apricot Seed
Prunus cerasus	Cherry
Prunus domestica	Prune
Prunus laurocerasus	Cherry Laurel
Prunus persica	Peach
Prunus serotina	Wild Cherry
Ptelea trifoliata	Wafer ash
Pterocarpus marsupium	Kino
Pterocarpus santalinus	Red Sandalwood
Pueraria tuberosa	Kudzu
Pulmonaria officinalis	Lungwort
Punica granatum	Pomegranate
Pyrola maculatum	Spotted pyrola
Pyrus aucuparia	Mountain ash
Quassia amara	Quassia
Quercus infectoria	Galls
Quercus robur	Oak
Quercus tinctoria	Black oak
Quillaja saponaria	Soap Bark
Ranunculus ficaria	Lesser Celendine
Rauwolfia serpentaria	Rauwolfia
Rehmannia glutinosa	Rehmannia
Rhamnus cathartica	Buckthorn
Rhamnus frangula	Alder Buckthorn
Rhamnus purshiana	Cascara Sagrada
Rheum officinale	Chinese Rhubarb
Rheum palmatum	Rhubarb Root
Rheum rhaponticum	English Rhubarb
Rhus aromatica	Sweet Sumach
Rhus glabra	Smooth Sumach
Rhus toxicodendron	Poison oak
Ribes nigrum	Blackcurrant
Ricinus communis	Castor Oil Plants
Rorippa nasturtium	Watercress
Rosa canina	Dog Rose
Rosa damascena	Damask Rose
Rosmarinus officinalis	Rosemary
Rubia cordifolia	Indian Madder
Rubia tinctorum	Prune
Rubus idaeus	Raspberry
Rubus trivialis	Dewberry
Rubus villosus	Blackberry
Rumex acetosa	Sorrel
Rumex acetosella	Sheep's Sorrel
Rumex aquatica	Water Dock
Rumex crispus	Yellow Dock
Ruscus aculeatus	Butcher's Broom
Ruta graveolens	Rue
Sabal serrulata	Saw Palmetto
Sabatia angularis	American centaury

Saccharum officinarum	Sugar
Sagus rumphii	Sago
Salix alba	White Willow
Salix cinerea	Willow
Salvia officinalis (var. *rubia*)	Red Sage
Salvia polystachya	Chia Seeds
Salvia sclarea	Clary
Sambucus ebulus	Dwarf Elder
Sambucus nigra	Elder
Sanguinaria canadensis	Bloodroot
Sanguisorba officinalis	Greater Burnet
Sanicula europaea	Sanicle
Santalum album	Sandalwood
Santolina chamaecyparissus	Lavender Cotton
Saponaria officinalis	Soapwort
Sarothamnus scoparius	Broom
Sarracenta purpurea	Pitcher Plant
Sassafras albidum	Sassafras
Satureja hortensis	Summer Savory
Satureja montana	Winter Savory
Schoenocaulon officinalis	Sabadilla
Scolopendrium vulgare	Hartstongue
Scopula carniolica	Scopolia
Scrophularia aquatica	Water Betony
Scrophularia nodosa	Figwort
Scutellaria laterifolia	Skullcap
Secale cornutum	Rye ergot
Selenicereus grandiflorus	Night-blooming Cereus
Sempervivum tectorum	Houseleek
Senecio aureus	Life Root
Senecio jacobaea	Ragwort
Serenoa serrulata	Saw Palmetto
Sesamum indicum	Sesame Seeds
Sesamum orientale	Sesame
Sida cordifolia	India Country mallow
Sida rhombifolia	Mahabala
Silphium laciniatum	Rosinweed
Silybum marianum	Milk Thistle
Simaba cedron	Cedron
Simaruba amara	Simaruba
Sinapis species	White Mustard
Sisymbrium officinale	Hedge Mustard
Smilax spp.	Sarsaparilla
Solanum carolinense	Horsenettle
Solanum dulcamara	Bittersweet
Solidago virgaurea	Golden Rod
Spigelia marilandica	Pink Root
Spirea tomentosa	Hardtack
Stachys officinalis	Wood Betony
Stachys palustris	Woundwort
Statice caroliniana	Marsh rosemary
Stellaria media	Chickweed
Stillingia sylvatica	Queen's Delight
Strophanthus gratus	Strophanthus

Strophanthus kombe	Strophanthus
Strychnos ignatii	Ignatius Beans
Strychnos nux vomica	Nux Vomica
Strychnos ignatia	Ignatia
Styrax benzoin	Benzoin
Swertia chirata	Chiretta
Symphytum officinale	Comfrey
Symplocarpus foetidus	Skunk Cabbage
Syzygium cumini	Jambul
Tabebuia avellanedae	Pau D'arco
Tamarindus indica	Tamarind
Tamus communis	Black Bryony
Tanacetum chrysanthemum	Feverfew
Tanacetum vulgare	Tansy
Taraxacum officinale	Dandelion
Taxus baccata	Yew
Terminalia belerica	Bibhitaki
Terminalia chebula	Myrobalan
Teucrium chamaedrys	Germander
Teucrium scordium	Water Germander
Teucrium scorodonia	Wood Sage
Theobroma cacao	Cocoa
Thuja occidentalis	Western Hemlock
Thymus spp.	Thyme
Tilia cordata	Linden
Tilia platyphylla	Linden
Tribulis terrestris	Goathead
Trifolium pratense	Red Clover
Trigonella foenum-graecum	Fenugreek
Trillium erectum	Beth Root
Trillium pendulum	Beth Root
Triosteum perfoliatum	Feverroot
Triticum vulgare	Wheat
Tropaeolum majus	Nasturtium
Tsuga canadensis	Pinus Bark
Turnera diffusa	Damiana
Tussilago farfara	Coltsfoot
Typha spp.	Cattail
Ulmus campestris	Elm
Ulmus rubra	Slippery Elm
Urginia maritima	Squill
Urtica dioica	Nettles
Usnea spp.	Spanish Moss
Ustilago maydis	Corn smut
Vaccinium myrtillus	Bilberry
Valeriana officinalis	Valerian
Vanilla aromatica	Vanilla
Veratrum album	White hellebore
Veratrum sabadilla	Cevadilla
Veratrum viride	American Hellebore
Verbascum thapsus	Mullein
Verbena officinalis	Vervain
Veronica beccabunga	Brooklime
Veronica officinalis	Speedwell

Veronicastrum virginicum	Black Root
Viburnum opulus	Cramp Bark
Viburnum prunifolium	Black Haw
Vinca major	Periwinkle
Viola odorata	Sweet Violet
Viola pedata	Pansy violet
Viola tricola	Heartsease
Viscum album	Mistletoe
Vitex agnus-castus	Chasteberry
Vitis vinifera	Grape
Wintera aromatica	Winter's bark
Withania somnifera	Ashwaganda
Xanthorrhiza apiifolia	Yellow root
Zanthoxylum americanum	Prickly Ash
Zea mays	Corn Silk
Zingiber officinale	Ginger
Zyzyphus jujube	Jujube

Herbs Listed by English Names

Abscess Root	*Polemonium reptans*
Acacia Gum	*Acacia senegal*
Acacia Bark	*Acacia arabica*
Acacia Bark	*Acacia decurrens*
Aconite	*Aconitum napellus*
Adder's Tongue, American	*Erythronium americanum*
Adder's Tongue, English	*Ophioglossum vulgatum*
Agar	*Gelidium amansii*
Agaric of oak	*Boletus ignarius*
Agaricus	*Fomes officinalis*
Agrimony	*Agrimonia eupatoria*
Alder	*Alnus glutinosa*
Alder Buckthorn	*Rhamnus frangula*
Alkanet root	*Anchusa tinctoria*
Alkanet	*Alkanna tinctoria*
Allspice	*Pimenta dioica*
Almond	*Prunus amygdalus*
Aloe	*Aloe spp.*
Alstonia Bark	*Alstonia scholaris*
Alum root	*Heuchera americana*
Amaranth	*Amaranthus hypochondriacus*
American Ginseng	*Panax quinquefolium*
American Ground Pine	*Lycopodium complanatum*
American Hellebore	*Veratrum viride*
American Ipecac	*Euphorbia ipecacuanha*
American Liverwort	*Hepatica nobilis*
American Mandrake	*Podophyllum peltatum*
American Pennyroyal	*Hedeoma pulegioides*
American Senna	*Cassia marilandica*
American Spikenard	*Aralia racemosa*
American White Pond Lily	*Nymphaea odorata*
Amla	*Emblica officinalis*
Ammoniacum	*Dorema ammoniacum*
Angelica	*Angelica archangelica*
Angelica tree	*Aralis spinosa*
Angostura	*Galipea officinalis*
Angustura	*Casparia febrifuga*
Aniseed	*Pimpinella anisum*
Annatto	*Bixa orellana*
Apricot Seed	*Prunus armeniaca*
Arbutus	*Epigaea repens*
Archangel	*Lamium album*
Arnica	*Arnica montana*
Arrowroot	*Maranta arundinacea*
Arum root	*Arum triphyllum*
Asafetida	*Ferula assa-foetida*
Ash	*Fraxinus excelsior*
Ashwaganda	*Withania somnifera*
Asparagus	*Asparagus officinalis*
Astragalus	*Astragalus membranaceus*
Atbala	*Abutilon indicum*
Avens	*Geum urbanum*

Azedarach	*Azadirachta indica*
Balm	*Melissa officinalis*
Balm of Gilead	*Populus candicans*
Balm of Gilead	*Populus gileadensis*
Balm of Gilead	*Populus nigra*
Balmony	*Chelone glabra*
Bamboo Manna	*Bambusa arundinacea*
Barberry	*Berberis vulgaris*
Barley	*Hordeum vulgare*
Basil	*Ocimum basilicum*
Bay	*Myrica acris*
Bayberry	*Myrica cerifera*
Bearberry	*Arctostaphylos uva-ursi*
Bearsfoot	*Polymnia uvedalia*
Bebeeru	*Nectandra rodiaei*
Beech	*Fagus sylvatica*
Belladonna	*Atropa belladonna*
Benzoin	*Styrax benzoin*
Betel	*Piper betle*
Beth Root	*Trillium erectum*
Bhringaraj	*Eclipta alba*
Bibhitaki	*Terminalia belerica*
Bilberry	*Vaccinium myrtillus*
Birch	*Betula spp.*
Birthwort	*Aristolochia spp.*
Bistort	*Polygonum bistorta*
Bitter polygala	*Polygala rubella*
Bitter Root	*Apocynum androsaemifolium*
Bittersweet	*Solanum dulcamara*
Bittersweet, American	*Celastrus scandens*
Black Bryony	*Tamus communis*
Black Catechu	*Acacia catechu*
Black Cohosh	*Cimicifuga racemosa*
Black Haw	*Viburnum prunifolium*
Black Hellebore	*Helleborus niger*
Black Horehound	*Ballota nigra*
Black Mustard	*Brassica nigra*
Black Oak	*Quercus tinctoria*
Black Root	*Leptandra virginicum*
Black Root	*Veronicastrum virginicum*
Blackberry	*Rubus villosus*
Blackcurrant	*Ribes nigrum*
Bladderwrack	*Fucus vesiculosus*
Blessed thistle	*Cnicus benedictus*
Bloodroot	*Sanguinaria canadensis*
Blue Cohosh	*Caulophylum thalictroides*
Blue Flag	*Iris caroliniana*
Blue Flag	*Iris versicolor*
Bogbean	*Menyanthes trifoliata*
Boldo	*Peumus boldus*
Boneset	*Eupatorium perfoliatum*
Borage	*Borago officinalis*
Box	*Buxus sempervirens*
Boxwood, American	*Cornus florida*

Brooklime	*Veronica beccabunga*
Broom	*Cytisus scoparius*
Broom	*Sarothamnus scoparius*
Buchu	*Agathosma betulina*
Buckwheat	*Fagopyrum esculentum*
Bugle	*Ajuga reptans*
Bugleweed	*Lycopus virginicus*
Bugloss	*Echium vulgare*
Burdock	*Arctium lappa*
Burgundy pitch	*Abies excelsa*
Burnet Saxifrage	*Pimpinella saxifraga*
Burr Marigold	*Bidens tripartita*
Butcher's Broom	*Ruscus aculeatus*
Butterburr	*Petasites hybridus*
Button snakeroot	*Eryngium aquaticum*
Cabbage Tree	*Andira araroba*
Cade oil	*Juniperus oxycedrus*
Cajaput	*Melaleuca leucadendron*
Calabar Bean	*Physostigma venenosum*
Calamint	*Calamintha ascendens*
Calendula	*Calendula officinalis*
Californian Poppy	*Eschscholzia californica*
Calumba	*Jateorhiza palmata*
Camphor	*Camphora officinalis*
Canadian Hemp	*Apocynum cannabinum*
Canella	*Canella winterana*
Caraway	*Carum carvi*
Cardamon	*Elattaria cardamomum*
Carnauba	*Copernicia cerifera*
Cascara	*Cascara sagrada*
Cascara Sagrada	*Rhamnus purshiana*
Cascarilla	*Croton eleuteria*
Cashew	*Anacardium occidentale*
Cassia	*Cinnamomum aromaticum*
Castor Oil Plants	*Ricinus communis*
Catmint	*Nepeta cataria*
Cattail	*Typha spp.*
Cayenne	*Capsicum minimum*
Cedron	*Simaba cedron*
Celery Seed	*Apium graveolens*
Centaury	*Centaurium erythraea*
Cevadilla	*Veratrum sabadilla*
Chamomile	*Anthemis nobilis*
Chamomile	*Matricaria recutita*
Chaparral	*Larrea divaricata*
Chasteberry	*Vitex agnus-castus*
Chaulmoogra	*Hydrocarpus spp.*
Cherry Laurel	*Prunus laurocerasus*
Cherry	*Prunus cerasus*
Chestnut	*Castanea sativa*
Chia Seeds	*Salvia polystachya*
Chickweed	*Stellaria media*
Chicory	*Cichorium intybus*
Chinese Foxnuts	*Euryale ferox*

Chinese Rhubarb	*Rheum officinale*
Chiretta	*Swertia chirata*
Chrysanthemum	*Chrysanthemum indicum*
Cinchona	*Cinchona spp.*
Cinnamon	*Cinnamomum verum*
Clary	*Salvia sclarea*
Cleavers	*Galium aparine*
Cloves	*Eugenia caryophillata*
Clubmoss	*Lycopodium clavatum*
Coca	*Erythroxylum coca*
Cocillana	*Guarea rusbyi*
Cocoa	*Theobroma cacao*
Coffee	*Caffea arabica*
Colchicum	*Colchicum autumnale*
Coleus	*Coleus forskohlii*
Colocynth	*Citrullus colocynthis*
Coltsfoot	*Tussilago farfara*
Columbo, American	*Frasera carolinensis*
Comfrey	*Symphytum officinale*
Common dogwood	*Cornus florida*
Condurango	*Marsdenia condurango*
Contrajerva	*Dorstenia contrajerva*
Copaiba	*Copaifera langsdorffi*
Coral Root	*Corallorhiza odontorhiza*
Coriander	*Coriandrum sativum*
Corn Silk	*Zea mays*
Corn smut	*Ustilago maydis*
Cornflower	*Centaurea cyanus*
Cotton Root	*Gossypium herbaceum*
Couch Grass	*Agropyron repens*
Cowhage	*Mucuna pruriens*
Cowslip	*Primula veris*
Cramp Bark	*Viburnum opulus*
Cranesbill	*Geranium maculatum*
Croton	*Croton tiglium*
Croton Seeds	*Croton tiglium*
Cubeb	*Piper cubeba*
Cuckoopint	*Arum maculatum*
Cudweed	*Gnaphalium uliginosum*
Cumin	*Cuminum cyminum*
Cupmoss	*Cladonia pyxidata*
Daisy	*Bellis perennis*
Damiana	*Turnera diffusa*
Dandelion	*Taraxacum officinale*
Date	*Phoenix dactylifera*
Devil's Claw	*Harpagophytum procumbens*
Dewberry	*Rubus trivialis*
Dill	*Anethum graveolens*
Dodder	*Cuscuta epithymum*
Dog Rose	*Rosa canina*
Dragon's Blood	*Daemonorops draco*
Dwarf chestnut	*Castanea pumila*
Dwarf Elder	*Sambucus ebulus*
Dwarf Pine	*Pinus Montana*

Dyer's Greenweed	*Genista tinctoria*
Echinacea	*Echinacea spp.*
Elder	*Sambucus nigra*
Elecampane	*Inula helenium*
Elm	*Ulmus campestris*
Embelia	*Embelia ribes*
English Horsemint	*Mentha longifolia*
English Liverwort	*Peltigera canina*
English Rhubarb	*Rheum rhaponticum*
Ergot	*Claviceps purpurea*
Eryngo	*Eryngium maritimum*
Eternal Flower	*Helichrysum stoechas*
Eucalyptus	*Eucalyptus spp.*
Euphorbia	*Euphorbia hirta*
Evening Primrose	*Oenothera biennis*
Eyebright	*Euphrasia spp.*
False Hellebore	*Adonis vernalis*
False sarsaparilla	*Aralia nudicaulis*
False Unicorn Root	*Chamaelirium luteum*
Fennel	*Foeniculum vulgare*
Fenugreek	*Trigonella foenum-graecum*
Feverbrush	*Garrya fremontii*
Feverfew	*Tanacetum chrysanthemum*
Feverroot	*Triosteum perfoliatum*
Fig	*Ficus carica*
Figwort	*Scrophularia nodosa*
Five-leaf-grass	*Potentilla reptans*
Flaxseed	*Linum usitatissimum*
Fleabane	*Erigeron canadense*
Fluellen	*Kickxia elatine*
Fo-ti	*Polygonum multiflorum*
Fetid Hellebore	*Helleborus foetidus*
Fool's Parsley	*Aethusa cynapium*
Foxglove	*Digitalis spp.*
Frankincense	*Boswellia thurifera*
Fringetree	*Chionanthus virginicus*
Frostwort	*Helianthemum canadense*
Fumitory	*Fumaria officinalis*
Galangal	*Alpinia officinarum*
Galbanum	*Ferula gummosa*
Galls	*Quercus infectoria*
Gamboge	*Garcinia hanburyi*
Garlic	*Allium sativum*
Gentian	*Gentiana spp.*
Germander	*Teucrium chamaedrys*
Ginger	*Zingiber officinale*
Ginkgo	*Ginkgo biloba*
Ginseng	*Panax ginseng*
Ginseng, American	*Panax quinquefolius*
Gladwin	*Iris foetidissima*
Goat's Rue	*Galega officinalis*
Goathead	*Tribulis terrestris*
Gold Thread	*Coptis trifolia*
Golden Rod	*Solidago virgaurea*

Golden Seal	*Hydrastis canadensis*
Goldenrod	*Solidago odora*
Gotu Kola	*Hydrocotyle asiatica*
Grains of Paradise	*Aframomum melegueta*
Grape	*Vitis vinifera*
Gravel Root	*Eupatorium purpureum*
Greater Burnet	*Sanguisorba officinalis*
Greater Celandine	*Chelidonium majus*
Grindelia	*Grindelia squarrosa*
Ground Elder	*Aegopodium podagraria*
Ground Ivy	*Glechoma hederacea*
Ground Pine	*Ajuga chamaepitys*
Guaiacum	*Guaiacum officinale*
Guarana	*Paullinia cupana*
Guggulu	*Commiphora mukul*
Gumweed	*Grindelia camporum*
Gutta-percha	*Isonandra gutta*
Hair cap moss	*Polystrichum juniperum*
Hardtack	*Spirea tomentosa*
Hartstongue	*Scolopendrium vulgare*
Hawthorn	*Crataegus monogyna*
Hawthorn	*Crataegus oxyacantha*
Heartsease	*Viola tricola*
Hedge Mustard	*Sisymbrium officinale*
Hedge Hyssop	*Gratiola officinalis*
Hemlock	*Conium maculatum*
Hemlock pitch	*Abies canadensis*
Hemp Agrimony	*Eupatorium cannabinum*
Henbane	*Hyoscyamus niger*
Henna	*Lawsonia inermis*
Holly	*Ilex aquifolium*
Honeysuckle	*Lonicera caprifolium*
Hops	*Humulus lupulus*
Horehound	*Marrubium vulgare*
Horse chestnut	*Aesculus hippocastanum*
Horsemint	*Monarda punctata*
Horsenettle	*Solanum carolinense*
Horseradish	*Armoracia rusticana*
Horsetail	*Equisetum arvense*
Houndstongue	*Cynoglossum officinale*
Houseleek	*Sempervivum tectorum*
Hydrangea	*Hydrangea arborescens*
Hyssop	*Hyssopus officinalis*
Iceland moss	*Cetraria islandica*
Ignatia	*Styrchnos ignatia*
Ignatius Beans	*Strychnos ignatii*
India Country Mallow	*Sida cordifolia*
Indian Hemp	*Cannabis sativa*
Indian Long Pepper	*Piper longum*
Indian Madder	*Rubia cordifolia*
Indian Physic	*Gillenia stipulata*
Ipecacuanha	*Cephaëlis ipecacuanha*
Irish Moss	*Chrondrus crispus*
Ivy	*Hedera helix*

Jaborandi	*Pilocarpus species*
Jacob's Ladder	*Polemonium caeruleum*
Jalap	*Exogonium purga*
Jalap	*Ipomoea purga*
Jamaican Dogwood	*Piscidia erythrina*
Jambul	*Syzgium cumini*
Jasmine	*Jasminum grandiflorum*
Jequirity	*Abrus precatorius*
Jewel Weed	*Impatiens biflora*
Jujube	*Zyzyphus jujube*
Juniper	*Juniperus communis*
Kamala	*Mallotus philippinensis*
Kava Kava	*Piper methysticum*
Kino	*Pterocarpus marsupium*
Knapweed	*Centaurea nigra*
Kola Nut	*Cola vera*
Kooso	*Brayers anthelmentica*
Kousso	*Hagenia abyssinica*
Kudzu	*Pueraria tuberosa*
Kumarhou	*Pomaderris elliptic*
Kutki	*Picrorhiza Kurroa*
Labrador Tea	*Ledum groenlandicum*
Lachnanthes	*Lachnanthes tinctoria*
Lady's Mantle	*Alchemilla arvensis*
Lady's Bedstraw	*Galium verum*
Lady's Slipper	*Cypripedium calceolus*
Larch	*Larix decidua*
Large flowering spurge	*Euphorbia corollata*
Larkspur	*Delphinium consolida*
Laurel	*Laurus nobilis*
Lavender Cotton	*Santolina chamaecyparissus*
Lavender	*Lavandula officinalis*
Lemon	*Citrus limon*
Lemon Grass	*Cymbopogon citratus*
Lemon Verbena	*Aloysia triphylla*
Lesser Celendine	*Ranunculus ficaria*
Life Everlasting	*Antennaria dioica*
Life Root	*Senecio aureus*
Lily of the Valley	*Convallaria majalis*
Lime	*Citrus aurantifolia*
Linden	*Tilia cordata, Tilia spp.*
Lippia	*Lippia dulas*
Liquorice	*Glycyrrhiza glabra*
Lobelia	*Lobelia inflata*
Logwood	*Haematoxylon campechianum*
Lomatium	*Lomatium dissectum*
Loosestrife	*Lysimachia vulgaris*
Lucern	*Medicago sativa*
Lungmoss	*Lobaria pulmonaria*
Lungwort	*Pulmonaria officinalis*
Ma Huang	*Ephedra sinica*
Magnolia	*Magnolia glauca*
Mahabala	*Sida rhombifolia*
Maidenhair Fern	*Adiantum capillus-veneris*

Malabar Nut	*Adhatoda vasica*
Male Fern	*Dryopteris felix-mas*
Mallow	*Malva sylvestris*
Manaca	*Brunfelsia hopeana*
Manna	*Fraxinus ornus*
Marjoram	*Origanum majorana*
Marsh rosemary	*Statice caroliniana*
Marshmallow	*Althaea officinalis*
Masterwort	*Heracleum lanatum*
Masterwort	*Peucedanum ostruthium*
Mastic	*Pistacia lentiscus*
Matico	*Piper angustifolia*
Mayweed	*Anthemis cotula*
Meadow Lily	*Lilium candidum*
Meadowsweet	*Filipendula ulmaria*
Mescal Buttons	*Lophophora williamsii*
Mexican Scammony Root	*Ipomoea orizabensis*
Mezereon	*Daphne mezereum*
Milk Thistle	*Silybum marianum*
Milkweed	*Asclepias syriaca*
Mistletoe	*Viscum album*
Monsonia	*Monsonia ovata*
Motherwort	*Leonurus cardiaca*
Mountain Ash	*Pyrus aucuparia*
Mountain Flax	*Linum catharticum*
Mountain Grape	*Berberis aquifolia*
Mountain Laurel	*Kalmia latifolia*
Mouse Ear	*Hieracium pilosella*
Mugwort	*Artemisia vulgaris*
Muira-Puama	*Liriosma ovata*
Mulberry	*Morus nigra*
Mullein	*Verbascum thapsus*
Muskseed	*Abelmoschus moschatus*
Mustard	*Brassica spp.*
Myrrh	*Commiphora mol-mol*
Myrobalan	*Terminalia chebula*
Myrtle	*Myrtus communis*
Nasturtium	*Tropaeolum majus*
Neem	*Azadiracta indica*
Nettles	*Urtica dioica*
Night-blooming Cereus	*Selenicereus grandiflorus*
Nikkar Nuts	*Caesalpinia bonducella*
Nutgrass	*Cyperus esculentus*
Nutmeg	*Myristica fragrans*
Nux Vomica	*Strychnos nux vomica*
Oak	*Quercus robur*
Oats	*Avena sativa*
Olive	*Olea europaea*
Onion	*Allium cepa*
Opium Poppy	*Papaver somniferum*
Orange	*Citrus aurantium*
Oregano	*Origanum vulgare*
Oregon Grape	*Mahonia repens*

Orris	*Iris germanica, Iris pallida, Iris florentina*
Osha	*Ligusticum porteri*
Osier, Red, American	*Cornus sericea*
Ox-Eye Daisy	*Chrysanthemum leucanthemum*
Pale catechu	*Ourouparia gambir*
Pansy violet	*Viola pedata*
Papaya	*Carica papaya*
Paraguay Tea	*Ilex paraguariensis*
Pareira-brava	*Chondodendron tomentosum*
Parsley	*Petroselinum crispum*
Partridge Berry	*Mitchella repens*
Pasque Flower	*Anemone pulsatilla*
Passion Flower	*Passiflora incarnata*
Patchouli	*Pogostemon cablin*
Pau D'arco	*Tabebuia avellanedae*
Peach	*Prunus persica*
Peanut	*Arachis hypogaea*
Pellitory of the Wall	*Parietaria officinalis*
Pennyroyal	*Mentha pulegioides*
Peony	*Paeonia officinalis*
Pepper	*Piper nigrum*
Peppermint	*Mentha piperita*
Periwinkle	*Vinca major*
Persimmon	*Diospyros virginiana*
Peruvian Balsam	*Myroxylon pereirae*
Pichi	*Fabiana imbricata*
Pill Bearing Spurge	*Euphorbia pilulifera*
Pink Root	*Spigelia marilandica*
Pitcher Plant	*Sarracenta purpurea*
Plantain	*Plantago media*
Pleurisy root	*Asclepias tuberosa*
Poison oak	*Rhus toxicodendron*
Poke	*Phytolacca decandra*
Polypody root	*Polypodium vulgare*
Pomegranate	*Punica granatum*
Poplar	*Populus alba*
Prickly Ash	*Zanthoxylum americanum*
Pride of India	*Melia azedarach*
Primrose	*Primula vulgaris*
Prune	*Prunus domestica*
Psyllium	*Plantago psyllium*
Puff Ball	*Calvatia species*
Pumpkin	*Cucurbita maxim*
Pumpkin	*Cucurbita pepo*
Punarnava	*Boerhaavia diffusa*
Purging Buckthorn	*Rhamnus catharticus*
Purging Cassia	*Cassia fistula*
Purple Loosestrife	*Lythrum salicaria*
Pyrethrum	*Chrysanthemum cinerariaefolium*
Quassia	*Quassia amara*
Quebracho	*Aspidosperma quebracho*
Queen's Delight	*Stillingia sylvatica*
Quince	*Cydonia oblonga*

Ragwort	*Senecio jacobaea*
Raspberry	*Rubus spp.*
Rauwolfia	*Rauwolfia serpentaria*
Red Cedar	*Juniperus virginiana*
Red Clover	*Trifolium pratense*
Red Maple	*Acer rubrum*
Red Poppy	*Papaver rhoeas*
Red Root	*Ceanothus americanus*
Red Sage	*Salvia officinalis*
Red Sandalwood	*Pterocarpus santalinus*
Rehmannia	*Rehmannia glutinosa*
Rest Harrow	*Onosis spinosa*
Rhatany	*Krameria triandra*
Rhubarb Root	*Rheum palmatum*
Rice	*Oryza sativa*
Rooibosch	*Cyclopia genistoides*
Rosemary	*Rosmarinus officinalis*
Rosinweed	*Silphium laciniatum*
Round-leaved dogwood	*Cornus circinata*
Rubber	*Hevea ssp.*
Rue	*Ruta graveolens*
Rupturewort	*Herniaria glabra*
Rye ergot	*Secale cornutum*
Sabadilla	*Schoenocaulon officinalis*
Safflower	*Carthamus tinctorius*
Saffron	*Crocus sativus*
Samphire	*Crithmum maritimum*
Sandalwood	*Santalum album*
Sanicle	*Sanicula europaea*
Sarsaparilla	*Smilax spp.*
Sassafras	*Sassafras albidum*
Savin	*Juniperus sabina*
Saw Palmetto	*Serenoa serrulata*
Scammony	*Convolvulus scammonia*
Scarlet Pimpernel	*Anagallis arvensis*
Scopolia	*Scopula carniolica*
Scurvy grass	*Cochlearia officinalis*
Self-heal	*Prunella vulgaris*
Senna	*Cassia angustifolia*
Senna	*Cassia senna*
Sesame	*Sesamum orientale*
Shatavari	*Asparagus racemosus*
Sheep's Sorrel	*Rumex acetosella*
Shepherd's Purse	*Capsella bursa-pastoris*
Silverweed	*Potentilla anserina*
Simaruba	*Simaruba amara*
Skullcap	*Scutellaria laterifolia*
Skunk Cabbage	*Symplocarpus foetidus*
Slippery Elm	*Ulmus rubra*
Smartweed	*Polygonum hydropiper*
Smooth Sumach	*Rhus glabra*
Snakeroot	*Aristolochia reticulata*
Snakeroot	*Polygala senega*
Sneezewort	*Achillea ptarmica*

Soap Bark	*Quillaja saponaria*
Soapwort	*Saponaria officinalis*
Solomon's Seal	*Polygonatum multiflorum*
Sorrel	*Rumex acetosa*
Southernwood	*Artemisia abrotanum*
Soybean	*Glycine Max*
Spanish Moss	*Usnea spp.*
Spearmint	*Mentha spicata*
Speedwell	*Veronica officinalis*
Spotted pyrola	*Pyrola maculatum*
Squill	*Urginia maritima*
St. John's Wort	*Hypericum perforatum*
Star Anise	*Ilicium verum*
Stavesacre	*Delphinium staphisagria*
Stone Root	*Collinsonia canadensis*
Storax	*Liquidambar orientalis*
Strawberry	*Fragaria vesca*
Strophanthus	*Strophanthus gratus,*
	Strophanthus kombe
Sugar	*Saccharum officinarum*
Sumbul	*Ferula sumbul*
Summer Savory	*Satureja hortensis*
Sundew	*Drosera rotundifolia*
Sunflower	*Helianthus annuus*
Swamp Milkweed	*Asclepias incarnata*
Sweet Birch	*Betula lenta*
Sweet Cicely	*Myrrhis odorata*
Sweet Flag	*Acorus calamus*
Sweet Gale	*Myrica gale*
Sweet Sumach	*Rhus aromatica*
Sweet Vernal Grass	Anthoxanthum odoratum
Sweet Violet	*Viola odorata,*
	T. pendulum
Tamarack	*Larix laricina*
Tamarind	*Tamarindus indica*
Tansy	*Tanacetum vulgare*
Tapioca	*Cassava ssp.*
Tarragon	*Artemisia dracunculus*
Tea	*Camellia sinensis*
Thorn apple	*Datura stramonium*
Thyme	*Thymus spp.*
Ti Tree	*Melaleuca alternifolia*
	Tilia platyphylla
Tobacco	*Nicotiana tabacum*
Tolu Balsam	*Myroxylon balsamum*
Tonka Beans	*Dipteryx odorata*
Tragacanth	*Astragalus gummifer*
Tree of Heaven	*Ailanthus altissima*
True Unicorn Root	*Aletris farinosa*
Tulip tree	*Liriodendron tulipifera*
Turkey Corn	*Dicentra canadensis*
Turmeric	*Curcuma longa*
Turpeth	*Ipomoea turpethum*
Valerian	*Valeriana officinalis*

Vanilla	*Vanilla aromatica*
Vervain	*Verbena officinalis*
Vetiverian	*Andrapogon muricatus*
Vidari Kanda	*Ipomemea digitata*
Virginia snakeroot	*Aristolochia serpentaria*
Wafer ash	*Ptelea trifoliata*
Wahoo	*Euonymus atropurpurea*
Walnut	*Juglans cinerea*
Walnut	*Juglans regia*
Water avens	*Gerum rivale*
Water Betony	*Scrophularia aquatica*
Water Dock	*Rumex aquatica*
Water Dropwort	*Oenanthe crocata*
Water Fennel	*Oenanthe aquatica*
Water Germander	*Teucrium scordium*
Watercress	*Rorippa nasturtium*
Western Hemlock	*Thuja occidentalis*
Wheat	*Triticum vulgare*
White Bryony	*Bryonia alba*
White hellebore	*Veratrum album*
White Mustard	*Brassica alba*
White Poplar	*Populus tremuloides*
Wild Carrot	*Daucus carrota*
Wild Cherry	*Prunus serotina*
Wild Cucumber	*Ecballium elaterium*
Wild Ginger	*Asarum canadense*
Wild Indigo	*Baptisia tinctoria*
Wild Lettuce	*Lactuca virosa*
Wild Mint	*Mentha aquatica*
Wild Yam	*Dioscorea villosa*
Willow	*Salix alba, S.cinerea, S.fragilis*
Winter Cherry	*Physalis alkekengi*
Winter Savory	*Satureja montana*
Winter's Bark	*Drimys winteri*
Wintergreen	*Gaultheria procumbens*
Witch Hazel	*Hamamelis virginiana*
Wood Betony	*Stachys officinalis*
Wood Sage	*Teucrium scorodonia*
Wood Sorrel	*Oxalis acetosella*
Woodruff	*Galium odoratum*
Wormseed	*Chenopodium ambrosioides*
Wormwood	*Artemisia absinthium*
Woundwort	*Stachys palustris*
Yarrow	*Achillea millefolium*
Yellow Dock	*Rumex crispus*
Yellow Flag	*Iris pseudacorus*
Yellow root	*Xanthorrhiza apiifolia*
Yellow Toadflax	*Linaria vulgaris*
Yerba Santa	*Eriodictyon californicum*
Yew	*Taxus baccata*
Yohimbé	*Pausinystalia yohimbe*
Zedoary	*Curcuma zedoaria*

Prefixes & Suffixes

a-	not, without	*cyt*	cell
ab-	away from	*cyto-*	cell
adeno-	gland	*dacryo-*	tears
-agra	seizure or pain	*dendr*	tree
algo-	pain	*dent*	tooth
andro-	male	*denti-*	tooth
angio-	box, vessel	*derm*	skin
anth-	flower	*dermato-*	skin
-antheros	flowery	*dextro-*	right side
anti-	against	*di*	two, separate
api-	tip, apex	*dichotomos*	cut into two
arterio-	artery	*dictyo*	net
arthro-	joint	*dys-*	ill, impaired
-ate	provided with, formed	*-ectomy*	surgical removal
	into	*el*	diminutive end-
auto-	self		ing
bacill-	rodlike	*-emia*	blood condition
bacteri-	bacteria	*encephalo-*	brain
basidio-	small base	*endo*	enclosure, in-
bi-	two, double		side
blepharo-	eyelid	*entero-*	intestine
brady-	slow	*epi*	upon
broncho-	windpipe, throat	*equinus*	horse
cap	head	*erythr*	red
capill-	hair	*erythro-*	red
carcino-	cancer	*eu*	true, good
cardio-	heart	*ex*	from, beyond
carp	fruit	*exo*	outside
caul	stem	*febri-*	fever
-cele	tumor	*fer*	bearer
cephal	head	*fibro-*	fibrous
cephalo-	head	*fil*	thread-like
cerebro-	brain	*fissio*	splitting
chilo-	lip	*flagellum*	whip
chiro-	hand	*flav*	yellow
chloro	green	*flor*	flower
cholo-	bile	*fol*	leaf
chondrio-	cartilage	*fungus*	mushroom
chrom	color	*funiculus*	a small cord
cid	cut, kill	*gamet*	spouse, sex cell
circ	circle	*gamo*	union, marriage
cleisto	closed	*gastro-*	stomach
-coccus	spherical bacterium	*gen*	origin, birth
coll	glue	*-genic*	producing or
colo-	lower intestine		causing, pro-
coma	hair		duced or
coro-	pupil of eye		caused by
cortico-	cortex	*genus*	race
costo-	rib	*geo*	earth
cyan	dark blue	*geronto-*	old age
cyst	bladder, bag	*glab*	bald
cysto-	bladder, cyst	*gland*	secretory spot

glosso-	tongue	ligne	wood
glut	glue	lipo-	fat
gymn	naked	lith	stone
gyn	female	litho-	stone, calcification
gyneco-	woman	loc	a small place, cell
habitus	condition, physique	logos	discourse, study
hal	salt	-lysis	breaking down,
hema-	blood		decomposing
hemi	half	macro	large, long
hemo-	blood	masto-	breast
hepato-	liver	mega	large
hetero	other, different	meiosis	reduction
hex	six	melano-	black, dark
histo-	tissue	meri	part, segment,
holo	entire		component
homo	same, alike	meso	middle
hydro	water	micro	small, tiny
hydro-	water	mitos	thread
hyper-	extreme, excessive	mono	one, single
hyph	web	morph	form, structure
hypno-	sleep	musculo-	muscle
hypo	below	myco	fungus, mushroom
hypo-	insufficient	myco-	fungus, mold
hystero-	uterus, womb	myelo-	marrow, spinal cord
-ia	name of disease	myo-	muscle
	or condition	myx	slime
-iasis	disease	narco-	stupor, drugged state
-iatrics	medical treatment	nat	born, borne
-iatrist	physician or healer	nephro-	kidney
iatro-	medicine	neuro-	nerve
-iatry	specific area of healing	nom	name
	or medical practice	ode	like
idion	diminutive ending	odonto-	tooth
il	diminutive ending	-odynia	pain
ilio-	flank, upper hipbone	oec	household
immuno-	immune	-oid	resembling or refer-
infra	below		ring to form
inter	between	ol	little
intra	within	-oma	tumor
iso	equal, homogenous	oon	egg
-itis	inflammation or	ophthalmo-	eye
	abnormal condition	-opia	eye, sight
karyon	nut, nucleus	-opsy	medical examination
kerato-	hornlike	orchido-	testes
lab	lip	orth	straight
labio-	lip	ortho-	erect, straight, normal
lamel	plate, layer	-osis	diseased or abnormal
lamin	blade		condition or state
lance	lance, blade	ossi-	bone
laparo-	flank, abdominal wall	osteo	bone
laryngo-	windpipe, larynx	ostiol	little door
leuco	white	oto-	ear
leuko-	white	ov	egg
lig	strap, ribbon	ovi-	egg

paleo	ancient	*pyle*	gate
palm	hand	*rad*	root
palustr	swamp	*reni-*	kidney
-pathy	suffering, disease, or treatment	*reticulum*	a small net
		rhap	needle
para	beside	*rhiz*	root
patho-	disease, sickness, suffering	*rhodon*	rose color
		-rrhagia	rupture, profuse flow or discharge
pect	comb		
ped, pod	foot, stalk	*-rrhaphy*	suture
pedii	foot	*-rrhea*	flow, discharge
pedo-	child	*-rrhexis*	rupture
pelt	shield	*ros*	rose
per	through, by means of	*sagitt*	arrow
peri	around	*sangui-*	blood
pharmaco-	drug or medication	*sapro*	rotten
pharyngo-	pharynx	*sarco-*	flesh
phellos	cork	*schiz*	deeply divided
phil	love	*schizo-*	split
phlebo-	vein	*scis*	cut
phloos	bark	*-scope*	instrument for viewing
phore	bearer		
phyco	seaweed	*-sect*	cut opening
phyle	tribe	*semi*	half
phyll	leaf	*septum*	partition, wall
phyte	plant	*sero-*	serum, blood
pinn	feather	*sessilis*	fit for sitting
-phasia	speech disorder	*soma*	body
-phrenia	lack, deficiency, disorder	*somato-*	body
		somni-	sleep
-plasia	growth	*soros*	heap
-plast	cell, living substance	*species*	kind
-plasty	surgical repair or molding formation	*sperm*	seed
		sphen	wedge
pleuro-	rib, side of body	*sporo*	seed, spore
ploid	fold	*stell*	star
plume	feather	*stoma*	mouth
pneum	lung, air, gas	*stomy*	surgical operation in-volving creation of artificial opening
pneumo-	lung, air		
podo-	foot		
polio-	gray matter	*strobilos*	twisted object, top
poly	many, much	*stroma*	cushion, mattress
por	small opening	*stylo*	pillar
prim	first	*sub*	under, less than
pro	before	*super, supra*	above, over
procto-	anus, rectum	*syn*	together, with
protiston	the very first	*tachy*	rapid
proto	first, original	*taxis*	arrangement, order
pseud	false	*terra*	earth
psilos	bare, mere	*tetra*	four
psycho-	mind	*thall*	shoot
pterid	fern	*thanato*	death
pulmo-	lung	*thrombo*	blood clot, coagulation
pyelo-	pelvis		

tome	cutting instrument
tonia	muscle or nerve tension
tomo	cut, section
tomy	surgical incision or excision
toxico	poison
tracheo	windpipe, trachea
tri	three
tricho	hair
trop	bend
tropho	nourishment
trophic	having nutritional requirements
tuber	knob, swelling
ul	little
uni	one
urino	urine
uro	urine
utero	womb, uterus
vaso	vessel
veno	vein
ventro	abdomen
vermi	worm
vor	eat
xanthos	yellow
xer	dry
xylon	wood
zygo	yoke, pair
zymo	fermentation

Glossary

Abortifacient: induces abortion or miscarriage.

Abscess: a localized collection of pus and liquefied tissue in a cavity.

Absolute: a highly concentrated viscous, semi-solid or solid perfume material, usually obtained by alcohol extraction from the concrete.

Acetylcholine: a neurotransmitter.

Achlorhydria: absence of hydrochloric acid in the stomach.

Acid: a compound producing hydrogen ions in aqueous solution. Acidic refers to a pH number below 7.0.

Acidosis: abnormal state of reduced alkalinity of blood and tissues.

Acrid: leaving a burning sensation in the mouth.

ACTH: adrenocorticotropic hormone.

Acupressure: manual application of pressure at points where acupuncture needles would be inserted.

Acupuncture: Chinese practice that involves insertion of needles into body at specific points along meridians to treat disease and reduce pain.

Acute: designating disease with rapid onset, severe symptoms, and brief duration, opposite of chronic.

Acute abdomen: emergency condition caused by damage to one or more abdominal organs that results in intense pain and shock.

Adaptogen: herbs that increase resistance and resilience to stress, enabling the body to avoid reaching collapse because it can adapt around the problem.

Addison's disease: condition marked by weakness, low blood pressure, and dark pigmentation due to inadequate hormone secretion by adrenal glands.

Adenitis: regional inflammation of gland or lymph node.

Adenocarcinoma: malignant epithelial tumor in glandular pattern.

ADH: antidiuretic hormone.

Adhesion: union by fibrous connective tissue of two normally separate parts.

Adipose: fat in connective tissue.

Adrenaline: hormone secreted by the adrenal gland which produces the "fight or flight" response. Also called epinephrine.

Adrenergic: compound that acts like epinephrine or norepinephrine.

Adrenocorticotropic hormone: ACTH; polypeptide secreted by anterior pituitary that stimulates adrenal cortex to secrete cortisol.

Aerophagy: swallowing of air.

Agar: polysaccharide derived from seaweed, used as culture medium for microorganisms; gelatinous natural laxative.

Agglutinin: substance, esp. antibody, that causes bacteria, blood cells, and antigens to clump together.

Agranulocytosis: acute illness caused by chemicals or drug reaction in which certain white blood cells disappear, causing rapid, massive infection.

Ague: malaria; general malaise marked by fever.

AIDS: acquired immune deficiency syndrome; severe weakening or destruction of body's immune system by human immunodeficiency virus.

AIDS related complex arc: chronic enlargement of lymph nodes and persistent fever caused by AIDS virus.

Albumin: most abundant protein found in blood plasma.

Albuminuria: presence of protein albumin in urine.

Aldosterone: a hormone secreted by the adrenal gland which causes the retention of sodium and water.

Algae: unicellular organisms distinguished from plants by having no true root stem.

Alkaline: solutions having a pH above 7.0.

Alkaloid: a large and varied group of nitrogen-containing compounds found in plants. Often alkaline, they react with acids to form soluble salts, many of which are physiologically active.

Alkalosis: abnormal state of increased alkalinity of blood and tissues.

Allergen: any substance which comes into contact with body tissue (by skin absorption, ingestion, or inhalation) and causes a specific reaction within the bloodstream.

Allergy: hypersensitivity to particular substance or antigen, such as pollens, furs, feathers, mold, dust, drugs, dyes, cosmetics, or foods, causing characteristic symptoms when encountered, ingested, or inhaled.

Alliaceous: garlic- or onion-like.

Allopathy: a term that describes the conventional method of medicine which combats disease by using substances and techniques specifically against the disease.

Alopecia: absence of hair from area where it normally grows, esp. progressive hair loss in men; baldness.

Alterative: herbs that gradually restore proper functioning of the body, increasing health and vitality. Some alteratives support natural waste elimination via the kidneys, liver, lungs, or skin. Others stimulate digestive function or are anti-microbial.

Alzheimer's disease: progressive dementia and brain degeneration.

Amebiasis: infection with or disease caused by amebas.

Amebic dysentery: severe dysentery caused by protozoan amebas.

Amenorrhea: absence or cessation of menstruation due to congenital defect, hormonal deficiency, hypothalamus disorder, or emotional problem.

Amino acid: any of twenty-five organic acids containing an amino group that link together into polypeptide chains to form proteins.

Amoebicidal: a substance with the power of destroying amoebae.

Amphoteric: having the ability to act either as an acid or a base.

Amylase: enzyme that breaks down starch into disaccharides.

Anabolism: constructive metabolism in which food is changed into living tissue.

Analgesic: a substance which reduces the sensation of pain.

Anaphrodisiac: reduces sexual desire.

Anaphylaxis: acute, allergic reaction to substance to which person has been previously sensitized, resulting in faintness, palpitations, loss of color, difficulty in breathing, and shock.

Androgen: male sex hormone.

Anemia: reduced hemoglobin in blood, causing fatigue, breathlessness, and pallor.

Anesthetic: agent that diminishes or abolishes sensation and can produce unconsciousness.

Aneurysm: balloon-like swelling of arterial wall.

Angina: feeling of suffocation; chest pain.

Angina pectoris: pain in center of chest that spreads to jaws and arms, due to insufficient blood supply to heart.

Angiosperm: flowering plant.

Annual: plant with life cycle of one year or season.

Anodyne: substance that soothes or relieves pain.

Anodynia: absence of pain.

Anorexia: the medical term for loss of appetite.

Anorexia nervosa: extreme loss of appetite, esp. in adolescent females, causing severe weight loss and starvation.

Anoxia: condition in which body tissues receive inadequate oxygen.

Antacid: substance that neutralizes acid.

Anthelmintic: a vermifuge, destroying or expelling intestinal worms.

Anther: part of stamen that produces and releases pollen.

Anthocyanidin: a particular class of flavonoids which gives plants, fruits and flowers colors ranging from red to blue.

Anthraquinones: glycoside compounds that produce dyes and purgatives.

Antianaemic: an agent which combats anemia.

Antiarthritic: an agent which combats arthritis.

Antibiotic: drugs that kill microorganisms.

Antibody: protein manufactured by lymphocytes that reacts with specific antigen to fight invasion as principal component of immunity.

Anticatarrhal: anticatarrhals help the body remove excess catarrh, whether in the sinus area or other parts of the body.

Anticoagulant: agent that prevents blood from clotting.

Anticonvulsant: helps arrest or prevent convulsions.

Antidepressant: helps alleviate depression.

Antidiarrhoeal: efficacious against diarrhoea.

Antidiuretic hormone: ADH; peptide hormone synthesized in hypothalamus and released from posterior pituitary, causing retention of more water in body.

Antidote: a substance which counteracts the effects of a poison.

Antiemetic: an agent which reduces the incidence and severity of nausea or vomiting.

Antifungal: a substance that inhibits the growth or multiplication of fungi.

Antigen: any substance or microorganism that, when introduced into the body, causes the formation of antibodies against it.

Antihaemorrhagic: an agent which prevents or combats hemorrhage or bleeding.

Antihepatotoxic: protects liver cells from chemical damage.

Antihistamine: chemical that blocks action of histamine.

Antihypertensive: blood pressure-lowering effect.

Antiinflammatory: soothes inflammations or reduces the inflammation of the tissue directly.

Antilithic: prevents the formation of a calculus or stone.

Antimicrobial: antimicrobials help the body destroy or resist pathogenic microorganisms. They help the body strengthen its own resistance to infective organisms and throw off the illness.

Antineuralgic: relieves or reduces nerve pain.

Antioxidant: a compound which prevents free radical or oxidative damage.

Antiphlogistic: checks or counteracts inflammation.

Antipruritic: relieves sensation of itching or prevents its occurrence.

Antiputrescent: an agent which prevents and combats decay or putrefaction.

Antipyretic: reduces fever; *see also* febrifuge.

Antirheumatic: helps prevent and relieve rheumatism.

Antisclerotic: helps prevent the hardening of tissue.

Antiscorbutic: a remedy for scurvy.

Antiseborrhoeic: helps control the production of sebum, the oily secretion from sweat glands.

Antiseptic: destroys and prevents the development of microbes.

Antispasmodic: drug that relieves smooth muscle spasms.

Antitoxic: an antidote or treatment that counteracts the effects of poison.

Antitumor: a substance which prevents or is effective against tumors.

Antitussive: substance that reduces coughing, esp. one that affects activity in the brain's cough center and depresses respiration.

Antiviral: substance which inhibits the growth of a virus.

Anxiety: an unpleasant emotional state ranging from mild unease to intense fear.

Aperient: a mild laxative.

Aperitif: a stimulant of the appetite.

Aphonia: loss of voice.

Aphrodisiac: increases or stimulates sexual desire.

Apnea: temporary cessation of breathing.

Apoplexy: sudden loss of consciousness, a stroke or sudden severe hemorrhage.

Appendicitis: acute inflammation of vermiform appendix.

Application: medication, remedy, or antiseptic placed externally on body part, as in compress.

Arbovirus: RNA-containing virus that can cause disease when transmitted from animals to humans by insects.

ARC: AIDS-related complex.

Aril: the husk or membrane covering the seed of a plant.

Aromatherapy: the therapeutic use of essential oils.

Aromatic: a substance with a strong aroma or smell.

Arrhythmia: irregularity or deviation from normal rhythm or force of heartbeat.

Arteriosclerosis: deposit of cholesterol on artery walls, hardening of the arteries.

Artery: a blood vessel which carries oxygen-rich blood away from the heart.

Arthritis: inflammation of joints.

Asbestosis: lung disease caused by inhalation of asbestos fibers, sometimes leading to lung cancer.

Asepsis: complete absence of disease-causing bacteria, viruses, fungi, or microorganisms.

Asthenia: *see* debility.

Asthma: paroxysmal attacks of bronchial spasms that cause difficulty in breathing, often hereditary, bronchial asthma.

Astigmatism: distortion of visual images due to failure of retina to focus light.

Astringent: astringents have a binding action on mucous membranes, skin and other tissue, due to tannins precipitating protein molecules thus reducing irritation and inflammation, creating a barrier against infection that is helpful in wounds and burns.

Asymptomatic: showing no evidence of a disease.

Ataxia: shaky movements and unsteady gait when brain fails to regulate posture or direction of limb movements.

Atheroma: degeneration of artery walls due to fatty plaques and scar tissue; common form of arteriosclerosis, atherosclerosis

Atherosclerosis: a process in which fatty substances (cholesterol and triglycerides) are deposited in the walls of medium to large arteries, eventually leading to blockage of the artery.

Athlete's foot: contagious fungal infection of skin between toes.

Atony: lessening or lack of muscular tone or tension.

Atopy: a predisposition to various allergic conditions including eczema and asthma.

Atresia: congenital absence or abnormal narrowing of body opening.

Atrophy: wasting away of normally developed organ or tissue due to degeneration of cells.

Atropine: belladonna extract that inhibits activity of autonomic nervous system and relaxes smooth muscle.

Attrition: normal wearing away of surface of teeth.

Autoimmune: designating disorder of body's defense mechanism in which antibodies are produced against the body's own tissues, treating them as foreign substances.

Autoimmune disease: disorder that permits destruction of tissue by body's own antibodies.

Autologous: derived from same individual or organism.

Autonomic: occurring involuntarily, controlled by autonomic nervous system.

Axil: upper angle between a stem and leaf or bract.

Ayurveda: highly developed system of therapeutics developed in the Hindu and Buddhist cultures of the Indian subcontinent.

Bacteremia: presence of bacteria in blood, indicating infection.

Bactericidal: an agent that destroys bacteria (a type of microbe or organism).

Bacteriostat: substance that retards growth of bacteria.

Balm: fragrant ointment or aromatic oil with medicinal value.

Balsam: a resinous semi-solid mass or viscous liquid exuded from a plant. A "true" balsam is characterized by its high content of benzoic acid, benzoates, cinnamic acid or cinnamates.

Baroreceptor: neural receptor sensitive to pressure and rate of change in pressure; stretch receptor.

Basal metabolic rate: the rate of metabolism when the body is at rest.

Basal cell carcinoma: common, usu. curable, slow-growing malignant tumor on skin.

Basal rosette: leaves radiating directly from the crown of the root.

Basophil: a type of white blood cell which is involved in allergic reactions..

Bechic: anything which relieves or cures coughs; or referring to cough.

Bedwetting: enuresis.

Bell's palsy: paralysis of muscles on one side of face and inability to close eye, sometimes with loss of taste and excess sensitivity to noise.

Benign: consisting of localized mass of nonmalignant specialized cells within connective tissue that do not invade and destroy tissue or spread throughout body.

Berry: small, fleshy fruit or dry seed or kernel of various plants.

Beta blocker: drug that decreases heart activity by affecting receptors of sympathetic nervous system.

Beta cells: the cells in the pancreas which manufacture insulin.

Beta-carotene: pro-vitamin A. A plant carotene which can be converted to two vitamin A molecules.

Biennial: plant with two-year life cycle in which the vegetative first-year growth is followed by fruiting and dying during second year.

Bile: greenish liver secretion that is stored in gallbladder until released to emulsify fats in small intestine.

Bile salts: steroid molecules in bile that promote solubilization and digestion of fats.

Bilirubin: the breakdown product of the haemoglobin molecule of red blood cells.

Bilirubinemia: excess bile pigment in blood that causes jaundice.

Binomial: standard scientific name for organism in Latin.

Biopsy: a diagnostic test in which tissue or cells are removed from the body for examination under a microscope.

Bitters: herbs with a bitter taste.

Blade: broad, expanded part of leaf.

Bleeding time: the time required for the cessation of bleeding from a small skin puncture as a result of platelet disintegration and blood vessel constriction. Ranges from 1 to 4 minutes.

Blennorrhagia: heavy discharge of mucus, esp. from urethra.

Blepharitis: inflammation, scaling, and crusting of eyelids.

Blister: external swelling that contains watery fluid and blood or pus, caused by friction.

Blocking antibody: antibody whose production is induced by cancer cells or tissue transplants and that blocks the killing of those cells by cytotoxic T cells.

Blood pressure: the force exerted by blood as it is pumped by the heart and presses against and attempts to stretch blood vessels.

Blood poisoning: prolonged invasion of bloodstream by pathogenic bacteria due to infectious disease or skin lesions; bacteremia; septicemia; toxemia.

Blood-brain barrier: group of anatomical barriers and transport systems that tightly controls types of substances entering extracellular space of brain.

Boil: tender, inflamed, pustulant area of skin, usu. due to staphylococcus infection; furuncle.

Bolus: single, large mass of substance.

Botany: branch of biology dealing with life, structure, growth, and classification of plants.

Bract: leaflike structure growing below or encircling flower cluster or flower.

Bradycardia: slowing of heart rate to under fifty beats per minute.

Bradykinin: peptide vasodilator that increases capillary permeability and probably stimulates pain receptors.

Bromeliad: member of the pineapple family of plants, usu. epiphytic, with stiff, leathery leaves and spikes of bright flowers.

Bronchial asthma: asthma.

Bronchitis: inflammation of walls of bronchi in lungs due to virus or bacteria, causing coughing and production of sputum.

Bronchodilator: drug that relaxes bronchial muscle to open air passages to lungs.

Bronchospasm: muscular contraction that narrows bronchi and causes difficulty esp. in exhalation.

Bruit: any abnormal sound or murmur heard with a stethoscope.

Bryophyte: any member of the division of nonvascular plants, including mosses and liverworts.

Bubo: swollen and inflamed lymph node in armpit or groin.

Bulb: dormant underground bud stage of some plants.

Bulimia: usu. psychogenic syndrome of overeating followed by vomiting, also caused by hypothalamus lesion; binge purge syndrome.

Bunion: swelling of joint between big toe and first metatarsal.

Bursa: a sac or pouch which contains a special fluid which lubricates joints.

Bursitis: inflammation of a bursa.

Cachexia: weight loss, weakness, and debility associated with chronic disease.

Calcinosis: abnormal deposit of calcium salts in tissue.

Calcitonin: peptide hormone secreted by thyroid that reduces excess of calcium in blood by depositing it in bone.

Calculus: pebblelike mass, such as gallstone or kidney stone, formed within body; hard tartar layer formed on teeth by plaque.

Callus: hard thickening of area of skin undergoing rubbing, on hands or feet; mass of tissue forming around fractured bone ends.

Calmative: a sedative.

Calorie: a unit of heat. A nutritional calorie is the amount of heat necessary to raise 1 kg of water 1° C.

Calyx: the sepals or outer layer of floral leaves.

Cambium: layer of formative cells beneath bark of tree.

Cancer: malignant tumor anywhere in body due to uncontrolled cell division, causing disruption of metabolism and invasion and destruction of neighboring tissue.

Cancrum: ulceration of lip or mouth; canker.

Candidiasis: yeast-like fungus infection in mouth and moist areas of body; thrush.

Canker: cancrum.

Capsule: a dry fruit, opening when ripe, composed of more than one carpel.

Carbohydrate: sugars and starches.

Carbuncle: staphylococcus infection of skin that causes boils with multiple drainage channels.

Carcinogen: any agent or substance capable of causing cancer.

Carcinogenesis: the development of cancer caused by the actions of certain chemicals, viruses and unknown factors on primarily normal cells.

Carcinoma: cancer in epithelium lining skin or internal organs.

Cardiac arrest: abrupt cessation of heartbeat, causing loss of pulse, consciousness, and breathing.

Cardiac output: volume of blood pumped by either ventricle per minute.

Cardiac remedies: herbal remedies that have a beneficial action on the heart. Some of the remedies in this group are powerful cardio-active agents such as foxglove, whereas others are gentler, safer herbs such as hawthorn and motherwort.

Cardiac stenosis: abnormal narrowing of heart valve.

Cardiomyopathy: chronic viral, congenital, or other disorder that affects heart muscle and causes heart failure, arrhythmias, or embolisms.

Cardiopulmonary: pertaining to the heart and lungs.

Cardiotonic: a compound which tones and strengthens the heart.

Carditis: inflammation of heart.

Caries: decay of bone tissue, esp. tooth; cavity.

Carminative: plants that are rich in aromatic volatile oils that stimulate the digestive system to work properly and with ease, soothing the gut wall, reducing any inflammation that might be present, easing griping pains and helping the removal of gas from the digestive tract.

Carotene: fat-soluble plant pigments, some of which can be converted into vitamin A by the body.

Carpal tunnel syndrome: compression of median nerve entering palm of hand that causes pain and numbing in middle and index fingers.

Cartilage: a type of connective tissue which acts as a shock absorber at joint interfaces.

Castor oil: unpleasant-tasting, irritant laxative or cathartic.

Catalyst: a chemical which increases the rate of a chemical reaction without itself being consumed.

Cataract: opacity of eye lens that causes blurred vision, esp. in elderly.

Catarrh: excessive secretion of thick phlegm or mucus by mucous membrane of nose.

Catecholamines: chemically similar neurotransmitters dopamine, epinephrine, and norepinephrine.

Cathartic: a substance which stimulates the movement of the bowels, more powerful than a laxative.

Cavity: hollow in tooth produced by carous decay.

Cell-mediated immunity: specific immune response mediated by cytotoxic T lymphocytes.

Cephalalgia: headache.

Cephalic: remedy for disorders of the head; referring or directed towards the head.

Cerebral hemorrhage: bleeding from cerebral artery into brain tissue.

Cerebral: pertaining to the largest part of the brain, the cerebrum.

Cervicitis: inflammation of cervix.

Chancre: painless ulcer on lips, genitals, urethra, or eyelid.

Chelating agents: organic compounds capable of binding metals.

Chemotype: the same botanical species occurring in other forms due to different conditions of growth, such as climate, soil, altitude, etc.

Cheyne Stokes respiration: cyclical slowing of breathing to cessation, then speeding up to peak.

Chilblain: red, round, itchy swelling of skin on fingers or toes due to exposure to cold.

Chiropractic: treatment method using manipulation of muscular and skeletal system, esp. the spine.

Chlamydia: sexually transmitted, virus-like microorganism causing conjunctivitis, urethritis, and cervicitis.

Chlorophyll: pigment in chloroplast, needed for photosynthesis.

Chloroplast: membrane-bound organelle that is site of photosynthesis.

Cholagogue: a compound which stimulates the contraction of the gallbladder.

Cholecystitis: inflammation of the gallbladder.

Cholecystokinetic: agent which stimulates the contraction of the gallbladder.

Cholecystokinin: CCK; peptide hormone secreted by small intestine.

Cholelithiasis: presence of gallstones.

Choleretic: aids excretion of bile by the liver, so there is a greater flow of bile.

Cholestasis: the stagnation of bile within the liver.

Cholesterol: steroid molecule that is precursor of steroid hormones and bile salts, component of plasma membranes, and present in fat and blood.

Cholinergic: pertaining to the parasympathetic portion of the autonomic nervous system and the release of acetylcholine as a transmitter substance.

Chromatography: separation of chemical compounds.

Chronic: long-term or frequently recurring.

Chronic fatigue syndrome: persistent, extreme exhaustion and weakness due to unknown causes.

Chyme: solution of partially digested food in lumen of stomach and intestines.

Cicatrizant: an agent which promotes healing by the formation of scar tissue.

Cicatrix: scar.

Cirrhosis: progressive liver condition from various causes.

Claudication: cramping pain from inadequate blood supply to muscle.

Climacteric: physical and emotional changes as sexual maturity gives way to cessation of reproductive function in female and testosterone decrease in male.

Clot: soft, thickened lump formed in liquid, esp. blood.

Club moss: any of various small, nonseed-bearing vascular plants with conelike, spore-bearing structures on top of stems.

Clubbing: thickening of tissue at base of fingernail or toenail, esp. enlargement of fingertip.

CNS: central nervous system.

Coccus: spherical bacterium.

Coenzyme: nonprotein organic molecule that temporally joins with enzyme during reaction, serves as a carrier molecule, is not consumed in reaction, and can be reused until degraded; cofactor.

Cofactor: coenzyme.

Cold sore: small swelling or eruption of skin around lips that dries to leave crusty patch; fever blister.

Colic: pain due to contraction of the involuntary muscle of the abdominal organs.

Colitis: any inflammation of colon, causing diarrhea and lower abdominal pain.

Collagen: extremely strong fibrous protein that functions as structural element in connective tissue, tendons, and ligaments.

Collagen diseases: various diseases characterized by changes in makeup of connective tissue: lupus, rheumatic fever, rheumatoid arthritis, and scleroderma.

Collodion: solution of nitrocellulose in alcohol or ether, applied to skin for protection of minor wounds.

Colloid: an extremely fine particle suspended in a surrounding medium.

Collyrium: medicated solution used to bathe eyes.

Coma: prolonged state of deep unconsciousness from which patient cannot be roused.

Comedo: blackhead.

Complement: set of enzymes in bloodstream that work with antibodies to attack foreign cells and bacteria.

Composite: one of a large family of herbaceous plants with flower heads of dense clusters of small florets surrounded by ring of small leaves or bracts.

Compress: moistened pad of folded cloth, often medicated, applied with heat, cold, or pressure to soothe body part.

Concrete: a concentrated, waxy, solid or semi-solid perfume material prepared from previously live plant matter, usually using a hydrocarbon type of solvent.

Cone: reproductive structure of certain non-flowering plants with overlapping scales or bracts containing pollen, ovules, or spores.

Congestion: accumulation of blood within an organ; clogging of upper respiratory system with mucus.

Congestive heart failure: inability of heart to adequately supply blood to body tissue, often due to weakening of cardiac muscle, causing body swelling and shortness of breath.

Conifer: cone-bearing gymnosperm, usu. with narrow, needle-like or small scale-like leaves.

Conjunctivitis: inflammation of mucous membrane covering front of eye, often with discharge of pus; pinkeye.

Connective tissue: the type of tissue which performs the function of providing support, structure and cellular cement to the body.

Constipation: infrequent, difficult, often painful bowel movements with hard feces; irregularity.

Contagious: a disease which can be transferred from one person to another by direct contact.

Contraceptive: medication or device to prevent conception.

Contusion: surface injury in which skin is not broken; bruise.

Convulsion: involuntary muscle contraction that causes contorted movements of body and limbs.

Cordial: a stimulant and tonic.

Corm: underground stem base that acts as reproductive structure.

Corn: area of hard or thickened skin on or between toes.

Corolla: the petals of a flower considered as a whole.

Coronary heart disease: serious condition affecting coronary artery.

Coronary: of or pertaining to arteries of heart.

Corpus luteum: the remains of the egg follicle after ovulation.

Cortical: involving external layers of brain.

Corticosteroid drugs: a group of drugs similar to natural corticosteroid hormones which are used predominantly in the treatment of inflammation and to suppress the immune system.

Corticosteroid hormones: a group of hormones produced by the adrenal glands that control the body's use of nutrients and the excretion of salts and water in the urine.

Cortisol: steroid hormone secreted by adrenal cortex that regulates organic metabolism by converting fats and proteins to glucose.

Cortisone: steroid hormone secreted by adrenal cortex that counteracts pain and swelling.

Coryia: catarrhal inflammation of mucous membrane in nose.

Corymb: flat-topped or convex cluster of flowers in which outer flowers open first.

Cotyledon: first or second leaf of seedling.

Cough: violent exhalation of irritant particles or congestive mucus from respiratory system; tussis.

Coumarins: glycoside compounds that are responsible for the "new mown hay" smell of many grasses.

Counter-irritant: applications to the skin which relieve deep-seated pain, usually applied in the form of heat; *see also* rubefacient.

Crab louse: crab-like louse that infests pubic regions, transmitted by sexual contact.

Cramp: prolonged painful contraction or spasm of muscle.

Crepitation: soft crackling sound heard in lungs through stethoscope; rale.

Crepitus: crackling sound made by grating of bone on bone or cartilage, esp. in arthritic joint.

CRH: corticotropin-releasing hormone.

Crick: painful muscle spasm or cramp in neck or upper back.

Crohn's disease: condition marked by chronic inflammation and thickening of alimentary tract.

Croup: inflammation and obstruction of larynx in young children due to viral respiratory infections, characterized by harsh cough.

Cushing's disease: syndrome due to excess corticosteroid hormone, causing weight gain, excess body hair, and high blood pressure.

Cutaneous: pertaining to the skin.

Cuticle: waxy layer on outer surface of plants.

Cyanosis: bluish discoloration of skin and mucous membrane due to inadequate oxygenation of blood.

Cycad: any of the order of gymnosperms intermediate between ferns and palms, often with thick, columnar trunk crowned by large, tough, pinnate leaves.

Cyme: inflorescence in which primary axis bears single central or terminal flower that blooms first.

Cyst: abnormal sac or cavity lined with epithelium and filled with liquid or semisolid substance.

Cyst: an abnormal lump or swelling, filled with fluid or semisolid material, in any body organ or tissue.

Cystic fibrosis: hereditary disease of exocrine glands that produces respiratory infections, malabsorption, and sweat with high salt content.

Cystitis: inflammation of the inner lining of the bladder. It is usually caused by a bacterial infection.

Cytokinin: plant hormone that promotes cell division.

Cytomegalovirus: a virus in herpes family that causes enlargement of epithelial cells and mononucleosis-like disease.

Cytophylactic: referring to cytophylaxis—the process of increasing the activity of leukocytes in defense of the body against infection.

Cytotoxic: toxic to all cells.

Cytotoxin: substance that has toxic effect on certain cells, used against some tumors.

Debility: weakness, lack of tone.

Deciduous: designating any plant that sheds all its leaves once each year.

Decoction: a herbal preparation, where the plant material (usually hard or woody) is boiled in water and reduced to make a concentrated extract.

Decongestant: substance used to reduce nasal mucus production and swelling.

Deficiency disease: any disease, such as beriberi, caused by nutritional deficiency.

Dehiscence: splitting open of a wound.

Dehydration: deficiency or loss of water in body tissues marked by thirst, nausea, and exhaustion.

Delirium: acute mental disorder due to organic brain disease, causing hallucinations, disorientation, and extreme excitation.

Dementia: senility. Loss of mental function.

Demineralization: loss of minerals from the bone.

Demulcent: herbs rich in mucilage that soothe and protect irritated or inflamed tissue.

Deodorant: an agent which corrects, masks or removes unpleasant odors.

Depressant: drug that lowers nervous or functional activity; sedative.

Depurative: helps combat impurity in the blood and organs; detoxifying.

Dermal: pertaining to the skin.

Dermatitis: skin inflammation.

Detumescence: reduction or subsidence of swelling.

Diabetes: diabetes mellitus.

Diabetes insipidus: rare deficiency of pituitary hormone that causes constant thirst and excessive urination.

Diabetes mellitus: common deficiency, possibly inherited, of the pancreatic hormone insulin, causing disorder in carbohydrate metabolism and inability to properly utilize sugars; diabetes.

Dialysis: a technique using sophisticated machinery to remove waste products from the blood and excess fluid from the body in the treatment of kidney failure.

Diaphoretic: promotes perspiration, helping the skin eliminate waste from the body, thus helping the body ensure a clean and harmonious inner environment.

Diarrhea: frequent bowel evacuation, esp. of soft or liquid feces.

Diastole: period of cardiac cycle in which ventricles are not contracting.

Diastolic pressure: minimum blood pressure during cardiac cycle.

Dicot: dicotyledon.

Dicotyledon: angiosperm having two seed leaves or cotyledons; dicot.

Digestion: process of breaking down large particles and high-molecular weight substances into small molecules.

Digestive: substance which promotes or aids the digestion of food.

Dioecious: having male and female organs on different individuals.

Diphtheria: acute, highly contagious bacterial infection of the throat that can cause death from respiratory obstruction or carditis.

Disaccharide: a sugar composed of two monosaccharide units.

Disinfectant: cleansing agent that destroys bacteria and other microorganisms, used on surfaces and surgical tools.

Diuretic: increases the production and elimination of urine.

Diverticuli: sac-like outpouchings of the wall of the colon.

Diverticulitis: colonic diverticulosis with inflammation.

Diverticulosis: condition characterized by existence of diverticular sacs at weak points in walls of alimentary tract, esp. intestine.

Dizziness: feeling off balance, unstable, confused, as though whirling in place.

Dopamine: catecholamine neurotransmitter, precursor of epinephrine and norepinephrine.

Dormancy period: of time in which growth ceases.

Double-blind study: a way of controlling against experimental bias by ensuring that neither the researcher nor the subject knows when an active agent or placebo is being used.

Douche: introduction of water and/or a cleansing agent into the vagina with the aid of a bag with tubing and nozzle attached.

Dressing: protective or healing material applied externally to wound or diseased body part.

Dropsy: excess of fluid in the tissues.

Drug: substance that affects structure or functional processes of an organism, esp. to prevent or treat diseases or relieve symptoms.

Drupe: a fleshy fruit, with one or more seeds, each surrounded by a stony layer.

Dumping syndrome: faintness, sweating, and paleness due to rapid emptying of stomach, esp. in one who has had gastrectomy.

Duodenal ulcer: ulcer in lining of duodenum caused by excess stomach acid.

Dysentery: infection of intestinal tract that causes severe diarrhea mixed with blood and mucus.

Dysfunction: abnormal function.

Dysmenorrhea: painful, difficult menstruation.

Dyspepsia: digestive disorder with abdominal pain and gas after eating, sometimes with nausea and vomiting; indigestion.

Dysplasia: any abnormality of growth.

Dyspnea: labored or difficult breathing; breathlessness.

Dystrophy: organ or muscle disorder caused by insufficient nourishment or hereditary disorder.

Ear, nose, and throat: ent; treatment of diseases of these parts; otorhinolaryngology.

Ecchymosis: bluish black mark on skin from release of blood into tissues, usu. due to injury; black-and-blue mark.

Eclampsia: convulsions, esp. due to toxemia during pregnancy.

Ectopic pregnancy: state in which fertilized egg implants at a site other than uterus.

Edema: excessive accumulation of fluid in tissues; dropsy.

Eicosapentaenoic acid (EPA): a fatty acid found primarily in cold-water fish.

Electrocardiogram (ECG): machine which measures and records the activity of the heart.

Electroencephalogram (EEG): a machine which measures and records brain waves.

Electrolyte: substance that ionizes in solution and conducts electric current.

Electuary: medication mixed with honey.

Elimination diet: a diet which eliminates allergic foods.

Elixir: substance that contains alcohol or glycerin, used as solution for bitter or nauseating drugs.

Elliptical: shaped like an ellipse, or regular curve.

Embolism: obstruction of artery by lodged blood clot, fat, air, or foreign body carried by circulating blood.

Embolus: mass of matter that obstructs blood flow.

Emesis: vomiting; vomited matter.

Emetic: substance that induces vomiting.

Emmenagogue: stimulates menstrual flow and activity.

Emollient: medical preparation that soothes and softens external tissue.

Emphysema: air in tissues; pulmonary disorder, characterized by increase in size of air sacs due to destruction of their walls, causing shortness of breath.

Empyema: accumulation of pus in body cavity, esp. pleural cavity.

Emulsification: maintenance of lipid droplets in solution.

Emulsify: the dispersement of large globules into smaller uniformly distributed particles. Usually refers to fat globules.

Encephalitis: viral or bacterial inflammation of brain, also caused by infection or allergic reaction; sleeping sickness.

Endemic: disease that is constantly present in particular region but generally under control.

Endocarditis: inflammation and damage to heart cavity lining due to bacterial infection or rheumatic fever.

Endocrine gland: ductless organ that synthesizes hormones and releases them directly into bloodstream.

Endocrine system: all ductless glands in body.

Endocrinology: study of endocrine glands and hormones.

Endometrium: the mucus membrane lining the uterus.

Endometriosis: a condition in which tissue similar to that normally lining the uterus is found outside of the uterus, usually the ovaries, fallopian tubes and other pelvic structures.

Endorphin: neurotransmitter that exhibits pain-killing activity.

Enervation: weakness, lack of energy.

Engorgement: congestion of a part of the tissues, or fullness (as in the breasts).

Enteric-coated: a special way of coating a tablet or capsule to ensure that it does not dissolve in the stomach and so can reach the intestinal tract.

Enteritis: viral or bacterial inflammation of small intestine, causing diarrhea.

Enuresis: involuntary urination, esp. at night, usu. functional in nature; bedwetting.

Enzyme: complex proteins that are produced by living cells, and catalyze specific biochemical reactions.

Ephedrine: widely used drug similar to epinephrine.

Epidemiology: study of causes and control of epidemics.

Epilepsy: one of various brain disorders that cause recurrent, sudden convulsive attacks.

Epinephrine: hormone released by adrenal medulla that elevates blood sugar and initiates fight-or-flight response; adrenaline.

Epiphyte: nonparasitic plant growing upon another plant for support.

Epistaxis: attack of bleeding from the nose.

Epithelium: the cells that cover the entire surface of the body and that line most of the internal organs.

Epstein-Barr syndrome: infectious mononucleosis caused by herpes-like virus; glandular fever.

Erysipelas: skin infection from streptococcus bacteria that causes inflammation, swelling, and fever.

Erythema: a superficial redness of the skin due to excess of blood.

Erythropoiesis: formation of erythrocytes.

Erythropoietin: hormone secreted mainly by kidney that stimulates erythrocyte production.

Essential fatty acid (EFA): fatty acids which the body cannot manufacture—linoleic and linolenic acids.

Essential oil: a volatile oil obtained from the leaves, stem, flower, other parts of plants, usually carrying the odor characteristic of the plant.

Estrogen: hormone produced by ovary that stimulates breast and uterine growth, used to treat amenorrhea and menopausal disorders and to inhibit lactation.

Etiology: science of causes and origins of diseases.

Evergreen: plant that maintains functional green foliage throughout year.

Excretion: the elimination of waste products from a cell, tissue or the entire body.

Exfolliant: a product or ingredient whose purpose is to remove unwanted tissue or waste products from the skin and other body surfaces.

Exocrine gland: gland that secretes through a duct.

Exophthalmic goiter: enlargement of thyroid gland accompanied by protrusion of eyeball from orbit.

Expectorant: soothes bronchial spasm and loosens mucous secretions, helping in dry, irritating coughs.

Extracellular: the space outside the cell, composed of fluid.

Exudate: escaping fluid or semifluid material that oozes from a space that may contain serum, pus and cellular debris.

Eyewash: medicinal solution that soothes eyes.

Fatty acid: organic compound whose carbon chain ends in a carboxyl group.

Febrifuge: substance that relieves or reduces fever.

Feces: digestive waste products.

Fern: non-flowering, vascular plant having roots, stems, and fronds and reproducing by spores instead of seeds.

Fever: rise in body temperature above normal 98.6 degrees.

Fibrillation: rapid, uncontrolled irregular twitching of heart muscle.

Fibroma: usu. benign tumor composed mainly of fibrous or connective tissue.

Fibrosarcoma: malignant tumor of connective tissue, esp. in legs.

Fibrocystic changes: formation of benign cysts of various sizes in the breast.

Fibrosis: thickening and scarring of connective tissue due to injury or inflammation.

First-degree burn: reddening of outer layer of skin.

Fissure: crack in membrane lining.

Fistula: abnormal passage that leads from abscess or cavity to skin or to another abscess or cavity, caused by disease or injury.

Fixative: a material which slows down the rate of evaporation of the more volatile components in a perfume composition.

Fixed oil: a name given to vegetable oils obtained from plants which, in contradistinction to essential oils, are fatty, dense and non-volatile, such as olive or sweet almond oil.

Flatulence: expulsion of intestinal gas through mouth by belching or through anus by passing flatus.

Flatus: intestinal gas.

Flavonoid: plant pigments which exert a wide variety of physiological effects in the human body.

Floret: small flower; one of individual flowers comprising the head of a composite plant.

Flowering plant: any angiosperm that produces flowers, fruit, and seeds in an enclosed ovary.

Foliage: leaves of plant or tree.

Follicle: saclike structure that forms inside an ovary when an egg is produced.

Free radicals: highly reactive molecules that can bind to and destroy cellular compounds.

Frond: fern or palm foliage.

Fructose: yellowish to white, crystalline, water-soluble sugar found in many fruits.

Fruit: mature ovary of flowering plant, sometimes edible.

Functional cyst: a benign cyst that forms on an ovary and usually resolves on its own without treatment.

Functional disorder: condition for which no physical cause can be found.

Fungicidal: prevents and combats fungal infection.

Fungus: unicellular or filamentous organism, formerly classified with plants.

Furuncle: boil.

Galactagogue: increases secretion of milk.

Gallstone: hard mass of bile pigments, cholesterol, and calcium salts in gall-bladder that causes pain or passes into and obstructs bile duct.

Gamma globulin: part of blood serum that contains antibodies, used in temporary prevention of infectious diseases.

Gargle: antiseptic, often medicated, liquid used to rinse mouth and throat; mouthwash.

Gastric ulcer: stomach ulcer caused by action of acid on stomach lining.

Gastrin: digestive system hormone that stimulates hydrochloric acid release by stomach and secretion of digestive enzyme by pancreas.

Gastritis: inflammation of stomach lining from an ingested substance, infection, or chronic inflammation.

Gastroenteritis: inflammation of stomach and intestine, due to virus, bacteria, or food poisoning, that causes vomiting.

Genital herpes: infection of genital area by herpes simplex virus.

Genus: category of closely related species ranking below family and above species.

German measles: rubella.

Germicidal: destroys germs or microorganisms such as bacteria, etc.

Germinate: sprout and start to grow from spore, seed, a bud.

Gingivitis: inflammation of gums, sometimes with bleeding.

Glandular fever: mononucleosis.

Glaucoma: abnormally high fluid pressure in the eye, often leading to loss of vision.

Glaucous: covered with a fine, white, often waxy film, which rubs off.

Glioma: cancer of nerve tissue.

Glomerular filtration rate: gfr; milliliters of plasma per minute filtered through kidney.

Glomerulonephritis: potentially fatal streptococcal infection of kidney.

Glucagon: pancreatic hormone that increases blood glucose levels.

Glucocorticoid: adrenal cortex hormone that affects salt and water metabolism and stimulates conversion of noncarbohydrates to carbohydrates.

Glucose: a monosaccharide which is found in the blood and is one of the body's primary energy sources.

Glutamic acid: amino acid that may be brain neurotransmitter.

Gluten: one of the proteins in wheat and certain other grains that give dough its tough, elastic character.

Glycerin: glycerol.

Glycerol: syrupy liquid prepared by hydrolysis of fats and oils for use as skin lotion.

Glycine: simplest amino acid, present in most proteins.

Glycogen: white polysaccharide sugar, derived from glucose, that is principal form in which carbohydrate is stored in tissue.

Glycoprotein: carbohydrate-protein complex.

Glycosides: these common plant chemicals consist of molecules made up of two sections, one of which is a sugar. Some have a strong effect on the heart and are known as cardio-active glycosides (e.g. foxglove/digitalis). Some are purgative (e.g. the anthraquinones in cascara, senna, rhubarb, buckthorn).

Glycosuria: excretion of excess sugar in urine, as in diabetes.

Goblet cell: a goblet-shaped cell which secretes mucus.

Goiter: swollen neck due to enlarged thyroid gland.

Gonorrhea: sexually transmitted bacterial disease that affects mucous membranes in genital tract, pharynx, or rectum.

Gout: accumulation of excess uric acid in bloodstream and joints that causes joint destruction, kidney stones, and arthritis.

Grand mal: generalized epileptic seizure with flexion and extension of extremities and loss of consciousness.

Granuloma: nodule of connective tissue and capillaries associated with tuberculosis, syphilis, or nonorganic foreign bodies.

Graves' disease: disease characterized by enlarged thyroid and increased basal metabolism, due to excessive thyroid secretion.

Grippe: influenza.

Ground substance: the thick, gel-like material in which the cells, fibers and blood capillaries of cartilage, bone and connective tissue are embedded.

Gum: a class of carbohydrates which swell in the presence of water and increase the thickness of water-based products.

Gymnosperm: member of the division of seed plants having ovules on open scales, esp. cones.

Haematuria: blood in the urine.

Haemostatic: arrests bleeding.

Halitosis: offensive breath, esp. from diseases of gums, teeth, throat, or lungs; bad breath.

Hallucinogenic: causes visions or delusions.

Hay fever: common, usu. seasonal allergy to plant pollen that causes sneezing, runny nose, and watery eyes.

HDL: high-density lipoprotein.

Headache: pain within skull, commonly due to stress or fatigue; cephalalgia.

Heart attack: myocardial infarction.

Heart failure: inadequate pumping of heart ventricle due to coronary thrombosis, hypertension, or arrhythmia; congestive heart failure.

Heart murmur: blowing or swishing noise produced by blood passing through defective heart valve.

Heartburn: pain rising from abdomen to throat, often accompanied by bitter fluid in mouth; pyrosis.

Heartwood: the central portion of a tree trunk.

Helper T cell: white blood cells which help in the immune response.

Hematoma: clotted accumulation of blood in tissue forming solid swelling.

Hemophilia: hereditary deficiency of one blood coagulant that causes slowness in clotting and prolonged or spontaneous bleeding.

Hemorrhage: outflow of blood from ruptured blood vessel, esp. internal bleeding.

Hemorrhoids: enlarged veins in anus walls, esp. due to prolonged constipation or diarrhea, characterized by fissure, painful swelling, and bleeding; piles.

Hemostatic: a substance which checks bleeding.

Heparin: natural anticoagulant produced by liver cells as a polysaccharide.

Hepatic: pertaining to the liver.

Hepatics: aid the liver. They tone, strengthen and in some cases increase the flow of bile. In a broad holistic approach to health they are of great importance because of the fundamental role of the liver in the working of the body.

Hepatitis: inflammation of liver, due to virus transmitted by food or drink (infectious hepatitis) or blood on needle or in transfusion (serum hepatitis), causing fever and jaundice.

Hepatomegaly: enlargement of the liver.

Herbaceous: non-woody.

Hernia: protrusion of tissue or organ outside cavity it normally occupies, esp. in lower abdomen, due to physical strain or coughing.

Herniated disk: slipped disk.

Herpes: herpes simplex; small viral blisters on skin.

Herpes simplex: virus in herpes family; non-venereal blisters on mucous membrane that can cause conjunctivitis, vaginal inflammation, or cold sores, herpes.

Herpes zoster: virus in herpes family characterized by vesicles, often with severe pain along distribution of nerve; shingles.

Hiccup: characteristic sound made by abrupt involuntary lowering of diaphragm and closing of upper end of trachea.

High density lipoprotein: hdl; lipid-protein aggregate with low proportion of lipid or cholesterol that removes cholesterol from arteries.

Histamine: amine derived from amino acid histidine that is released in allergic reaction, causing dilation of blood vessels.

HIV: human immunodeficiency virus.

Hives: round, red itching wheals up to several inches across on skin, caused by acute or chronic allergic reaction; urticaria.

Hodgkin's disease: condition marked by malignancy in lymphatic tissue that causes enlarged lymph nodes, fever, and profuse sweating.

Holistic medicine: a form of therapy aimed at treating the whole person, not just the part or parts in which symptoms occur.

Homeostasis: maintenance of constant internal environment.

Hormone: a secretion of an endocrine gland that controls and regulates functions in other parts of the body.

Housemaid's knee: fluid-filled swelling of bursa in front of kneecap, often caused by prolonged kneeling.

Human immunodeficiency virus: HIV; virus that causes AIDS.

Humoral immunity: defense against disease by antibodies in body fluids.

Hybrid: a plant originating by fertilization of one species or subspecies by another.

Hydrocarbon: compounds containing only hydrogen and carbon.

Hydrocele: accumulation of watery fluid, esp. about testis.

Hydrocephalus: excess of cerebrospinal fluid in brain ventricles that causes enlargement of head in children and pressure and drowsiness in adults.

Hydrochloric acid: acid secreted by stomach during digestion.

Hyperglycaemia: high blood sugar level.

Hyperinsulinism: overproduction of insulin, due to glandular disturbance or poor nutrition, producing symptoms of hypoglycemia.

Hyperlipidaemic: elevation of cholesterol and triglycerides in the blood.

Hyperplasia: increase in number of fat cells, causing obesity.

Hypersecretion: excessive secretion.

Hypersensitivity: allergic reaction.

Hypertension: high blood pressure.

Hypertensive: a substance that causes a rise in blood pressure.

Hyperthermia: exceptionally high body temperature of 105 degrees F. or above; fever induced as treatment.

Hyperthyroidism: overactivity of thyroid gland that causes rapid heartbeat, sweating, tremors, weight loss, and anxiety.

Hypertrophy: increase in size of tissue or organ due to enlargement of cells.

Hyperventilation: abnormally rapid breathing that lowers carbon dioxide concentration in blood.

Hypochlorhydria: insufficient gastric acid output.

Hypochondria: obsession with real and imagined physical ailments.

Hypoglycemia: low blood sugar.

Hypoglycemic: plant remedies that lower abnormally elevated blood sugar.

Hypopraxia: listlessness, enfeeblement, or lack of interest in activity.

Hypotension: low blood pressure.

Hypotensive: plant remedies that lower abnormally elevated blood pressure.

Hypothermia: dropping of body temperature below normal range.

Hypothyroidism: subnormal thyroid gland activity that can lead to cretinism if present at birth.

Hypoxia: an inadequate supply of oxygen.

Hysterectomy: surgical removal of the uterus.

Hysteria: extreme emotional excitation, sensory and motor disturbances, and outbursts of uncontrolled feeling.

Iatrogenic: meaning literally "physician-produced"; the term can be applied to any medical condition, disease or other adverse occurrence that results from medical treatment.

Idiopathic: of unknown cause.

Ig: immunoglobulin.

Ileitis: inflammation of ileum in small intestine.

Immune responses: body's defense reaction through dual modes of antibody and cellular response.

Immunity: ability of body to recognize and neutralize foreign matter, either natural or acquired.

Immunoglobulin: any of five classes of antibodies: Ig, Igg, Igm, Iga, and Igf.

Immunomodulator: a plant that affects immune system functioning in some positive way.

Immunostimulant: a plant that stimulates some aspect of immune system functioning.

Impairment: damage to or weakening of body part or function.

Impetigo: contagious skin infection from streptococcal or staphylococcal bacteria, esp. in children, causing crusty yellow blisters.

Inborn immunity: congenital resistance to specific disease.

Incidence: the number of new cases of a disease that occur during a given period (usually years) in a defined population.

Incontinence: involuntary passage or leakage of urine.

Incubation period: time between entry of disease organisms into body and onset of disease symptoms.

Infarction: death of tissue due to oxygen deprivation.

Infestation: attack on body by parasitic microorganism.

Inflorescence: flowering structure above the last stem leaves (including bracts and flowers).

Influenza: highly contagious viral infection of respiratory system, transmitted by coughing or sneezing, that causes headache, fever, general aches and pains—flu; grippe.

Infusion: a herbal remedy prepared by steeping the plant material in water.

Inorganic: in chemistry the term inorganic refers to compounds which do not contain carbon.

Insomnia: inability to fall asleep or remain asleep.

Insulin: pancreatic hormone that regulates blood sugar level.

Interferon: substance produced by infected cells that inhibits specific viral growth.

Intramuscular: situated in or administered by entering a muscle, used esp. of injections.

Irreversible: impossible to halt or reverse by treatment.

Irritable bowel syndrome: recurrent chronic abdominal pain with constipation and/or diarrhea caused by abnormal contractions of colon muscles; spastic colon.

Irritant: a substance which produces redness, itching, swelling or blisters on the skin.

Ischemia: reduced blood supply to organ or tissue.

Jaundice: a condition caused by elevation of bilirubin in the body and characterized by yellowing of the skin.

Keratin: an insoluble protein found in hair, skin and nails.

Ketone: product of lipid metabolism.

Kidney stone: hard, pebble-like mass in kidney that causes pain and blood in urine; nephrolithiasis; renal calculus.

Kinin: vasodilatory polypeptide.

Laceration: tear in flesh, esp. with irregular edges.

Lactase: an enzyme which breaks down lactose into the monosaccharides glucose and galactose.

Lactose: one of the sugars present in milk. It is a disaccharide.

Lanceolate: lance-shaped, oval and pointed at both ends (usually a leaf shape).

Laparoscopy: a surgical procedure in which a slender, light-transmitting telescope, the laparoscope, is used to view the pelvic organs.

Larvicidal: an agent which prevents and kills larvae.

Laryngitis: inflammation of larynx and vocal cords, due to bacterial or viral infection, causing coughing, husky voice, or complete voice loss.

Laxative: stimulates bowel movements. Stimulating laxatives should not be used long term. If this appears to be necessary then diet, general health and stress should all be closely considered.

LDL: low-density lipoprotein.

Lecithin: phospholipid in nerve tissue and blood.

Legume: a fruit consisting of one carpel, opening on one side, such as a pea.

Lenticel: spongy area of bark on woody plant that allows exchange of gases between stem and atmosphere.

Lesion: any localized, abnormal change in tissue formation.

Lethargy: a feeling of tiredness, drowsiness or lack of energy.

Leukocyte: white blood cell responsible for fighting disease.

Leucocytosis: an increase in the number of white blood cells above the normal limit.

Leucoplakia: a precancerous lesion usually seen in the mouth that is characterized by a white-colored patch.

Leukemia: overproduction of abnormal white blood cells by bone marrow and other blood-forming organs, usu. causing fatal systemic malignancy.

Leukocytosis: abnormal level in number of white blood cells, usu. due to infection.

Leukopenia: reduction in number of white blood cells to below normal level.

Leukotrienes: inflammatory compounds produced when oxygen interacts with polyunsaturated fatty acids.

Lichen: fungus in symbiotic union with an alga.

Lignin: organic substance that serves as binder for cellulose fibers in wood and certain plants.

Ligulet: a narrow projection from the top of a leaf sheath in grasses.

Liniment: soothing camphor and alcohol preparation rubbed into skin or applied on surgical dressing.

Lipase: fat-splitting enzyme.

Lipid: fat, phospholipid, steroid or prostaglandin.

Lipolytic: causing lipolysis, the chemical disintegration or splitting of fats.

Lipoprotein: molecule combining protein and lipid.

Lipotropic: promoting the flow of lipids to and from the liver.

Liverwort: any of various small, flat bryophytes, usu. on logs, rocks, or soil in moist areas.

Lotion: an emollient emulsion, usually of the water in oil type.

Low density lipoprotein: LDL; protein-lipid aggregate that is major cholesterol carrier in plasma.

Lozenge: medicated tablet with sugar that is dissolved in the mouth to soothe throat.

Lubricant: greasy substance applied to reduce friction on body surface.

Lumbago: lower backache due to injury or sciatica.

Lumen: cavity within tubular structure.

Lung cancer: malignancy in epithelium of air passages or lung, esp. due to smoke or other outside agents.

Lupus erythematosus: chronic inflammation of connective tissue that causes red scaly rash on face, arthritis, and organ damage.

Lycopod: club moss.

Lyme disease: spirochetal infection transmitted by a tick that causes skin rash, headache, fever, and sometimes arthritis and heart damage.

Lymph: colorless fluid derived from blood and carried in special ducts of lymphatic vessels.

Lymphatic: pertaining to the lymph system.

Lymphocyte: a type of white blood cell found primarily in lymph nodes.

Lymphoid tissue: connective tissue containing lymphocytes.

Lymphoma: malignant tumor of lymph nodes that is not Hodgkin's disease.

Macerate: soak until soft.

Macule: discoloration or thickening of skin in contrast to surrounding area.

Malabsorption: impaired absorption of nutrients, most often due to diarrhea.

Malaise: general sense of being unwell, often accompanied by physical discomfort and weakness.

Malignant: a term used to describe a condition that tends to worsen and eventually causes death.

Malnutrition: insufficient food consumption to satisfy bodily needs over prolonged period.

Mammogram: an X-ray of the breast, used to detect breast cancer.

Mania: excessive activity and euphoria.

Manipulation: as a therapy, the skillful use of the hands to move a part of the body or a specific joint or muscle.

Mast cell: a cell found in many tissues of the body which contributes greatly to allergic and inflammatory processes by secreting histamine and other inflammatory chemicals.

Mastitis: inflammation of breasts due to bacterial infection often through damaged nipples.

Measles: highly infectious viral epidemic disease, mainly in children, that causes high fever and elevated pink rash; rubeola.

Melanoma: malignant tumor of melanin-forming cells, esp. in skin.

Meniere's syndrome: disease of labyrinth of inner ear, causing deafness and vertigo.

Meningitis: inflammation of membranes lining skull and vertebral canal, due to viral or bacterial infection, causing fever, intense headache, muscular rigidity, and sometimes convulsion, delirium, or death; spinal meningitis.

Menorrhagia: excessive loss of blood during periods.

Menstruation: the discharge of blood and tissue from the uterus that occurs when an egg is not fertilized.

Metabolic rate: level of energy expenditure.

Metabolism: a collective term for all the chemical processes that take place in the body.

Metabolite: a product of a chemical reaction.

Metallo-enzyme: an enzyme which contains a metal at its active site.

Metastasis: spread of malignant tumor far from site of origin, usu. through vascular system.

Microflora: the microbial inhabitants of a particular region, e.g. colon.

Microorganism: any living organism too small to be viewed by unaided eye, including bacteria, viruses, protists, and some algae and fungi.

Migraine: recurrent, intense headache, often accompanied by blurred vision and vomiting, caused by contraction and dilation of arteries in brain.

Mineral oil: colorless, tasteless petroleum derivative used as laxative.

Mineralocorticoid: steroid salt-retaining hormone of adrenal cortex.

Miscible: the ability of a gas or liquid to mix uniformly with another gas or liquid. All gases are completely miscible in other gases.

Mitogenic: an agent that effects cell division.

Mold: multicellular filamentous fungus.

Mole: flat or raised area of brown pigment in skin.

Molecule: the smallest complete unit of a substance that can exist independently and still retain the characteristic properties of the substance.

Monoclonal antibodies: genetically engineered antibodies specific for one particular antigen.

Monocotyledon: angiosperm having only one seed leaf cotyledon.

Mononuclear phagocyte system: monocytes and macrophages.

Mononucleosis: infectious disease that manifests a high number of monocytes in blood, enlarged lymph nodes, prolonged fever, appetite loss, and malaise, esp. in young adults; glandular disease caused by Epstein-Barr virus; glandular fever.

Monosaccharide: a simple one-unit sugar like fructose and glucose.

Moss: any of various small bryophytes without true stems reproducing by spores, and growing in velvety clusters in moist areas on rocks, trees, and the ground.

Motion sickness: nausea, vomiting, dizziness, and headache caused by motion.

Motor: designating muscular activity stimulated by impulses from central nervous system.

Mouthwash: gargle.

Moxa: a dried herb (usually mugwort) burnt on or above the skin to stimulate an acupuncture point or serve as a counterirritant.

Mucilage: a substance containing gelatinous constituents which are demulcent.

Mucin: protein that forms mucus when mixed with water.

Mucolytic: dissolving or breaking down mucous.

Mucosa: another term for mucous membrane.

Mucous membrane: mucus-secreting membrane lining body cavities and canals connecting with external air.

Mucus: viscid watery lubricating solution secreted by mucus membranes.

Multiple sclerosis: ms; chronic nervous system disease with recurrent symptoms of unsteady gait, shaky limb movements, rapid involuntary eye movements, and speech defects.

Mumps: viral infection that causes fever and swelling of parotid salivary glands, esp. among children.

Muscle-relaxer: depressant or tranquilizer that acts to relieve tension in muscles.

Muscular dystrophy: inherited muscle disease marked by degeneration of muscle fiber.

Mutagen: external agent that increases mutation rate in cells.

Myasthenia gravis: muscular weakness that has its onset with repetitive activity and leads to paralysis.

Mycelium: mass of threadlike tubes forming the vegetative parts of a fungus.

Mycorrhiza: close symbiosis between mycelia of certain fungi and root cells of some vascular plants.

Mycosis: fungus infection.

Mycotoxins: toxins from yeast and fungi.

Myelin sheath: a white fatty substance which surrounds nerve cells and aids in nerve impulse transmission.

Myeloma: malignancy of bone marrow.

Myocardial infarction: death of portion of heart muscle due to interrupted blood supply; heart attack; coronary infarction.

Myocarditis: acute or chronic inflammation of heart muscle.

Myxedema: dry, firm, waxy swelling of skin and subcutaneous tissue, also characterized by labored speech and blunted senses.

Narcotic: a substance which induces sleep; intoxicating or poisonous in large doses.

Natural immunity: inborn lack of susceptibility to specific disease.

Naturopathy: treatment of disease that employs no surgery or synthetic drugs.

Nausea: feeling that one is about to vomit.

Necrosis: death of cells in organ or tissue.

Nectary: organ of plant that secretes nectar.

Neoplasia: a medical term for a tumor formation, characterized by a progressive, abnormal replication of cells.

Neoplasm: new tumor caused by uncontrolled reproduction of abnormal cells.

Nephralgia: pain in kidney and loin area.

Nephritis: inflammation of kidney; Bright's disease.

Nephrosis: syndrome characterized by edema, excess albumin in urine, and cholesterol in blood.

Nervine: nervines help the nervous system and can be meaningfully subdivided into three groups. Nervine tonics strengthen and restore the nervous system. Nervine relaxants ease anxiety and tension by soothing both body and mind. Nervine stimulants directly stimulate nerve activity.

Neuralgia: a stabbing pain along a nerve pathway.

Neurasthenia: outdated or non-technical term for fatigue, irritability, headache, dizziness, anxiety, and intolerance to noise due to head injury or mental illness.

Neurasthenia: nervous exhaustion.

Neuritis: inflammation of nerves; neuropathy.

Neurodermatitis: localized skin disease with itching and thickening of skin.

Neurofibrillary tangles: clusters of degenerated nerves.

Neurofibromatosis: congenital disease that causes growth on fibrous nerve coverings of benign tumors that may become malignant.

Neuron: functional unit of a nerve, including cell body, axon, and dendrites.

Neuropathy: neuritis.

Neurotransmitters: substances which modify or transmit nerve impulses.

Night sweats: copious perspiration while sleeping.

Nit: Louse egg that attaches to body

Nocturia: the disturbance of a person's sleep at night by the need to pass urine.

Nonvascular plant: bryophyte nut dry, single-seeded fruit of various trees and shrubs consisting of kernel enclosed in hard or tough shell.

Norepinephrine: commercial form of neurotransmitter used for emergency treatment of lowered blood pressure.

Obovate: oval, but broader towards the apex; refers to leaf shape.

Occlusion: closing or obstruction of hollow organ or body part.

Ointment: fatty substance used to soothe or heal skin; salve; unguent.

Oleo gum resin: a natural exudation from trees and plants that consists mainly of essential oil, gum and resin.

Oleoresin: a natural resinous exudation from plants, or an aromatic liquid preparation, extracted from botanical matter using solvents. They consist almost entirely of a mixture of essential oil and resin.

Olfaction: the sense of smell.

Opiate: derivative of opium that depresses central nervous system, relieves pain, and induces sleep.

Opportunistic: designating disease or infection occurring only under certain conditions, as when immune system is impaired.

Orchitis: inflammation of testis that causes pain, redness, and swelling of scrotum, usu. due to infection such as mumps.

Organ: collection of tissues joined in structural unit to serve a common function.

Organic disorder: disorder associated with physiological changes in structure of organ or tissue.

Organic: in the chemical sense organic refers to all compounds containing carbon.

Osteoarthritis: joint cartilage disease that causes pain and impaired joint function and occurs in later life, due to overuse of joint or as a complication of rheumatoid arthritis.

Osteomyelitis: inflammation of bone marrow and adjacent bone, mostly from infection, esp. after compound fractures where marrow is exposed.

Osteopathy: treatment of disease by manipulation and massage of musculoskeletal system.

Osteoporosis: loss of bony matrix that causes brittle bones due to injury, infection, or old age.

Otalgia: earache.

OTC: over the counter; medication available without doctor's prescription.

Otitis: inflammation of ear, due to viral or bacterial infection, causing severe pain and high fever.

Otosclerosis: disease of bone surrounding inner ear, causing impaired hearing.

Ovate: egg-shaped.

Ovulation: the release of an egg from one of the ovaries.

Oxytocic: an agent that stimulates labor contractions.

Pack: folded, moistened, often medicated pad of cotton or cloth applied to body or inserted in cavity.

Pain: sensation of strong discomfort in bodily part.

Painkiller: agent that relieves or inhibits pain, analgesic.

Palisade cell: chloroplast-containing cell just below surface of a leaf.

Palliative: medicine that relieves symptoms but does not cure disease.

Palmate: with 3 or more leaflets, nerves, or lobes radiating from a central point.

Palpitation: abnormally rapid or violent heartbeat, esp. due to fear, exertion, neurosis, or arrhythmia.

Panacea: a cure-all.

Pancreatitis: inflammation of pancreas with sudden, severe pain.

Pandemic: epidemic disease that spreads to different countries over large region.

Panicle: loose, diversely branching flower clusters.

Papain: the protein-digesting enzyme of papaya.

Pappus: the calyx in a composite flower having feathery hairs, scales or bristles.

Papule: small, superficial bump or spot on skin, often part of rash.

Parahormone: chemical control agent that can be synthesized by more than one cell type.

Parasite: organism that lives in or on another living organism while contributing nothing to host's welfare, often causing irritation or interfering with function.

Parasiticide: prevents and destroys parasites such as fleas, lice, etc.

Parathyroid hormone: pth; hormone that promotes vitamin D synthesis and elevates blood calcium

Paregoric: camphorated tincture of opium used to relieve diarrhea, formerly used as painkiller.

Parenchyma: soft tissue forming chief substance of leaves and roots, fruit pulp, and center of stems.

Parkinson's disease: neurological disorder of late middle age characterized by tremor, rigidity, and little spontaneous movement.

Parkinsonism: Parkinson's disease.

Paroxysm: sudden, violent spasm or convulsion; abrupt worsening of symptom.

Parturient: aiding childbirth.

Passive immunity: short-term resistance to disease from injection of another's antibodies.

Pathogen: any agent, particularly a microorganism, that causes disease.

Pathogenesis: the process by which a disease originates and develops, particularly the cellular and physiologic processes.

Pathogenic: causing or producing disease.

Pectin: white, colloidal carbohydrate, found in certain ripe fruits, that has thickening properties.

Pedicel: stalk of single flower, fruit, or leaf.

Pediculicide: an agent which destroys lice.

Pediculosis: infestation of body and/or scalp by lice, causing itching and sometimes bacterial infection with weeping lesions.

Peduncle: stalk supporting flower or flower cluster of an angiosperm or bearing the fruiting body of a fungus.

Pellagra: B-vitamin nutritional deficiency that causes scaly dermatitis, diarrhea, and depression.

Pepsin: stomach enzyme that degrades proteins.

Peptic ulcer: breach in lining of digestive tract due to excess acid, occurring in esophagus, stomach, or duodenum.

Peptic: applied to gastric secretions and areas affected by them.

Peptide: compound of two or more amino acids.

Perennial: plant that lives more than two years, esp. herbaceous plant that produces flowers from the same root structure several years in a row.

Perfoliate: A leaf that appears to be perforated by the stem.

Perfusion: passage of fluid through tissue, esp. blood through lungs.

Pericarditis: acute or chronic inflammation of sac surrounding heart, due to viral infection, uremia, or cancer, often causing fever, chest pain, and fluid accumulation.

Periodontal disease: disease of gums, mouth lining, and bony structures supporting teeth, caused by plaque; pyorrhea.

Peripheral resistance: opposition to flow of blood in vessels.

Peristalsis: successive muscular contractions of the intestines which move food through the gastrointestinal tract.

Peristaltic waves: successive contractions of tubular wall.

Peritonitis: inflammation of abdominal cavity membrane, often due to bacteria spread in bloodstream or perforation or rupture of abdominal organ, causing pain, swelling, fever, and shock.

Pertussis: whooping cough.

Pessary: vaginal appliance or medicated suppository.

Petal: one of the circle of flower parts inside the sepals.

Petiole: the stalk of a leaf.

Petit mal: lesser epileptic seizure characterized by brief spells of sleepiness or unconsciousness.

pH: a scale from 0 to 14 used in measuring the acidity or alkalinity of solutions. Pure water, at pH 7.0, is considered neutral. Acidity increases as the numbers decrease. Alkalinity increases as the numbers increase.

Pharmaceutical: drug or medication manufactured and sold by pharmacy.

Pharmacology: medical science of drugs which deals with their actions, properties and characteristics.

Pharmacopoeia: an official publication of drugs in common use, in a given country.

Pharmacy: preparation and dispensing of drugs; place where this is done.

Pharyngitis: inflammation of pharynx that causes sore throat or tonsillitis.

Phenol: natural or synthetic aromatic compounds containing a hydroxide (—oh) ring.

Phlebitis: inflammation of vein wall, esp. in legs as complication of varicose veins, causing extreme tenderness.

Phlegm: sputum.

Phospholipid: lipid compound containing water-soluble phosphate group.

Photosynthesis: production of organic substances from carbon dioxide and water in green plant cells which chemically transform the energy of sunlight.

Physic: medicine or remedy, esp. laxative or cathartic.

Physiological: describes the natural biological processes of a living organism.

Physiology: the study of the functioning of the body, including the physical and chemical processes of its cells, tissues, organs and systems.

Physostigmine: a drug which blocks the breakdown of acetylcholine.

Phytoestrogen: plant compound which exerts estrogen-like effects.

Phytohormones: plant substances that mimic the action of human hormones.

Phytotherapy: the treatment of disease by plants; herbal medicine.

Picolinic acid: an amino acid secreted by the pancreas that facilitates zinc absorption and transport.

Piles: hemorrhoids.

Pill: small ball or tablet of medicine to be swallowed whole; oral contraceptive.

Pinkeye: conjunctivitis.

Pinnate: a leaf composed of more than three leaflets arranged in two rows along a common stalk.

Placebo: inactive substance taken by patient who believes that it is an effective drug, which often causes improvement in condition.

Plaque: sticky, colorless mixture of saliva, bacteria, and carbohydrates on surface of teeth that causes tartar and caries.

Plasma: fluid portion of blood and lymph.

Plaster: pasty medicinal dressing applied to body part on cloth as curative counterirritant.

Pleurisy: inflammation of pleurae that cover lungs, usu. due to pneumonia or other lung disease, causing painful breathing.

Pneumoconiosis: black lung.

Pneumonia: inflammation or infection of lungs in which air sacs fill with pus, causing coughing and chest pain.

Pneumothorax: collapsed lung.

Pod: vessel enclosing one or more seeds.

Podagra: gout of foot, esp. big toe.

Poliomyelitis: infectious viral disease of central nervous system, formerly epidemic, causing stiffness and paralysis of muscles, esp. respiratory system muscles.

Pollen: fine, dust-like grains containing male sexual cells, produced in anthers or similar structures of seed plants.

Polymer: natural or synthetic macromolecules formed by the repetition of an identical small molecule.

Polyp: benign growth on mucous membrane, esp. in nose, ear, or stomach.

Polypeptide: protein, polymer of amino acid subunits.

Polysaccharide: a molecule composed of many sugar molecules linked together.

Pomade: a prepared perfume material obtained by the enfleurage process.

Poultice: the therapeutic application of a soft moist mass (such as fresh herbs) to the skin, to encourage local circulation and to relieve pain.

Prednisone: synthetic steroid, administered orally, used to treat leukemia and Hodgkin's disease.

Press: device for drying and flattening botanical specimens.

Priapism: persistent erection of penis due to blood clottage.

Progesterone: hormone that prepares uterus to receive and develop fertilized egg.

Prognosis: assessment of future course and outcome of patient's disease.

Prophylactic: preventive of disease or infection.

Proptosis: forward displacement of an organ, esp. eyeball.

Prostaglandin: hormone-like compounds manufactured from essential fatty acids.

Prostatitis: inflammation of prostate gland, due to bacterial infection, sometimes causing urinary obstruction.

Prostration: total exhaustion.

Protease: protein-splitting enzyme.

Protein: any of a large class of organic nitrogenous substances containing amino acids.

Pruritis: itching.

Psoriasis: condition characterized by chronic, itchy, scaly silvery patches of skin, esp. on elbows, forearms, knees, and scalp, of unknown cause but sometimes due to anxiety.

Psychomotor: relating to disorders of muscular activity affected by cerebral disturbances.

Puerperal fever: blood poisoning in mother shortly after childbirth due to infection of womb lining or vagina.

Pulmonary embolism: obstruction by blood clot of artery that conveys blood from heart to lungs.

Purgative: laxative purge, purgative or cathartic medication.

Purpura: skin rash due to bleeding into skin from defective capillaries or blood platelet deficiency.

Pus: thick yellow or green liquid containing blood cells and dead cells, formed at site of infection or inflammation.

Pustule: small, pus-containing blister.

Putrescence: foul smell caused by decomposition of tissue.

Pyorrhea: periodontal disease.

Pyrexia: fever.

Pyrosis: heartburn.

Quinine: alkaloid drug used to treat malaria.

Quinsy: pus-discharging inflammation of tonsils.

Raceme: diversely branching flowers.

Radiation sickness: acute disease caused by exposure to radioactive emissions, causing nausea, vomiting, diarrhea, bleeding, hair loss, and death.

Rale: crepitation.

Raynaud's disease: disorder, esp. in women, in which spasms of arteries to extremities cause fingertips and toes to turn pale, blue, and numb.

Rays (ray flowers): The strap-like, often sterile flowers commonly called "petals" surrounding the flowerhead of a plant in the composite family.

Receptacle: the upper part of the stem from which the floral parts arise.

Rectification: the process of redistillation applied to essential oils to rid them of certain constituents.

Referred pain: pain felt in unexpected part of body separate from its source.

Reflex: automatic, involuntary activity caused by simple nervous circuits.

Refrigerant: cooling—reduces fever.

Regurgitation: vomiting.

Rejection: immune reaction to transplanted organ or foreign substance.

REM sleep: rapid eye movement sleep.

Renal calculus: kidney stone.

Renal colic: severe pain in kidney.

Renin: enzyme secreted by kidneys.

Resinoids: a perfumery material prepared from natural resinous matter, such as balsams, gum resins, etc.

Resins: a natural or prepared product, either solid or semi-solid in nature. Natural resins are exudations from trees, such as mastic; prepared resins are oleoresins from which the essential oil has been removed.

Resolvent: an agent which disperses swelling, or affects absorption of a new growth.

Respiration: exchange of gases between body tissues and surrounding environment.

Respiratory arrest: cessation of breathing.

Restorative: an agent that helps strengthen and revive the body systems.

Reticulosis: abnormal malignant overgrowth of cells of lymphatic glands or immune system.

Retinitis pigmentosa: hereditary condition that causes progressive degeneration of retina of eye.

Revulsive: relieves pain by means of the diversion of blood or disease from one part of the body to another.

Reye's syndrome: acute disorder primarily in children after viral infections such as chicken pox or influenza, associated with aspirin use, causing brain swelling and affecting organs.

Rheum: watery discharge from mucous membrane of mouth, eyes, or nose.

Rheumatic fever: delayed complication of upper respiratory streptococcus infection, esp. in young.

Rheumatic heart disease: scarring and chronic heart inflammation from progressive state of rheumatic fever.

Rheumatism: any disorder causing aches and pains in muscles or joints.

Rheumatoid arthritis: common form of arthritis that affects extremities, digits, and hips.

Rhizome: creeping horizontal stem lying at or just beneath soil surface, which bears leaves at its tip and roots from its underside.

Rickettsiae: group of parasitic organisms similar to bacteria that infest body through ticks or mites.

Ringworm: highly contagious fungal infection of skin, esp. scalp and feet or under beard.

Root: underground part of plant that functions in absorption, aeration, food storage, and as support system.

Rosacea: chronic acne characterized by red, pustular lesions about nose, cheeks, and forehead.

Roseola: rubella.

Rosette: leaves which are closely arranged in a spiral.

Rubefacient: they generate a localized increase in blood flow when applied to the skin, helping healing, cleansing and nourishment. They are often used to ease the pain and swelling of arthritic joints.

Rubella: highly contagious viral infection, primarily in children, causing enlarged lymph nodes in neck and pink rash; German measles; roseola.

Rubeola: measles.

Saccharide: a sugar molecule.

Saliva: watery, slightly acidic secretion of salivary glands that moistens food and initiates its breakdown.

Salmonella poisoning: food poisoning caused by aerobic intestinal bacteria.

Salt: the chemical combination of an acid and a base yields a salt plus water.

Salve: medicinal ointment used to soothe or heal skin irritations, burns, or wounds; ointment; unguent.

Saponins: these glycosides form a soap-like lather when shaken in water. There are two broad groups: the steroidal saponins, which seem to mimic the precursors of female sex hormones, and the tri-terpenoid saponins, which mimic the adrenal hormone ACTH.

Saprophyte: free-living organism that lives on dead or putrefying tissues.

Sarcoma: tumor of connective tissue.

Saturated fat: fat in which carbon chains are bonded by single bonds while simultaneously bound to as much hydrogen as possible.

Scab: hard crust of blood, serum, or pus over healing wound.

Scabies: skin infection from infestation of mites that causes severe itching, esp. around groin, nipples, and between fingers.

Scar: mark left on skin by healing wound where connective tissues replace damaged tissues; cicatrix.

Scarlatina: scarlet fever.

Scarlet fever: highly contagious childhood disease caused by streptococcus bacteria, characterized by sore throat and widespread rash; scarlatina.

Schistosomiasis: intestinal disease in tropics, due to infestation of blood flukes, that causes anemia, diarrhea, dysentery, and cirrhosis; snail fever.

Sciatica: condition marked by pain down back of thigh, due to disintegration of intervertebral disk, accompanied by numbness and stiff back.

Scleroderma: thickening and hardening of tissues beneath skin, causing rigidity of skin.

Sclerosis: hardening of tissue due to inflammation.

Scopolamine: belladonna derivative.

Scrape: abrasion.

Scurvy: vitamin C deficiency from absence of fresh fruit and vegetables in diet that causes swollen, bleeding gums, subcutaneous bleeding, and death when prolonged.

Seborrhea: excessive secretion by sebaceous glands in face, esp. at puberty.

Seborrheic dermatitis: skin eruption due to excess secretion of sebum, common on face at puberty.

Second-degree burn: blistering of surface skin and damage to underlying dermis.

Secretion: synthesis and release of substance by cell or organ.

Sedative: an agent which reduces functional activity; calming.

Seed: fertilized plant ovule containing embryo, capable of germinating to produce new plant.

Seizure: sudden attack of disease or condition.

Senescence: bodily degeneration after maturity.

Senile dementia: mental deterioration associated with aging.

Senility: loss of intellectual faculties in old age.

Sepal: leaflike, usu. green outer circle of calyx.

Septic: affected with putrefactive destruction by disease-carrying bacteria or their toxins.

Septicemia: tissue destruction by disease-causing bacteria or toxins absorbed from bloodstream; blood poisoning.

Serum: liquid portion of the blood.

Serum hepatitis: liver inflammation that causes fever and jaundice, transmitted by infected hypodermic needle or blood transfusion.

Sessile: Lacking a stalk; such as a leaf or flower with no obvious stalk.

Shingles: herpes zoster.

Sialogogue: an agent that stimulates the secretion of saliva.

SIDA: common name for AIDS outside U.S., based on Spanish sindromo inmuno-deficiencia adquirido or French syndrome immuno-deficitaire acquis.

Silique: a term applied to the peculiar seedpod structure of plants in the mustard family.

Slipped disk: abnormal protrusion of disk between abutting vertebrae, esp. in lumbar region, causing painful pressure against spinal cord; herniated disk.

Sinusitis: inflammation or infection of sinus sacs behind and around nose, causing headache and discharge through nose.

Soporific: a substance which induces sleep.

Spadix: a thick, fleshy flower spike usually enveloped by a spathe.

Spasm: sustained involuntary muscular contraction.

Spasmolytic: *see* antispasmodic.

Spastic colon: irritable bowel syndrome.

Spasticity: resistance to passive movement of limb; lack of motor coordination.

Spathe: A modified, leaflike structure surrounding a spadix.

Species: basic unit of biological classification ranking below genus, including similar organisms capable of interbreeding.

Spike: inflorescence in which flowers bloom along entire length of single stalk.

Spinal meningitis: meningitis.

Spirillum: spiral bacterium.

Splenic: relating to the spleen, the largest endocrine gland.

Spondylosis: degeneration of intervertebral disks in backbone, causing pain and restricting movement.

Sprue: deficient absorption of food due to intestinal disease that causes diarrhea, anemia, and inflamed tongue; psilosis.

Sputum: mucus coughed up from respiratory tract; phlegm.

Stamens: the pollen-bearing anthers with attached filaments (sometimes without filaments).

Stenosis: abnormal narrowing of blood vessel or heart valve.

Steroid: any of large family of chemical compounds including hormones produced by adrenal glands, ovaries, and testes; medication used for immunosuppression and hormone replacement.

Stimulant: an agent which quickens the physiological functions of the body.

Stipule: appendages resembling small leaves at the base of leaves of certain plants.

Stitch: sudden, sharp pain, usu. in muscle between ribs.

Stolon: stem that takes root at intervals along ground, forming new plants.

Stomachic: digestive aid and tonic; improving appetite.

Strangury: painful urination in which the urine is emitted in droplets due to muscle spasms.

Strep throat: infection of throat by streptococcus bacteria.

Stridor: loud, harsh breathing noise due to partial obstruction of trachea or larynx.

Stroke: sudden weakness or paralysis, often on one side of body, due to interruption of blood flow to brain caused by thrombosis, embolus, or hemorrhage; apoplexy; cerebrovascular accident.

Sty: acute bacterial infection of gland at base of eyelash.

Styptic: an astringent agent which stops or reduces external bleeding.

Subclinical: designating suspected disease or injury that is not developed enough to produce definite signs and symptoms.

Submucosa: the tissue just below the mucous membrane.

Succulent: plant with thick, fleshy tissues that store starch.

Sudorific: an agent which causes sweating.

Suppressor T cell: lymphocytes controlled by the thymus gland which suppress the immune response.

Suppuration: formation and discharge of pus.

Surfactant: a compound which reduces the surface tension in water, between water and another liquid, or between liquid and a solid.

Sycosis: inflammation and itching of hair follicles.

Sympatholytic: drug that affects sympathetic nervous system.

Symptom: characteristic indication of disease or disorder.

Synapse: junction between two excitable cells.

Syncope: fainting.

Syndrome: set of signs and symptoms indicative of particular disease or condition.

Syphilis: bacterial sexually transmitted disease that causes a chancre in acute stage and may lead to blindness or paralysis in chronic stage and insanity in advanced stage.

Systemic: affecting entire body, not just one part.

Systole: contraction of heart muscle.

Systolic: the first number in a blood pressure reading. The pressure in the arteries during the contraction phase of the heart beat.

T cell: a lymphocyte which is under the control of the thymus gland.

Tablet: small disk, made from compressed powders of one or more drugs, that is swallowed whole.

Tachycardia: abnormally increased heartbeat and pulse rate.

Tachypnea: rapid breathing.

Tampon: plug of absorbent material used to absorb blood or secretions, esp. in vagina for menstrual discharge.

Tannins: these are compounds that react with protein to produce a leather-like coating on animal tissue (as in the process of tanning). They promote healing and numbing (to reduce irritation), reduce inflammation, and halt infection.

Taproot: deep main root from which lateral roots develop.

Tartar: calcareous deposit and encrustation on teeth.

Taxonomy: system of classifying organisms into natural related groups based on shared features or traits.

Tendonitis: inflammation of bands of connective tissue that join muscle to bones and joints, due to physical trauma or hereditary disease.

Tendril: threadlike, often spiral part of climbing plant which clings to or coils around objects.

Teratogen: substance that can cause birth defects.

Teratoma: tumor composed of tissues not normally found at site.

Testosterone: principal male sex hormone produced by testes, used in replacement therapy and as an anabolic steroid.

Tetany: spasm and twitching of muscles of face, hands, and feet.

Thalassemia: genetic, anemic condition characterized by deficiency of hemoglobin in blood.

Thallus: nonvascular plant body without clear differentiation into stems, leaves, or roots.

Third-degree burn: total destruction of skin and damage to tissue beneath.

Thrombocytosis: condition marked by increase in number of platelets in blood.

Thromboembolism: condition in which blood clot forms at one point in circulation, dislodges, and moves to another point.

Thrombophlebius: inflammation of a vein and formation of blood clot that adheres to its wall.

Thrombosis: formation of a thrombus or blood clot.

Thrush: whitish spots and ulcers on mouth due to parasite, esp. in children; candidiasis.

Thyroid hormone: TH; thyroxine.

Tic douloureux: neuralgia of facial nerves.

Tincture: a herbal remedy, or perfumery material prepared in an alcohol base.

Tinea: athlete's foot.

Tinnitus: ringing in the ears.

Tissue: group of similar cells that performs particular function.

Tonic: tonics nurture and enliven.

Tonsillitis: inflammation of tonsils, due to bacterial or viral infection, causing sore throat and fever.

Topical: (of a drug) applied directly to skin surface, not taken internally.

Torpor: sluggishness, unresponsiveness to stimuli.

Torsion: twisting of a bodily organ or mass.

Toxemia: accumulation of toxins in blood.

Toxic: poisonous.

Toxicosis: any disease caused by toxic effect of a substance.

Toxin: poisonous substance.

Trifoliate: a plant having three distinct leaflets.

Triglyceride: neutral fat lipid molecule composed of glycerol and three fatty acids.

Troche: small, medicinal lozenge that soothes mouth and throat.

Tuber: fat underground stem from which some plants grow, similar to but shorter and thicker than a rhizome.

Tularemia: disease transmitted to humans from rabbits by deer flies or direct contamination, characterized by infection with ulcers, fever, aches, and enlarged lymph nodes.

Tumescence: swelling, esp. due to accumulation of blood or other fluid in tissue.

Tumor: abnormal growth of tissue in or on body part.

Tussis: cough.

Typhoid fever: bacterial infection of digestive system, transmitted through contaminated food or water, that causes high fever, red rash on stomach, chills, sweating, and sometimes intestinal hemorrhage.

Typhus: one of various infections caused by parasitic Rickettsiae that results in high fever, severe headache, widespread rash, and delirium.

Ulcer: open, inflamed, nonhealing sore in skin or mucous membrane, esp. in lining of alimentary canal.

Ulcerative colitis: inflammation and ulceration of colon and rectum.

Ultrasound: a test in which sound waves are used to examine the fetus or view the internal organs.

Umbel: umbrella-like; a flower where the petioles all arise from the top of the stem.

Unguent: fatty substance used to soothe and heal skin; ointment; salve.

Unsaturated fat: fat in which some carbons are linked by double bonds.

Uraemia: the retention of urine by the body and the presence of high levels of urine components in the blood.

Urea: nitrogenous waste product of kidneys.

Urethritis: inflammation of urethra, esp. among males, due to bacterial or viral infection or obstruction.

Urinalysis: the analysis of urine.

Urticaria: hives.

Uterine: pertaining to the uterus.

Vaginitis: irritation of vagina, due to inflammation or infection, causing burning pain and discharge.

Vapors: mentholated salve applied to chest and nose to relieve congestion.

Varicella: chicken pox.

Varicose veins: bulging, distended, sometimes painful veins in legs, rectum, or scrotum due to obstruction of blood flow.

Vascular plant: any plant, such as the angiosperms, gymnosperms, or ferns, in which the xylem and phloem conduct water and organic nutrients.

Vasoconstrictor: an agent which causes narrowing of blood vessels.

Vasoconstriction: the constriction of blood vessels.

Vasodilator: an agent which dilates the blood vessels.

Vector: any agent, such as insect or tick, that transmits parasitic microorganisms and infectious diseases from host to host.

Venereal disease: VD; any infectious disease transmitted by sexual contact, now usu. caused sexually transmitted disease; social disease.

Vermicide: chemical agent that kills parasitic worms in intestine.

Vermifuge: chemical agent used to expel parasites from intestine; anthelmintic.

Verruca: wart.

Vertigo: feeling that one's surroundings are in motion, esp. spinning, due to disease of inner ear or vestibular nerve.

Vesicant: causing blistering to the skin; a counterirritant.

Vesicle: very small skin blister containing clear serum.

Vesicle: a small blister or sac containing fluid.

Virulent: disease-producing.

Vitamin: an essential compound necessary to act as a catalyst in normal processes of the body.

Volatile oils: these complex compounds are chemical mixtures of hydrocarbons and alcohols in the plants.

Volatile: unstable, evaporates easily, as in "volatile oil"; *see* essential oil.

Vulnerary: remedies that promote wound healing. Used mainly to describe herbs for skin lesions, the action is just as relevant for wounds such as stomach ulcers.

Wart: small, hard, benign growth in skin, caused by virus.

Welt: raised ridge on skin caused by slash or blow.

Wheal: temporary, itching, red or pale raised area of skin due to abrasion or allergy.

Whooping cough: acute contagious bacterial infection of mucous membrane lining air passages, esp. in children, causing fever and paroxysmal cough with bleeding from mouth and nose; pertussis.

Whorl: a circle of leaves around a node.

Xanthoma: skin condition characterized by raised patches.

Xerostomia: diminished secretion of saliva that causes abnormally dry mouth, esp. as drug reaction.

Examples of Citations from the MEDLINE Database

The MEDLINE database has a wealth of material that relates to both specific medicinal plants and also the practice of phytotherapy. The examples given here have been selected to reflect the clinical interests of the practitioner, excluding those papers that are purely pharmacological.

Citations from the MEDLINE Database for the Genus *Achillea* (Yarrow)

Barel S Segal R Yashphe J
The antimicrobial activity of the essential oil from Achillea fragrantissima.
J Ethnopharmacol 1991 May-Jun;33(1-2):187-91

Chandler RF Hooper SN Hooper DL Jamieson WD Flinn CG Safe LM
Herbal remedies of the Maritime Indians: sterols and triterpenes of Achillea millefolium L. (Yarrow).
J Pharm Sci 1982 Jun;71(6):690-3

Goldberg AS Mueller EC Eigen E Desalva SJ
Isolation of the anti-inflammatory principles from Achillea millefolium (Compositae).
J Pharm Sci 1969 Aug;58(8):938-41

Ibragimov DI Kazanskaia GB
[Antimicrobial action of cranberry bush, common yarrow and Achillea biebersteinii]
Antibiotiki 1981 Feb;26(2):108-9 (Published in Russian)

Kelley BD Appelt GD Appelt JM
Pharmacological aspects of selected herbs employed in Hispanic folk medicine in the San Luis Valley of Colorado, USA: II. Asclepias asperula (inmortal) and Achillea lanulosa (plumajillo).
J Ethnopharmacol 1988 Jan;22(1):1-9

Peng Y Yan H Wang SQ Liu XT
65 cases of urinary tract infection treated by total acid of Achillea alpina.
J Tradit Chin Med 1983 Sep;3(3):217-8

Tewari JP Srivastava MC Bajpai JL
Phytopharmacologic studies of Achillea millefolium Linn.
Indian J Med Sci 1974 Aug;28(8):331-6

Citations from the MEDLINE Database for the Genus *Aesculus* (Horse Chestnut)

Boiadzhiev Ts Tomov T
[Experimental studies on the action of total extracts of Aesculus hippocastanum L. (horse chestnut) on cellular respiration]
Eksp Med Morfol (1973) 12(1):11-4 (Published in Bulgarian)

Hagen B
[The action mechanism of aesculus extract]
Med Klin (1970 Aug 28) 65(35):1534-7 (Published in German)

Konoshima T Lee KH
Antitumor agents, 82. Cytotoxic sapogenols from Aesculus hippocastanum.
J Nat Prod (1986 Jul-Aug) 49(4):650-6

Kronberger L Golles J
[On the prevention of thrombosis with aesculus extract]
Med Klin (1969) 64(26):1207-9 (Published in German)

Kunz K Schaffler K Biber A Wauschkuhn CH
[Bioavailability of beta-aescin after oral administration of two preparations containing aesculus extract to healthy volunteers]
Pharmazie (1991 Feb) 46(2):145 (Published in German)

Senatore F Mscisz A Mrugasiewicz K Gorecki P
Steroidal constituents and anti-inflammatory activity of the horse chestnut (Aesculus hippocastanum L.) bark.
Boll Soc Ital Biol Sper (1989 Feb) 65(2):137-41

Sokolova VE
[Effects of horse chestnut (Aesculus hippocastanum) on the course of experimental arteriosclerosis in rabbits]
Patol Fiziol Eksp Ter (1969 Jan-Feb) 13(1):84-6 (Published in Russian)

Tsutsumi S Ishizuka S
[Anti-inflammatory effects of the extract of Aesculus hippocastanum L. (horse chestnut) seed]
Shikwa Gakuho (1967 Nov) 67(11):1324-8 (Published in Japanese)

Tsutsumi S Ishizuka S
[Anti-inflammatory effect of Aesculus extract]
Shikwa Gakuho (1967 Oct) 67(10):1249-54 (Published in Japanese)

Citations from the MEDLINE Database for the Genus *Agrimonia* (Agrimony)

Giachetti D Taddei E Taddei I
[Diuretic and uricosuric activity of Agrimonia eupatoria L.]
Boll Soc Ital Biol Sper 1986 Jun 30;62(6):705-11 (Published in Italian)

Koshiura R Miyamoto K Ikeya Y Taguchi H
Antitumor activity of methanol extract from roots of Agrimonia pilosa Ledeb.
Jpn J Pharmacol 1985 May;38(1):9-16

Peter HM
[Antibiotic effect of extracts from Agrimonia-variety]
Pharmazie 1969 Oct;24(10):632-5 (Published in German)

Wang JP Hsu MF Teng CM
Antihemostatic effect of Hsien-Ho-T'sao (Agrimonia pilosa).
Am J Chin Med 1984 Summer;12(1-4):116-23

Wang JP Hsu MF Teng CM
Antiplatelet effect of hsien-ho-t'sao (Agrimonia pilosa).
Am J Chin Med 1985;13(1-4):109-18

Citations from the MEDLINE Database for *Allium sativum* (Garlic)

Aboul-Enein AM
Inhibition of tumor growth with possible immunity by Egyptian garlic extracts.
Nahrung 1986; 30(2):161-9

Garlic bulbs (*Allium sativum*) were extracted with distilled water or ethanol. The extracts were then incubated with Ehrlich ascites carcinoma cells at 37 degrees C for 1 h. These pretreated cells were injected into Swiss albino mice which survived over 12 weeks. To the contrary, tumor cells which were pretreated with garlic extracts produced ascites tumor in all mice that died 2 or 4 weeks after intraperitoneal injection. When mice were treated twice at intervals of 7 days with freshly prepared tumor cells exposed to watery or ethanolic extracts of fresh garlic, they acquired resistance against a challenge with Ehrlich ascites tumor cells. Administration of garlic extracts to mice for at least 2 weeks before tumor transplantation caused a slight delay of 10-20 days in tumor growth and animal death. Generally, the ethanolic extract of garlic gave more pronounced effect as tumor inhibitor as well as immunity induction than watery extract. No change in serum electrophoretic pattern was detected in mice, whether the tumor cells injected were incubated or not with garlic extract. In animals treated with unincubated tumor cells, albumin and globulin percentages as well as albumin: globulin ratios (A/G) were decreased as compared to normal mice. A/G ratio was also decreased in immunized mice, pretreated with garlic extract, due to the increase of gamma globulin and unchanging of albumin.

Adoga GI
Effect of garlic oil extract on glutathione reductase levels in rats fed on high sucrose and alcohol diets: a possible mechanism of the activity of the oil.
Biosci Rep 1986 Oct; 6(10):909-12

The effect on glutathione reductase activities of feeding garlic oil to white albino rats maintained on high sucrose and alcohol diets was studied. Whereas high sucrose and alcohol diets resulted in significant increases in the activity of glutathione reductase in liver, kidneys and serum, the presence of garlic oil restored the levels to near normal. It is proposed that the mechanism of this action of garlic oil involves the active principle, diallyl disulphide, which interacts in an exchange reaction with enzymes and substrates such as glutathione reductase and glutathione which contain thiol groups.

Adoga GI Osuji J
Effect of garlic oil extract on serum, liver and kidney enzymes of rats fed on high sucrose & alcohol diets.
Biochem Int 1986 Oct; 13(4):615-24

High levels of alkaline phosphatase and alcohol dehydrogenase were observed in the serum, liver and kidneys of rats fed on high sucrose and high alcohol diets over a period of 75 days. Garlic oil extract fed with any of the diets significantly lowered the high levels of the two enzymes in the serum, liver and kidneys. This effect may be due to reduced biosynthesis of fatty acids as NADPH, required for the process, is utilised for the metabolism of the oil.

Ali M Mohammed SY
Selective suppression of platelet thromboxane formation with sparing of vascular prostacyclin synthesis by aqueous extract of garlic in rabbits.
Prostaglandins Leukotrienes Med 1986 Dec; 25(2-3):139-46

It has been suggested that a drug which selectively inhibits platelet thromboxane synthesis, sparing vascular synthesis of prostacyclin, would be more effective as an anti-thrombotic agent. We studied the effect of an aqueous extract of garlic on the production of thromboxane and prostacyclin by rabbit whole blood and aorta in vitro and ex vivo. A dose-dependent inhibition of thromboxane production was observed during blood clotting. Synthesis of prostacyclin was not affected by any concentration of garlic extract used in the experiment. A slight but insignificant reduction in the vascular synthesis of prostacyclin was observed at the highest concentration of garlic used in in vitro experiments. The synthesis of thromboxane by aorta was completely suppressed at all the concentrations of garlic tested. A similar pattern of results was observed after intraperitoneal administration of garlic (1 ml/kg) for one week on the enzymatic synthesis of thromboxane and prostacyclin of these tissues ex-vivo. Aortic synthesis of prostacyclin was significantly increased in the garlic treated rabbits compared to the controls. The data obtained from these rabbit experiments suggested that it may be possible to achieve a selective suppression of thromboxane formation by platelets with sparing of vascular synthesis of prostacyclin by garlic treatment.

Apitz-Castro R Cabrera S Cruz MR Ledezma E Jain MK
Effects of garlic extract and of three pure components isolated from it on human platelet aggregation, arachidonate metabolism, release reaction and platelet ultrastructure.
Thromb Res 1983 Oct 15; 32(2):155-69

We studied the effect of the methanol extract of garlic bulbs (EOG) and of three pure components isolated from it (F1, F2, F3), on human platelet aggregation induced by ADP, epinephrine, collagen, thrombin, arachidonate, PAF, and the ionophore A-23187. Incubation of PRP with EOG, either in methanol or in homologous PPP, inhibits platelet aggregation induced by all of the above mentioned agonists. F1, F2, and F3 also inhibit platelet aggregation, however, F3 was about four times more potent. Addition of EOG or F3 to platelets that have already been irreversibly aggregated by 10 microM ADP induces rapid deaggregation. Inhibition of aggregation was still present after three hours. The inhibitory effect persisted even after the treated platelets were Gel-Filtered (GFP) or separated from plasma through a metrizamide gradient and resuspended in new homologous PPP. Thrombin-induced release of ATP from GFP was inhibited by 75-80% after EOG or F3 treatment. Incorporation of [3-H]-arachidonate by intact platelets was decreased by 50-60% in treated platelets. However, platelets incubated with the inhibitors after incorporation of radiolabeled arachidonate, although they did not aggregate, produced, after thrombin activation, similar amounts of radiolabeled TXB2 and lipoxygenase products as the controls. Electron microscopy of inhibited platelets, in the presence of thrombin, showed no degranulation but an increase of spherical forms. Our results suggest that the effects described might be mediated by a perturbation of the physicochemical properties of the plasma membrane rather than by affecting arachidonate or calcium metabolism in the cells. Chemical structures of F1, F2 and F3 have been provisionally assigned: F1 is diallyltrisulfide, F2 is 2-vinyl-1,3-dithiene, and F3 is most probably allyl 1,5-hexadienyltrisulfide.

Ariga
Platelet aggregation inhibitor in garlic.
Lancet (1981 Jan 17) 1(8212):150-1

Bakhsh R Chughtai MI
Influence of garlic on serum cholesterol, serum triglycerides, serum total lipids and serum glucose in human subjects.
Nährung 1984; 28(2):159-63

Human subjects were used for a garlic experiment. The subjects were given a fat-rich diet for 7 days and on the 8th day the fasting blood was analyzed for serum cholesterol, serum triglycerides, serum total lipids and serum glucose. The human subjects were then given a fat-rich diet with 40 g of garlic for 7 days and on the 15th day the fasting blood was analyzed for the above investigations. On a fat-rich diet the serum cholesterol, serum triglycerides and serum total lipids were significantly increased as compared to normally fed diet. When 40 g of garlic was substituted in fat-rich diet for 7 days, the garlic significantly reduced the serum cholesterol and serum triglycerides.

Bhushan S Sharma SP Singh SP Agrawal S Indrayan A Seth P
Effect of garlic on normal blood cholesterol level.
Indian J Physiol Pharmacol 1979 Jul-Sep; 23(3):211-4

The effect of raw garlic on normal blood cholesterol level in males of the age group of 18-35 years was studied. The subjects, who never ingested garlic before, were given 10 g of garlic daily with their diet for two months. Fasting blood samples were investigated in respect of cholesterol before and after two months of garlic intake. Initially the blood cholesterol level ranged between 160-250 mg which decreased significantly in all the subjects of experimental group after two months of ingestion of garlic. The slight decrease or increase in the blood cholesterol level of control group was not significant. The raw garlic can be advocated for daily ingestion in order to lower one's blood cholesterol level even if it is within normal limits.

Bordia A
Effect of garlic on blood lipids in patients with coronary heart disease. Am J Clin Nutr 1981 Oct; 34(10):2100-3

The study was conducted on two groups of individuals. Group A consisted of 20 healthy volunteers who were fed garlic for 6 months and then followed for another 2 months without garlic. Garlic administration significantly lowered the serum cholesterol and triglycerides while raising the high-density lipoproteins. Group B consisted of 62 patients with coronary heart disease with elevated serum cholesterol. They were randomly divided into two subgroups: B1 was fed garlic for 10 months while B2 served as a control. Garlic decreased the serum cholesterol (p less than 0.05), triglycerides (p less than 0.05) and low density lipoprotein (p less than 0.05) while increasing the high-density fraction (p less than 0.001). The change reached statistically significant levels at the end of 8 months and persisted for the next 2 months of follow-up. Thus, the essential oil of garlic has shown a distinct hypolipidemic action in both healthy individuals and patients with coronary heart disease.

Boullin
Garlic as a platelet inhibitor.
Lancet (1981 Apr 4) 1(8223):776-7

Chutani SK Bordia A
The effect of fried versus raw garlic on fibrinolytic activity in man.
Atherosclerosis 1981 Feb-Mar; 38(3-4):417-21

The effect of fried and raw garlic on blood fibrinolytic activity has been compared in 20 patients with ischaemic heart disease. Three blood samples were collected on the first day of the study and similarly on the 2nd and 7th days after garlic administration, either in raw or fried form. Fibrinolytic activity increased by 72% and 63% within 6 h of administration of raw or fried garlic, respectively. The elevated levels were maintained up to 12 h. In the second part of the study, raw or fried garlic was administered for 4 weeks to patients with ischaemic heart disease and fibrinolytic activity was measured at weekly intervals. It showed a sustained increase, rising to 84.8% at the end of 28th day when raw garlic was administered. Similarly, with fried garlic the rise was 72%. The study shows that: (i) both raw and fried garlic significantly enhance fibrinolytic activity (FA); (ii) garlic enhances FA within hours of administration; (iii) FA continues to rise with continued administration of garlic; (iv) frying removes the strong acrid smell of garlic, but preserves its useful effect on FA.

Foushee DB Ruffin J Banerjee U
Garlic as a natural agent for the treatment of hypertension: a preliminary report.
Cytobios 1982; 34(135-36):145-52

The major objective of this study was to re-evaluate the effects of garlic on blood pressure with respect to its ability to provoke a decrease in blood pressure and to determine the length of time that this decrease would require. Spontaneously hypertensive rats were given three doses of garlic extract (0.1 ml/kg, 0.25 ml/kg, and 0.5 ml/kg) by oral injection. The blood pressures of these ether-anaesthetized rats were measured immediately before the extract was given, and then 0.5, 2, 4, 6, and 24 h after the extract was given. A blood pressure measurement was also taken at 48 h after extract administration for the 0.5 ml/kg dose. The Gilson Duograph System was used to measure blood pressure by the tail-cuff method. There was a marked decrease in the systolic blood pressure of all of the rats after three doses and the decrease occurred within 30 min in each case. Even though the average decreases for the 0.1 ml/kg and the 0.25 ml/kg doses were calculated as 51.25 mm Hg and 56.25 mm Hg, respectively, these doses were not sufficient to sustain the blood pressure in a normal range for more than 1 or 2 h. The 0.5 ml/kg dose, showing an average decrease of 65.7 mm Hg, was sufficient to provoke a decrease to a normal level and to sustain this decrease for up to 24 h. The results indicate that garlic is effective as a natural agent for the treatment of hypertension.

Jain
Effect of garlic oil in experimental cholesterol atherosclerosis.
Atherosclerosis 1978 Feb; 29(2):125-9

Addition of cholesterol in the diet of male albino rabbits produced hypercholesterolaemia, increased tissue cholesterol, and atheromatous changes in the aorta. Supplementation of garlic oil along with cholesterol significantly inhibited the hypercholesterolaemia, decreased tissue cholesterol and minimised the atheromatous changes in the aorta. These results show that the active constituent(s) in garlic responsible for its anti-atherogenic action is present in the oily fraction of garlic.

Kagawa K Matsutaka H Yamaguchi Y Fukuhama C
Garlic extract inhibits the enhanced peroxidation and production of lipids in carbon tetrachloride-induced liver injury.
Pn J Pharmacol 1986 Sep; 42(1):19-26

Carbon tetrachloride (CCl4) enhances lipid peroxidation, resulting in triglyceride accumulation in the liver. In this report, we studied the therapeutic, but not the preventive, effect of garlic extract on CCl4-intoxicated liver, in comparison to the effect of vitamin E. Garlic extract was given orally to mice in the dose of 10, 100 or 500 mg/kg at 6 hr after CCl4 administration. The increased conjugated-diene level was diminished significantly to 82% by the 100 mg/kg extract, and also thiobarbituric acid-reactivity was inhibited by all the doses of the extract. In addition to the above mentioned effects, the high doses of garlic extract lowered hepatic triglyceride and lipid contents. Highly significant and positive correlation was observed between hepatic triglyceride content and conjugated-diene level in the lipid fraction of the liver. Besides, vitamin E at the dose of 25 mg/kg inhibited only lipid peroxidation. We, therefore, conclude that not only is garlic extract effective on diminution of lipid peroxide and on alteration of peroxidative status to more reductive condition like the effect of vitamin E, but it also inhibits hepatic triglyceride accumulation in injured liver.

Morowitz
Between gargoylism and gas gangrene.
Hosp Pract (1981 Sep) 16(9):173, 176

Mohammad SF Woodward SC
Characterization of a potent inhibitor of platelet aggregation and release reaction isolated from *allium sativum* (garlic).
Thromb Res 1986 Dec 15; 44(6):793-806

When added to platelet-rich plasma, aqueous extracts of garlic inhibited platelet aggregation and the release reaction. Subsequent experiments designed to characterize the inhibitory component revealed that the inhibitory activity was i) associated with small molecular-weight components, ii) the inhibitory component possessed the typical garlic odor and contained an abundance of sulfur, iii) the inhibitory activity could be extracted with organic solvents, and iv) temperatures above 56 degrees C and alkaline pH above 8.5 quickly destroyed the inhibitory activity. The Rf value of the major inhibitory component after thin-layer chromatographic separation was similar to that of allicin, a unique thiosulfinate in garlic previously shown to possess strong antibiotic and antifungal properties. Allicin was synthesized. On thin-layer chromatographic plates, allicin co-migrated with the inhibitory component in garlic. At 10 microM concentration, allicin inhibited completely platelet aggregation and the release reaction. Comparative studies suggest that the major platelet aggregation and release inhibitor in garlic may be allicin.

Osler
Garlic—natural remedy for atherosclerosis-related symptoms?
Ugeskr Laeger (1985 Jan 14) 147(3):151-5

Sainani GS Desai DB Natu MN Katrodia KM Valame VP Sainani PG
Onion, garlic, and experimental atherosclerosis.
Jpn Heart J 1979 May; 20(3):351-7

Forty-two healthy male albino rabbits weighing around 1 Kg were divided into 4 groups. Group I (8)-fed on normal stock diet, Group II (8)-fed on stock diet plus cholesterol (0.5 gm in 5 ml of olive oil). Group III (15)-received stock diet plus cholesterol plus garlic (0.25 gm) juice. Group IV (11)-received stock diet plus cholesterol plus onion (2.5 gm) juice. The animals were closely observed and followed for 16 weeks. Approximately every 4 weeks, blood samples were collected for estimation of various parameters (S. cholesterol, S. triglycerides, S. lipoproteins, S. phospolipids, and fibrinolytic activity). At the end of experiment, animals were sacrificed and degree of aortic atherosclerosis was graded (grade 0 to 4) in different groups and compared. Experimental study revealed that both garlic and onion (garlic more than onion) had significant effect in inhibiting the rise in S. cholesterol, S. triglycerides, S. beta lipoproteins, and S. phospolipids and significant effect in enhancing the fibrinolytic activity. The beta: alpha ratio was altered favourably and the ratio was kept close to normal. As regards the degree of aortic atherosclerosis as seen on post mortem, it was significantly less in garlic and onion group when compared with pure cholesterol group.

Sharma
Effects of garlic extract and of three pure components isolated from it on human platelet aggregation, arachidonate metabolism, release reaction and platelet ultrastructure—comments
Thromb Res (1985 Feb 1) 37(3):489-90

Shoetan A Augusti KT Joseph PK
Hypolipidemic effects of garlic oil in rats fed ethanol and a high lipid diet.
Experientia 1984 Mar 15; 40(3):261-3

Feeding of ethanol and a high fat-high cholesterol diet to rats markedly increased the total lipids in the liver, and cholesterol and triglyceride levels in the serum, liver and kidneys. However, when ethanol mixed with 0.5% garlic oil was fed to animals maintained on the high fat-high cholesterol diet, these lipid levels were significantly reduced to levels near to those seen in untreated control rats. Garlic oil did not reduce the serum albumin or the total proteins of liver, kidneys or serum when fed along with ethanol. Probably the garlic oil enhances the catabolism of dietary cholesterol and fatty acids.

Citations from the MEDLINE Database for the Genus *Angelica* (Angelica, Dong Quoi)

Feng Y Lian NJ Jia ZL
[Clinical observations on the treatment of sudden deafness with concentrated Angelica injection]
Chung Hsi I Chieh Ho Tsa Chih 1986 Sep;6(9):536-7, 516 (Published in Chinese)

Guo TL Zhou XW
[Clinical observations on the treatment of the gestational hypertension syndrome with Angelica and Paeonia powder] Chung Hsi I
Chung Hsi I Chieh Ho Tsa Chih 1986 Dec;6(12):714-6, 707 (Published in Chinese)

Harada M Suzuki M Ozaki Y
Effect of Japanese Angelica root and peony root on uterine contraction in the rabbit in situ.
J Pharmacobiodyn 1984 May;7(5):304-11

He ZP Wang DZ Shi LY Wang ZQ
Treating amenorrhea in vital energy-deficient patients with angelica sinensis-astragalus membranaceus menstruation-regulating decoction.
J Tradit Chin Med 1986 Sep;6(3):187-90

Hikino H
Recent research on Oriental medicinal plants.
Economic Medical Plant Research 1:53-85, 1985

Kimura Y Ohminami H Arichi H Okuda H Baba K Kozawa M Arichi S
Effects of various coumarins from roots of Angelica dahurica on actions of adrenaline, ACTH and insulin in fat cells.
Planta Med 1982 Jul;45(3):183-7

Kimura Y Okuda H
Effects of active compounds isolated from Angelica shikokiana on lipid metabolism in fat cells.
J Ethnopharmacol 1989 May;25(3):269-80

Kimura Y Okuda H Baba K Kozawa M Arichi S
Effects of an active substance isolated from the roots of Angelica shikokiana on leukotriene and monohydroxyeicosatetreaenoic acid biosyntheses in human polymorphonuclear leukocytes.
Planta Med 1987 Dec;53(6):521-5

Ko FN Wu TS Liou MJ Huang TF Teng CM
Inhibition of platelet thromboxane formation and phosphoinositides breakdown by osthole from Angelica pubescens.
Thromb Haemost 1989 Nov 24;62(3):996-9

Kosuge T Yokota M Sugiyama K Yamamoto T Mure T Yamazawa H
Studies on bioactive substances in crude drugs used for arthritic diseases in traditional Chinese medicine. II. Isolation and identification of an anti-inflammatory and analgesic principle from the root of Angelica pubescens Maxim.
Chem Pharm Bull (Tokyo) 1985 Dec;33(12):5351-4

Kumazawa Y Mizunoe K Otsuka Y
Immunostimulating polysaccharide separated from hot water extract of Angelica acutiloba Kitagawa (Yamato tohki).
Immunology 1982 Sep;47(1):75-83

Kumazawa Y Nakatsuru Y Fujisawa H Nishimura C Mizunoe K Otsuka Y Nomoto K
Lymphocyte activation by a polysaccharide fraction separated from hot water extracts of Angelica acutiloba Kitagawa.
J Pharmacobiodyn 1985 Jun;8(6):417-24

Mei QB Tao JY Cui B
Advances in the pharmacological studies of radix Angelica sinensis (Oliv) Diels (Chinese Danggui).
Chin Med J (Engl) 1991 Sep;104(9):776-81

Mei QB Tao JY Zhang HD Duan ZX Chen YZ
[Effects of Angelica sinensis polysaccharides on hemopoietic stem cells in irradiated mice]
Chung Kuo Yao Li Hsueh Pao 1988 May;9(3):279-82 (Published in Chinese)

Okuyama T Takata M Takayasu J Hasegawa T Tokuda H Nishino A Nishino H Iwashima A
Anti-tumor promotion by principles obtained from Angelica keiskei.
Planta Med 1991 Jun;57(3):242-6

Sung CP Baker AP Holden DA Smith WJ Chakrin LW
Effect of extracts of Angelica polymorpha on reaginic antibody production.
J Nat Prod 1982 Jul-Aug;45(4):398-406

Tanaka S Ikeshiro Y Tabata M Konoshima M
Anti-nociceptive substances from the roots of Angelica acutiloba.
Arzneimittelforschung 1977;27(11):2039-45

Tao JY Ruan YP Mei QB Liu S Tian QL Chen YZ Zhang HD Duan ZX
[Studies on the antiasthmatic action of ligustilide of dang-gui, Angelica sinensis (Oliv.) Diels]
Yao Hsueh Hsueh Pao 1984 Aug;19(8):561-5 (Published in Chinese)

Yan TY Hou AC Sun BT
[Injection of Angelica sinensis in treating infantile pneumonia and its experimental study in rabbits]
Chung His I Chieh Ho Tsa Chih 1987 Mar;7(3):161-2, 133 (Published in Chinese)

Yoshiro K
The physiological actions of tang-kuei and cnidium.
Bull Oriental Healing Arts Inst USA 10:269-78, 1985

Zhang YK Wang HY Wang SX
[The effect of the Chinese medical herbs Astragalus membranaceus and Angelica sinensis on 3 kinds of experimental nephritis]
Chung Hua Nei Ko Tsa Chih 1986 Apr;25(4):222-5, 254 (Published in Chinese)

Zhou JZ
[Various pharmacological actions of Angelica extracts]
Chung Yao Tung Pao 1985 Apr;10(4):39-41 (Published in Chinese)

Citations from the MEDLINE Database for the Genus *Arnica* (Arnica)

Duquenois P
[A still mysterious medicinal plant, Arnica montana L]
Pharm Weekbl 1971 Mar 19;106(12):190-7 (Published in French)

Hofmeyr GJ Piccioni V Blauhof P
Postpartum homeopathic Arnica montana: a potency-finding pilot study.
Br J Clin Pract 1990 Dec;44(12):619-21

Kaziro GS
Metronidazole (Flagyl) and Arnica montana in the prevention of post-surgical complications, a comparative placebo controlled clinical trial.
Br J Oral Maxillofac Surg 1984 Feb;22(1):42-9

Labadie RP
[Arnica montana L.]
Pharm Weekbl 1968 Jun 21;103(25):769-81 (Published in Dutch)

Schroder H Losche W Strobach H Leven W Willuhn G Till U Schror K
Helenalin and 11 alpha,13-dihydrohelenalin, two constituents from Arnica montana L., inhibit human platelet function via thiol-dependent pathways.
Thromb Res 1990 Mar 15;57(6):839-45

Tveiten D Bruseth S Borchgrevink CF Lohne K
[Effect of Arnica D 30 during hard physical exertion. A double-blind randomized trial during the Oslo Marathon 1990]
Tidsskr Nor Laegeforen 1991 Dec 10;111(30):3630-1 (Published in Norwegian)

Willuhn G
[New findings from research on arnica]
Pharm Unserer Zeit 1981 Jan;10(1):1-7 (Published in German)

Citations from the MEDLINE Database for the genus *Arctium* (Burdock)

Dombradi CA Foldeak S
Screening report on the antitumor activity of purified Arctium Lappa extracts.
Tumori (1966 May-Jun) 52(3):173-5

Morita K Kada T Namiki M
A dysmutagenic factor isolated from burdock (Arctium Lappa Linne).
Mutat Res (1984 Oct) 129(1):25-31

Citations from the MEDLINE Database for the Genus *Arctostaphylos* (Bearberry, Uva-Ursi)

Jahodar L Jilek P Paktova M Dvorakova V
[Antimicrobial effect of arbutin and an extract of the leaves of Arctostaphylos uva-ursi in vitro]
Cesk Farm 1985 Jun;34(5):174-8 (Published in Czech)

Jahodar L Leifertova I Lisa M
Investigation of iridoid substances in Arctostaphylos uva-ursi.
Pharmazie 1978 Aug;33(8):536-7

Kubo M Ito M Nakata H Matsuda H
[Pharmacological studies on leaf of Arctostaphylos uva-ursi (L.) Spreng. I. Combined effect of 50% methanolic extract from Arctostaphylos uva-ursi (L.) Spreng. (bearberry leaf) and prednisolone on immuno-inflammation]
Yakugaku Zasshi 1990 Jan;110(1):59-67 (Published in Japanese)

Matsuda H Nakata H Tanaka T Kubo M
[Pharmacological study on Arctostaphylos uva-ursi (L.) Spreng. II. Combined effects of arbutin and prednisolone or dexamethazone on immuno-inflammation]
Yakugaku Zasshi 1990 Jan;110(1):68-76 (Published in Japanese)

Matsuda H Tanaka T Kubo M
[Pharmacological studies on leaf of Arctostaphylos uva-ursi (L.) Spreng. III. Combined effect of arbutin and indomethacin on immuno-inflammation]
Yakugaku Zasshi 1991 Apr-May;111(4-5):253-8 (Published in Japanese)

Citations from the MEDLINE Database for the genus *Astragalus* (Astragalus)

Chai ZN
[Effects of Codonopsis pilosular-Astragalus injection on the cyclic nucleotide levels and phosphodiesterase activity in platelets]
Chung Hsi I Chieh Ho Tsa Chih (1984 Aug) 4(8):486-7 (Published in Chinese)

Chai ZN
[Effects of Codonopsis pilosulae-Astragalus injection on superficial activity and ultrastructure of platelets]
Chung Hsi I Chieh Ho Tsa Chih (1984 Aug) 4(8):484-5 (Published in Chinese)

Chang CY Hou YD Xu FM
[Effects of Astragalus membranaceus on enhancement of mouse natural killer cell activity]
Chung Kuo I Hsueh Ko Hsueh Yuan Hsueh Pao (1983 Aug) 5(4):231-4

Chen LJ Shen ML Wang MY Zhai SK Liu MZ
[Effect of Astragalus polysaccharides on phagocytic function in mice (author's transl)]
Chung Kuo Yao Li Hsueh Pao (1981 Sep) 2(3):200-4 (Published in Chinese)

Chu DT Lepe-Zuniga J Wong WL LaPushin R Mavligit GM
Fractionated extract of Astragalus membranaceus, a Chinese medicinal herb, potentiates LAK cell cytotoxicity generated by a low dose of recombinant interleukin-2.
J Clin Lab Immunol (1988 Aug) 26(4):183-7

Chu DT Wong WL Mavligit GM
Immunotherapy with Chinese medicinal herbs. II. Reversal of cyclophosphamide-induced immune suppression by administration of fractionated Astragalus membranaceus in vivo.
J Clin Lab Immunol (1988 Mar) 25(3):125-9

Chu DT Wong WL Mavligit GM
Immunotherapy with Chinese medicinal herbs. I. Immune restoration of local xenogeneic graft-versus-host reaction in cancer patients by fractionated Astragalus membranaceus in vitro.
J Clin Lab Immunol (1988 Mar) 25(3):119-23

Dong DC Zhou LF Chen JX
[Changes in proteinuria, renal function and immunity after treatment with injections of a solution of Astragalus membranaceus]
Chung Hsi I Chieh Ho Tsa Chih (1987 Jul) 7(7):403-4, 388 (Published in Chinese)

Geng CS
[Advances in immuno-pharmacological studies on Astragalus membranaceus]
Chung Hsi I Chieh Ho Tsa Chih (1986 Jan) 6(1):62-4 (Published in Chinese)

He ZP Wang DZ Shi LY Wang ZQ
Treating amenorrhea in vital energy-deficient patients with angelica sinensis-astragalus membranaceus menstruation-regulating decoction.
J Tradit Chin Med (1986 Sep) 6(3):187-90

Hikino H Funayama S Endo K
Hypotensive principle of Astragalus and Hedysarum roots.
Planta Med (1976 Dec) 30(4):297-302

Li WS Liao JZ Yue ZS Liu XF Wu ZM Kang TP
Effects of codonopsis pilosula-astragalus injection on platelet aggregation and activity of PGI2-like substance.
J Tradit Chin Med (1986 Mar) 6(1):9-12

Liao JZ Chai ZN Li WS Liu XF Wang S Qin L Guo WQ
Pharmacologic effects of codonopsis pilosula-astragalus injection in the treatment of CHD patients.
J Tradit Chin Med (1988 Mar) 8(1):1-8

Pan SY
[Pharmacological action of Astragalus membranaceus on the central nervous system in mice]
Chung Yao Tung Pao (1986 Sep) 11(9):47-9

Ponomarenko AP
[The effect of astragalus on the functional status of the liver in patients with chronic circulatory insufficiency]
Vrach Delo (1966 Apr) 4:72-4 (Published in Russian)

Qian ZW Li YY
[Synergism of Astragalus membranaceus with interferon in the treatment of cervical erosion and their antiviral activities]
Chung Hsi I Chieh Ho Tsa Chih (1987 May) 7(5):268-9, 287, 259

Shen ML
[Biological activities of Astragalus polysaccharides]
Chung Hsi I Chieh Ho Tsa Chih (1984 Oct) 4(10):615-7, 581

Skakun NP Blikhar EI Oleinik AN
[Use of Astragalus dasyanthus in lesions of the liver in patients with pulmonary tuberculosis]
Vrach Delo (1988 Jun) (6):51-4 (Published in Russian)

Sun Y Hersh EM Lee SL McLaughlin M Loo TL Mavligit GM
Preliminary observations on the effects of the Chinese medicinal herbs Astragalus membranaceus and Ligustrum lucidum on lymphocyte blastogenic responses.
J Biol Response Mod (1983) 2(3):227-37

Wang DY Yang WY
[Effect of Astragalus polysaccharides on ribonucleic acid metabolism of spleen and liver cells of mice]
Chung Kuo Yao Li Hsueh Pao (1982 Sep) 3(3):204-7 (Published in Chinese)

Wang DY Zhang W Xu GY
[Protective effect of Astragalus polysaccharides on ribonucleases and the ribonuclease inhibitor system]
Chung Hsi I Chieh Ho Tsa Chih (1987 Feb) 7(2):93-6, 70 (Published in Chinese)

Zhang YD Shen JP Song J Wang YL Shao YN Li CF Zhou SH Li YF Li DX
[Effects of Astragalus saponin 1 on cAMP and cGMP levels in plasma and DNA synthesis in the regenerating liver]
Yao Hsueh Hsueh Pao (1984 Aug) 19(8):619-21

Zhang YK Wang HY Wang SX
[The effect of the Chinese medical herbs Astragalus membranaceus and Angelica sinensis on 3 kinds of experimental nephritis]
Chung Hua Nei Ko Tsa Chih (1986 Apr) 25(4):222-5, 254

Zhao YH
[Preliminary observation on the therapeutic effect of Astragalus membranaceus in experimental anti-glomerular basement membrane nephritis in rabbits]
Chung Hsi I Chieh Ho Tsa Chih (1983 Sep) 3(5):302-3 (Published in Chinese)

Citations from the MEDLINE Database for the Genus *Baptisia* (Wild Indigo)

Beuscher N Kopanski L
[Stimulation of immunity by the contents of Baptisia tinctoria]
Planta Med (1985 Oct) (5):381-4

Beuscher N Scheit KH Bodinet C Kopanski L
[Immunologically active glycoproteins of Baptisia tinctoria]
Planta Med (1989 Aug) 55(4):358-63

Citations from the MEDLINE Database for the Genus *Calendula* (Calendula, Marigold)

Bogdanova NS Nikolaeva IS Shcherbakova LI Tolstova TI Moskalenko NIu Pershin GN
[Study of antiviral properties of Calendula officinalis]
Farmakol Toksikol (1970 May-Jun) 33(3):349-55

Boucaud-Maitre Y Algernon O Raynaud J
Cytotoxic and antitumoral activity of Calendula officinalis extracts.
Pharmazie (1988 Mar) 43(3):220-1

Chakurski I Matev M Koichev A Angelova I Stefanov G
[Treatment of chronic colitis with an herbal combination of Taraxacum officinale, Hypericum perforatum, Melissa officinalis, Calendula officinalis and Foeniculum vulgare]
Vutr Boles (1981) 20(6):51-4

A total of 170 patients were treated—137 only with the herb combination (78 with duodenal ulcer and 59 with gastroduodenitis), 33 with the herb combination together with antacid (21 with duodenal ulcer and 12 with gastroduodenitis). As a result from the treatment, the spontaneous pains disappeared in 90 percent of the patients—in the group with and in the group without antacid, the dyspeptic complaints faded in over 85 percent but in the patients treated with herbs and antacid the mentioned complaints disappeared several days earlier. The palpitation pains, in both groups, disappeared in more than 90 percent of the patients within the same time. Gastric acidity, in both groups, showed a statistically insignificant tendency to decrease prior and post treatment. The gastroscopically control revealed that the ulcer niche, in both groups, was healed in almost the same percentage of the patients.

Dumenil G Chemli R Balansard C Guiraud H Lallemand M
[Evaluation of antibacterial properties of marigold flowers (Calendula officinalis L.) and mother homeopathic tinctures of C. officinalis L. and C. arvensis L. (author's transl)]
Ann Pharm Fr (1980) 38(6):493-9

Elias R De Meo M Vidal-Ollivier E Laget M Balansard G Dumenil G
Antimutagenic activity of some saponins isolated from Calendula officinalis L., C. arvensis L. and Hedera helix L.
Mutagenesis (1990 Jul) 5(4):327-31

Fleischner AM
Plant extracts: to accelerate healing and reduce inflammation.
Cosmet. Toilet. 100:45-46, 48-51, 54-55, 58 (Oct) 1985
Potential anti-inflammatory constituents from the extracts of Calendula officinalis, Anthemis nobilis, Tilia sylvestris, Centaurea cyanus, Matricaria chamomilla and Hypericum perforatum are described, and an evaluation of wound healing activity in 5 healthy subjects with artificially induced skin abrasions is discussed. In all 5 volunteers the extracts accelerated healing time an average of 16% (3.4 days) vs. the control.

Gasiorowska I Jachimowicz M Patalas B Mlynarczyk A
[The use of Calendula officinalis in the treatment of periodontopathies]
Czas Stomatol (1983 Apr) 36(4):307-11

Kartikeyan S Chaturvedi RM Narkar SV
Effect of calendula on trophic ulcers [letter; comment]
Lepr Rev (1990 Dec) 61(4):399

Klouchek-Popova E Popov A Pavlova N Krusteva S
Influence of the physiological regeneration and epithelialization using fractions isolated from Calendula officinalis.
Acta Physiol Pharmacol Bulg (1982) 8(4):63-7

Marinchev VN Bychkova LN Balvanovich NV Giraev AN
[Use of calendula for therapy of chronic inflammatory diseases of eyelids and conjunctiva]
Oftalmol Zh (1971) 26(3):196-8

Mozherenkov VP Shubina LF
[Treatment of chronic conjunctivitis with Calendula]
Med Sestra (1976 Apr) 35(4):33-4

Samochowiec E Urbanska L Manka W Stolarska E
[Evaluation of the effect of Calendula officinalis and Echinacea angustifolia extracts of Trichomonas vaginalis in vitro]
Wiad Parazytol (1979) 25(1):77-81 (Published in Polish)

Citations from the MEDLINE Database for the Genus *Capsella* (Shepherd's Purse)

Iurisson SM
[Vitamin content in shepherd's purse (Capsella bursa pastoris (L.) Medic.)]
Farmatsiia (1976 Jul-Aug) 25(4):66-7

Kuroda K Akao M
Effect of Capsella bursa-pastoris on liver catalase activity in rats fed 3-methyl-4-(dimethylamino)azobenzene.
Gann (1975 Aug) 66(4):461-2

Kuroda K Akao M Kanisawa M Miyaki K
Inhibitory effect of Capsella bursa-pastoris extract on growth of Ehrlich solid tumor in mice.
Cancer Res (1976 Jun) 36(6):1900-3

Kuroda K Akao M Kanisawa M Miyaki K
Inhibitory effect of Capsella bursa-pastoris on hepatocarcino-genesis induced by 3-methyl-4-(dimethylamino)azobenzene in rats.
Gann (1974 Aug) 65(4):317-21

Kuroda K Kaku T
Pharmacological and chemical studies on the alcohol extract of Capsella bursa-pastoris.
Life Sci (1969 Feb 1) 8(3):151-5

Kuroda K Takagi K
Physiologically active substance in Capsella bursa-pastoris.
Nature (1968 Nov 16) 220(168):707-8

Kuroda K Takagi K
Studies on capsella bursa pastoris. I. General pharmacology of ethanol extract of the herb.
Arch Int Pharmacodyn Ther (1969 Apr) 178(2):382-91

Kuroda K Takagi K
Studies on capsella bursa pastoris. II. Diuretic, anti-inflammatory & anti-ulcer action of the herb.
Arch Int Pharmacodyn Ther (1969 Apr) 178(2):392-9

Citations from the MEDLINE Database for the Genus *Capsicum* (Cayenne)

Buzzanca G Laterza S
[Clinical trial with an antirheumatic ointment]
Clin Ter 1977 Oct 15;83(1):71-83 (Published in Italian)

Coleridge HM Coleridge JC Luck JC
Pulmonary afferent fibres of small diameter stimulated by capsaicin and by hyperinflation of the lungs.
J Physiol (Lond) 1965 Jul;179(2):248-62

Collier HO McDonald-Gibson WJ Saeed SA
Letter: Stimulation of prostaglandin biosynthesis by capsaicin, ethanol, and tyramine.
Lancet 1975 Mar 22;1(7908):702

de Smet PA
A multidisciplinary overview of intoxicating snuff rituals in the western hemisphere.
J Ethnopharmacol 1985 Mar;13(1):3-49

Desai HG Venugopalan K Philipose M Zaveri MP Kalro RH Antia FP
Effect of red chilli powder on gastric mucosal barrier and acid secretion.
Indian J Med Res 1977 Sep;66(3):440-8

Escobar CH
[Relationship between habitual consumption of chile and the presence of submucous fibrosis]
Rev ADM 1988 Nov-Dec;45(6):369-72 (Published in Spanish)

Gabor M Endrenyi F
[Changes in capillary resistance in inflammation caused by red paprika (Capsicum annum L. Solanaceae)]
Orv Hetil 1970 Aug 2;111(31):1818-9 (Published in Hungarian)

Gill E
[Percutaneous treatment of functional and organic cardialgia]
Med Welt 1974 Dec 13;25(50):2127-9 (Published in German)

Glatzel H
[Treatment of dyspeptic disorders with spice extracts]
Hippokrates 1969 Dec 15;40(23):916-9 (Published in German)

Glatzel H
[Blood circulation effectiveness of natural spices]
Med Klin 1967 Dec 22;62(51):1987-9 (Published in German)

Glatzel H
[Spice therapy of dyspeptic disorders. Experiences with a combination of spice extracts]
Z Allgemeinmed 1973 Oct 31;49(30):1456-60 (Published in German)

Glatzel H Hackenberg K
[Radiologic studies on the effect of capsicum spice and mustard on the motility and secretion of the digestive tract]
Dtsch Z Verdau Stoffwechselkr 1966 Dec;26(3):113-21(Published in German)

Glatzel H Ruberg-Schweer M
[Modification of blood coagulation and fibrinolysis by common spices]
Med Klin 1967 Jul 14;62(28):1086-8 (Published in German)

Glatzel H Ruberg-Schweer M
Regional influence on cutaneous blood flow effected by oral spice intake.
Nutr Dieta Eur Rev Nutr Diet 1968;10(3):194-214

Govindarajan VS
Capsicum—production, technology, chemistry, and quality. Part III. Chemistry of the color, aroma, and pungency stimuli.
Crit Rev Food Sci Nutr 1986;24(3):245-355

Hartwell JL
Plants used against cancer. A survey.
Lloydia 1971 Jun;34(2):204-55

Henkin R
Cooling the burn from hot peppers.
JAMA 1991 Nov 20;266(19):2766

Henry CJ Emery B
Effect of spiced food on metabolic rate.
Hum Nutr Clin Nutr 1986 Mar;40(2):165-8

Horowitz M Wishart J Maddox A Russo A
The effect of chilli on gastrointestinal transit.
J Gastroenterol Hepatol 1992 Jan-Feb;7(1):52-6

Hot peppers and substance P [editorial]
Lancet 1983 May 28;1(8335):1198

Jancso N Jancso-Gabor A Szolcsanyi J
Direct evidence for neurogenic inflammation and its prevention by denervation and by pretreatment with capsaicin.
Br J Pharmacol 1967 Sep;31(1):138-51

Johnson LP Girma B Zenabett HL Wondemu M Worku S
The effect of red pepper on gastric secretion in Ethiopia.
Ethiop Med J 1978 Jul;16(3):111-3

Ketusinh O Dhorranintra B Juengjaroen K
Influence of capsicum solution on gastric acidities. A preliminary report.
Am J Proctol 1966 Dec;17(6):511-5

Klemm C
[Clinical experiences with an anti-rheumatic ointment treatment (Exrheudon-ointment)]
Z Allgemeinmed 1973 Aug 10;49(22):1049-52 (Published in German)

Kumar N Vij JC Sarin SK Anand BS
Do chillies influence healing of duodenal ulcer?
Br Med J (Clin Res Ed) 1984 Jun 16;288(6433):1803-4

Lawless H Stevens DA
Effects of oral chemical irritation on taste.
Physiol Behav 1984 Jun;32(6):995-8

Lembeck F
Columbus, Capsicum and capsaicin: past, present and future.
Acta Physiol Hung 1987;69(3-4):265-73

Makara GB Stark E Mihaly K
Sites at which formalin and capsaicin act to stimulate corticotropin secretion.
Can J Physiol Pharmacol 1967 Jul;45(4):669-74

Meyer-Bahlburg HF
Pilot studies on stimulant effects of capsicum spices.
Nutr Metab 1972;14(4):245-54

Myers BM Smith JL Graham DY
Effect of red pepper and black pepper on the stomach.
Am J Gastroenterol 1987 Mar;82(3):211-4

Ogston D
Nutritional influences on the fibrinolytic system.
Proc Nutr Soc 1985 Sep;44(3):379-84

Rozin P Ebert L Schull J
Some like it hot: a temporal analysis of hedonic responses to chili pepper.
Appetite 1982 Mar;3(1):13-22

Saber MS
Antimicrobial substances in certain members of Solanaceae. IV. Detection of active principles in pepper plant.
Zentralbl Bakteriol Parasitenkd Infektionskr Hyg 1976;131(2):110-2

Solanke TF
The effect of red pepper (Capsicum frutescens) on gastric acid secretion.
J Surg Res 1973 Dec;15(6):385-90

Sreenivasan VR Boese RA
Identification of lachrymators.
J Forensic Sci 1970 Jul;15(3):433-42

Viranuvatti V Kalayasiri C Chearani O Plengvanit U
Effects of capsicum solution on human gastric mucosa as observed gastroscopically.
Am J Gastroenterol 1972 Sep;58(3):225-32

Visudhiphan S Poolsuppasit S Piboonnukarintr O Tumliang S
The relationship between high fibrinolytic activity and daily capsicum ingestion in Thais.
Am J Clin Nutr 1982 Jun;35(6):1452-8

Wasantapruek S Poolsuppasit S Pibolnukarintr O
Letter: Enhanced fibrinolytic activity after capsicum ingestion.
N Engl J Med 1974 May 30;290(22):1259-60

Webb-Peploe MM Brender D Shepherd JT
Vascular responses to stimulation of receptors in muscle by capsaicin.
Am J Physiol 1972 Jan;222(1):189-95

Citations from the MEDLINE Database for the genus *Caulophyllum* (Blue Cohosh)

Anisimov MM Strigina LI Baranova SI Kul'ga AL Chetyrina NS
[The antimicrobial activity of the triterpene glycosides of Caulophyllum robustum maxim]
Antibiotiki (1972 Sep) 17(9):834-7

Chandrasekhar K Sarma GH
Proceedings: Observations on the effect of low and high doses of Caulophyllum on the ovaries and the consequential changes in the uterus and thyroid in rats.
J Reprod Fertil (1974 May) 38(1):236-7

Chandrasekhar K Vishwanath
CR Proceedings: Studies on the effect of Caulophyllum on implantation in rats.
J Reprod Fertil (1974 May) 38(1):245-6

Citations from the MEDLINE Database for the genus *Centella* (Gotu Cola)

Allegra C
[Comparative capillaroscopic study of certain bioflavonoids and total triterpenic fractions of Centella asiatica in venous insufficiency]
Clin Ter (1984 Sep 30) 110(6):555-9

Allegra C Pollari G Criscuolo A Bonifacio M Tabassi D
[Centella asiatica extract in venous disorders of the lower limbs. Comparative clinico-instrumental studies with a placebo]
Clin Ter (1981 Dec 15) 99(5):507-13

Arpaia MR Ferrone R Amitrano M Nappo C Leonardo G del Guercio R
Effects of Centella asiatica extract on mucopolysaccharide metabolism in subjects with varicose veins.
Int J Clin Pharmacol Res (1990) 10(4):229-33

Benedicenti A Galli D Merlini A
[The clinical therapy of periodontal disease, the use of potassium hydroxide and the water-alcohol extract of Centella in combination with laser therapy in the treatment of severe periodontal disease]
Parodontol Stomatol (Nuova) (1985 Jan-Apr) 24(1):11-26

Darnis F Orcel L de Saint-Maur PP Mamou P
[Use of a titrated extract of Centella asiatica in chronic hepatic disorders (author's transl)]
Sem Hop Paris (1979 Nov 8-15) 55(37-38):1749-50

Del Vecchio A Senni I Cossu G Molinaro M
[Effect of Centella asiatica on the biosynthetic activity of fibroblasts in culture]
Farmaco [Prat] (1984 Oct) 39(10):355-64

Dutta T Basu UP
Crude extract of Centella asiatica and products derived from its glycosides as oral antifertility agents.
Indian J Exp Biol (1968 Jul) 6(3):181-2

Fam A
Use of titrated extract of Centella asiatica (TECA) in bilharzial bladder lesions.
Int Surg (1973 Jul) 58(7):451-2 passim

Huriez C
[Action of the titrated extract of Centella asiatica in the cicatrization of leg ulcers (10 mg. tablets). Apropos of 50 cases]
Lille Med (1971) 17:Suppl 3:574-9

Maquart FX Bellon G Gillery P Wegrowski Y Borel JP
Stimulation of collagen synthesis in fibroblast cultures by a triterpene extracted from Centella asiatica.
Connect Tissue Res (1990) 24(2):107-20

Marastoni F Baldo A Redaelli G Ghiringhelli L
[Centella asiatica extract in venous pathology of the lower limbs & its evaluation compared with tribenoside]
Minerva Cardioangiol (1982 Apr) 30(4):201-7

Montecchio GP Samaden A Carbone S Vigotti M Siragusa S Piovella F
Centella Asiatica Triterpenic Fraction (CATTF) reduces the number of circulating endothelial cells in subjects with post phlebitic syndrome.
Haematologica (1991 May-Jun) 76(3):256-9

Nebout M
[Results of a controlled experiment of the titrated extract of Centella asiatica in a leper population with perforative foot lesions]
Bull Soc Pathol Exot Filiales (1974 Sep-Oct) 67(5):471-8

Pointel JP Boccalon H Cloarec M Ledevehat C Joubert M
Titrated extract of Centella asiatica (TECA) in the treatment of venous insufficiency of the lower limbs.
Angiology (1987 Jan) 38(1 Pt 1):46-50

Tenni R Zanaboni G De Agostini MP Rossi A Bendotti C Cetta G
Effect of the triterpenoid fraction of Centella asiatica on macromolecules of the connective matrix in human skin fibroblast cultures.
Ital J Biochem (1988 Mar-Apr) 37(2):69-77

Citations from the MEDLINE Database for the Genus *Cimicifuga* (Black Cohosh)

Duker EM Kopanski L Jarry H Wuttke W
Effects of extracts from Cimicifuga racemosa on gonadotropin release in menopausal women and ovariectomized rats.
Planta Med 1991 Oct;57(5):420-4

Ito M Kondo Y Takemoto T
Spasmolytic substances from Cimicifuga dahurica maxim.
Chem Pharm Bull (Tokyo) 1976 Apr;24(4):580-3

Jarry H Harnischfeger G
[Endocrine effects of constituents of Cimicifuga racemosa. 1. The effect on serum levels of pituitary hormones in ovariectomized rats]
Planta Med 1985 Feb(1):46-9 (Published in German)

Jarry H Harnischfeger G Duker E
[The endocrine effects of constituents of Cimicifuga racemosa. 2. In vitro binding of constituents to estrogen receptors]
Planta Med 1985 Aug(4):316-9 (Published in German)

Shibata M Ikoma M Onoda M Sato F Sakurai N
[Pharmacological studies on the Chinese crude drug "Shoma." III. Central depressant and antispasmodic actions of Cimicifuga rhizoma, Cimicifuga simplex Wormsk (author's transl)]
Yakugaku Zasshi 1980 Nov;100(11):1143-50 (Published in Japanese)

Shibata M Sakurai N Onoda M
[Pharmacological studies on the Chinese crude drug "Shoma." II. Anti-inflammatory action of Cimicifuga rhizoma, Cimicifuga simplex Wormsk (author's transl)]
Yakugaku Zasshi 1977 Aug;97(8):911-5 (Published in Japanese)

Shibata M Yamatake Y Amagaya Y Fukushima M
[Pharmacological studies on the Chinese crude drug "Shoma." I. Acute toxicity and anti-inflammatory action of Cimicifuga rhizoma, Cimicifuga dahurica Maxim. (author's transl)]
Yakugaku Zasshi 1975 May;95(5):539-46 (Published in Japanese)

Citations from the MEDLINE Database for the Genus *Commiphora* (Myrrh)

Amma MK Malhotra N Suri RK Arya OP Dani HM Sareen K
Effect of oleoresin of gum guggul (Commiphora mukul) on the reproductive organs of female rat.
Indian J Exp Biol (1978 Sep) 16(9):1021-3

Arora RB Das D Kapoor SC Sharma RC
Effect of some fractions of Commiphora mukul on various serum lipid levels in hypercholesterolemic chicks and their effectiveness in myocardial infarction in rats.
Indian J Exp Biol (1973 May) 11(3):166-8

Baldwa VS Bhasin V Ranka PC Mathur KM
Effects of Commiphora Mukul (Guggul) in experimentally induced hyperlipemia and atherosclerosis.
J Assoc Physicians India (1981 Jan) 29(1):13-7

Dixit VP Joshi S Sinha R Bharvava SK Varma M
Hypolipidemic activity of guggal resin (Commiphora mukul) and garlic (Alium sativum linn.) in dogs (Canis familiaris) and monkeys (Presbytis entellus entellus Dufresne).
Biochem Exp Biol (1980) 16(4):421-4

Kuppurajan K Rajagopalan SS Rao TK Sitaraman R
Effect of guggulu (Commiphora mukul—Engl.) on serum lipids in obese, hypercholesterolemic and hyperlipemic cases.
J Assoc Physicians India (1978 May) 26(5):367-73

Lata S Saxena KK Bhasin V Saxena RS Kumar A Srivastava VK
Beneficial effects of Allium sativum, Allium cepa and Commiphora mukul on experimental hyperlipidemia and atherosclerosis—a comparative evaluation.
J Postgrad Med (1991 Jul) 37(3):132-5

Malhotra SC Ahuja MM
Comparative hypolipidaemic effectiveness of gum guggulu (Commiphora mukul) fraction "A," ethyl-P-chlorophenoxyisobutyrate and Ciba-13437-Su.
Indian J Med Res (1971 Oct) 59(10):1621-32

Malhotra SC Ahuja MM Sundaram KR
Long term clinical studies on the hypolipidaemic effect of Commiphora mukul (Guggulu) and clofibrate.
Indian J Med Res (1977 Mar) 65(3):390-5

Nityanand S Kapoor NK
Hypocholesterolemic effect of Commiphora mukul resin (guggal).
Indian J Exp Biol (1971 Jul) 9(3):376-7

Satyavati GV
Gum guggul (Commiphora mukul)—the success story of an ancient insight leading to a modern discovery.
Indian J Med Res (1988 Apr) 87:327-35

Satyavati GV Dwarakanath C Tripathi SN
Experimental studies on the hypocholesterolemic effect of Commiphora mukul. Engl. (Guggul).
Indian J Med Res (1969 Oct) 57(10):1950-62

Sharma JN
Comparison of the anti-inflammatory activity of Commiphora mukul (an indigenous drug) with those of phenylbutazone and ibuprofen in experimental arthritis induced by mycobacterial adjuvant.
Arzneimittelforschung (1977 Jul) 27(7):1455-7

Tariq M Ageel AM Al-Yahya MA Mossa JS Al-Said MS Parmar NS
Anti-inflammatory activity of Commiphora molmol.
Agents Actions (1986 Jan) 17(3-4):381-2

Tripathi YB Malhotra OP Tripathi SN
Thyroid stimulating action of Z-guggulsterone obtained from Commiphora mukul.
Planta Med (1984 Feb) (1):78-80

Verma SK Bordia
Effect of Commiphora mukul (gum guggulu) in patients of hyperlipidemia with special reference to HDL-cholesterol.
Indian J Med Res (1988 Apr) 87:356-60

Citations from the MEDLINE Database for the Genus *Crataegus* (Hawthorn)

Ammon HP Handel M
[Crataegus, toxicology and pharmacology. Part III: Pharmacodynamics and pharmacokinetics (author's transl)]
Planta Med (1981 Dec) 43(4):313-22 (Published in German)

Ammon HP Handel M
[Crataegus, toxicology and pharmacology. Part II: Pharmacodynamics (author's transl)]
Planta Med (1981 Nov) 43(3):209-39 (Published in German)

Ammon HP Handel M
[Crataegus, toxicology and pharmacology. Part I: Toxicity (author's transl)]
Planta Med (1981 Oct) 43(2):105-20 (Published in German)

Beier A Konigstein RP Samec V
[Clinical experiences with a crataegus pentaerythrityl-tetranitrate combination drug in heart diseases due to coronary sclerosis in old age]
Wien Med Wochenschr (1974 Jun 15) 124(24):378-81 (Published in German)

Blesken R
[Crataegus in cardiology]
Fortschr Med (1992 May 30) 110(15):290-2 (Published in German)

The fact that the effectiveness of numerous phyto-preparations, so-called, has been demonstrated to the satisfaction of traditional medicine has led to increasing interest in phytotherapy. This also applies to Crataegus (whitethorn), the effects of which have been demonstrated in numerous pharmacological studies. These effects, produced mainly by the flavonoids, indicate a simultaneous cardiotropic and vasodilatory action, as confirmed clinically in controlled double-blind studies. This means that Crataegus can be employed for cardiological indications for which digitalis is not (yet) indicated. Prior to use, however, a Crataegus preparation must meet certain preconditions with respect to dosage, pharmaceutical quality of the preparation, and an accurate definition of the latter.

Ciplea AG Richter KD
The protective effect of Allium sativum and crataegus on isoprenaline-induced tissue necroses in rats.
Arzneimittelforschung (1988 Nov) 38(11):1583-92

Di Renzi L Cassone R Lucisano V Leggio F Gambelli G
[On the use of injectable crataegus extracts in therapy of disorders of peripheral arterial circulation in subjects with obliterating arteriopathy of the lower extremities]
Boll Soc Ital Cardiol (1969) 14(4):577-85 (Published in Italian)

Hammerl H Kranzl C Pichler O Studlar M
[Clinico-experimental metabolic studies using a Crataegus extract]
Klinisch-experimentelle Stoffwechseluntersuchungen mit einem Crataegus-Extrakt.
Arztl Forsch (1967 Jul 10) 21(7):261-4 (Published in German)

Kharchenko NS
[Medicinal value of Crataegus ucrainica]
Lekarstvennoe znachenie boiaryshnika ukrainskogo.
Vrach Delo (1965 Jan) 1:116-7 (Published in Russian)

Massoni G
[On the use of hawthorn extract (Crataegus) in the treatment of certain ischemic myocardial diseases in old age]
G Gerontol (1968 Sep) 16(9):979-84 (Published in Italian)

Muth HW
[Indications for treatment with crataegus]
Ther Ggw (1976 Feb) 115(2):242-55 (Published in German)

O'Conolly M Jansen W Bernhoft G Bartsch G
[Treatment of decreasing cardiac performance. Therapy using standardized crataegus extract in advanced age]
Fortschr Med (1986 Nov 13) 104(42):805-8 (Published in German)

Thompson EB Aynilian GH Gora P Farnworth NR
Preliminary study of potential antiarrhythmic effects of Crataegus monogyna.
J Pharm Sci (1974 Dec) 63(12):1936-7

Wolkerstorfer H
[Treatment of heart disease with a digoxin-crataegus combination]
Munch Med Wochenschr (1966 Feb 25) 108(8):438-41 (Published in German)

Citations from the MEDLINE Database for the Genus *Echinacea* (Echinacea)

Bauer R Foster S
Analysis of alkamides and caffeic acid derivatives from Echinacea simulata and E. paradoxa roots.
Planta Med 1991 Oct;57(5):447-9

Bauer VR Jurcic K Puhlmann J Wagner H
[Immunologic in vivo and in vitro studies on Echinacea extracts]
Arzneimittelforschung 1988 Feb;38(2):276-81 (Published in German)

Ethanolic extracts of Echinacea purpurea, E. pallida and E. angustifolia roots were examined for immunological activity in the carbon clearance test with mice and in the granulocyte test. In the in vivo experiment all extracts, administered orally, were found to enhance phagocytosis significantly. These results correlate with the stimulation of phagocytosis in the in vitro granulocyte test. The lipophilic fractions of the extracts appeared to be more active than the polar fractions. All extracts were analyzed by HPLC in order to correlate the chemical constituents with the immunological activities.

Coeugniet EG Elek E
Immunomodulation with Viscum album and Echinacea purpurea extracts.
Onkologie 1987 Jun;10(3 Suppl):27-33

Extracts of Viscum album (Plenosol) and Echinacea purpurea (Echinacin) are used clinically for their non-specific action on cell-mediated immunity. In vitro we could prove that these two extracts have a stimulating effect on the production of lympho-kines by lymphocytes and in the transformation test. A toxic effect on cells was pro-duced only with very high, clinically irrelevant concentrations. Clinical application of these extracts can produce a stimulation of cell-mediated immunity (one therapeutic administration followed by a free interval of one week) or can have a depressive action (daily administrations of higher doses). These observations were confirmed by lymphokine production and assay, 3H-thymidine incorporation and a skin test with recall antigens (Multitest Merieux).

Gaisbauer M Schleich T Stickl HA Wilczek I
[The effect of Echinacea purpurea Moench on phagocytosis in granulocytes mea-sured by chemiluminescence]
Arzneimittelforschung 1990 May;40(5):594-8 (Published in German)

Chemiluminescence was used as an indicator for phagocytic activity of granulocytes induced by zymosan in whole blood. Luminol was used to amplify the luminescence measured. Methods and conditions of the trial were varied and the dependence on the methods applied became evident. The effects of echinacea-extract (Echinacin) and phorbolester (PMA) in various concentrations on phagocytic activity of whole blood heparinized with 10 I.E./ml heparin as well as on phagocytic activity of erythrocytolized blood were investigated. The reaction of the granulocytes—phago-cytic and therefore chemiluminescence—under the influence of echinacea extract depends on the doses and methods applied. Therefore standardized methods and investigations of various immunoparameters as well as clinical investigations are nec-essary to prove the immunostimulative effect of so-called immunotherapeutics. This has not been undertaken up to now. Dose and method dependent single results cannot be a convincing justification for specific therapeutic medication.

Heinzer F Chavanne M Meusy JP Maitre HP Giger E Baumann TW
[The classification of therapeutically used species of the genus Echinacea]
Pharm Acta Helv 1988;63(4-5):132-6 (Published in German)

Lersch C Zeuner M Bauer A Siebenrock K Hart R Wagner F Fink U Dancygier H Classen M
Stimulation of the immune response in outpatients with hepatocellular carcino-mas by low doses of cyclophosphamide (LDCY), echinacea purpurea extracts (Echinacin) and thymostimulin.
Arch Geschwulstforsch 1990;60(5):379-83

Outpatients with inoperable far advanced hepato-cellular carcinomas (n = 5) were treated with LDCY—300 mg/m2 i.v. every 28 days, echinacin—60 mg/m2 i.m.—and thymostimulin—30 mg/m2 i.m., day 3-10 after LDCY, then twice a week. Therapy was well tolerated by all patients. Their Karnofsky index increased for 10% in the mean. A stable disease for more than 8 weeks was documented by abdominal ultrasonography in one patient. Serum levels of Alpha-Fetoprotein (AFP), Carcinoembryonic Antigen (CEA) and Tissue Polypeptide Antigen (TPA) did not in-crease in 2 patients. Median survival time was 2.5 months. One patient is still alive after 8 months. Absolute numbers of CD8+ cells significantly (p less than 0.02) de-creased for 7% 1 day after LDCY, whereas CD4+ cells increased (p less than 0.02) from day 1-7. Numbers of natural killer (NK-) cells increased for 17% (p less than 0.05), their activity for 90% (p less than 0.05). Activities of peripheral polymorphs (p less than 0.05) increased for 27% and of Lymphokine Activated Killer (LAK-) cells for 180% (p less than 0.05).

Luettig B Steinmuller C Gifford GE Wagner H Lohmann-Matthes ML
Macrophage activation by the polysaccharide arabinogalactan isolated from plant cell cultures of Echinacea purpurea.
J Natl Cancer Inst 1989 May 3;81(9):669-75

In this study, acidic arabinogalactan, a highly purified polysaccharide from plant cell cultures of Echinacea purpurea, with a molecular weight of 75,000, was effective in activating macrophages to cytotoxicity against tumor cells and micro-organisms (Leishmania enriettii). Furthermore, this polysaccharide induced macrophages to produce tumor necrosis factor (TNF-alpha), interleukin-1 (IL-1), and interferon-beta 2. Arabinogalactan did not activate B cells and did not induce T cells to produce interleukin-2, interferon-beta 2, or interferon-gamma, but it did induce a slight increase in T-cell proliferation. When injected ip, this agent stimulated macrophages, a finding that may have therapeutic implications in the defense against tumors and infectious diseases.

Mose J
Effect of echinacin on phagocytosis and natural killer cells.
Med Welt 34: 1463-7, 1983

Orinda D Diederich J Wacker A
[Antiviral activity of components of Echinacea purpurea]
Arzneimittelforschung 1973 Aug;23(8):1119-20 (Published in German)

Roesler J Emmendorffer A Steinmuller C Luettig B Wagner H Lohmann-Matthes ML
Application of purified polysaccharides from cell cultures of the plant Echinacea purpurea to test subjects mediates activation of the phagocyte system.
Int J Immunopharmacol 1991;13(7):931-41

Polysaccharides purified from large-scale cell cultures of the plant Echinacea purpurea were tested for their ability to activate human phagocytes in vitro and in vivo. These substances enhanced the spontaneous motility of PMN under soft agar and increased the ability of these cells to kill staphylococci. Monocytes were activated to secrete TNF-alpha, IL-6 and IL-1 whereas class II expression was unaffected. Intravenous application of the polysaccharides to test subjects immediately induced a fall in the number of PMN in the peripheral blood, indicating activation of adherence to endothelial cells. This fall was followed by a leukocytosis due to an increase in the number of PMN and a lesser increase of monocytes. The appearance of stab cells and some juvenile forms and even myelocytes indicated the migration of cells from the bone marrow into the peripheral blood. The acute phase C-reactive protein (CRP) was induced, probably due to activation of monocytes and macrophages to produce IL-6. In addition a moderate acceleration of the erythrocyte sedimentation rate was observed. Altogether, as in mice, the polysaccharides could induce acute phase reactions and activation of phagocytes in humans. The possibility of clinical use is discussed.

Roesler J Steinmuller C Kiderlen A Emmendorffer A Wagner H Lohmann-Matthes ML
Application of purified polysaccharides from cell cultures of the plant Echinacea purpurea to mice mediates protection against systemic infections with Listeria monocytogenes and Candida albicans.
Int J Immunopharmacol 1991;13(1):27-37

Purified polysaccharides from cell cultures of the plant Echinacea purpurea were investigated for their ability to enhance phagocytes' activities regarding nonspecific immunity in vitro and in vivo. Macrophages (M phi) from different organ origin could be activated to produce IL-1, TNF alpha and IL-6, to produce elevated amounts of reactive oxygen intermediates and to inhibit growth of Candida albicans in vitro.

Furthermore, in vivo the substances could induce increased proliferation of phago-cytes in spleen and bone marrow and migration of granulocytes to the peripheral blood. These effects indeed resulted in excellent protection of mice against the consequences of lethal infections with one predominantly M phi dependent and one predominantly granulocyte dependent pathogen, Listeria monocytogenes and C. albicans, respectively. Specific immune responses to sheep red blood cells (antibody production) and to Listeria (DTH) were not affected by the polysaccharides. The possibility of clinical use is discussed.

Samochowiec E Urbanska L Manka W Stolarska E
[Evaluation of the effect of Calendula officinalis and Echinacea angustifolia extracts of Trichomonas vaginalis in vitro]
Wiad Parazytol 1979;25(1):77-81 (Published in Polish)

Schumacher A Friedberg KD
[The effect of Echinacea angustifolia on non-specific cellular immunity in the mouse]
Arzneimittelforschung 1991 Feb;41(2):141-7 (Published in German)

Echinacea belongs to the most usable plants in medical treatment since many years. It is applicable in the fields of homeopathy and allopathy, however, there are many different ways of treatment. Two species are listed in the European Pharmacopoeia: Echinacea angustifolia and Echinacea purpurea. They differ in morphology and their chemical composition. There have been chemical and biological analyses of Echinacea for about 80 years. After exact investigations of these reports, the following results were found: Most chemical analyses were done with Echinacea angustifolia, especially the older ones, whereas biological activity was tested with Echinacea purpurea. In almost all of these experiments, proprietaries were preferred to use in contrast to any plant extracts. Most of the reports which declared the stimulating biological activity of Echinacea could not resist any critical opinion. So the frequency of medical application of this drug is mainly due to delivered practical knowledge. The experiments described in this study were practised with a water-soluble plant extract of Echinacea angustifolia, Echinacosid, one of its low-molecular compounds and proprietaries which contains this plant. Their influence on the unspecified cellular immunity of the mouse after intraperitoneal, intravenous or peroral application was investigated. Under various conditions no effects on the immune system could be found using the carbon clearance test.

Stimpel M Proksch A Wagner H Lohmann-Matthes ML
Macrophage activation and induction of macrophage cytotoxicity by purified polysaccharide fractions from the plant Echinacea purpurea.
Infect Immun 1984 Dec;46(3):845-9

Purified polysaccharides (EPS) prepared from the plant Echinacea purpurea are shown to strongly activate macrophages. Macrophages activated with these substances develop pronounced extracellular cytotoxicity against tumor targets. The activation is brought about by EPS alone and is independent of any cooperative effect with lymphocytes. Also the production and secretion of oxygen radicals and interleukin 1 by macrophages is increased after activation with EPS. Cells of the macrophages lineage seem to be the main target for the action of these polysaccharides. EPS has no effect on T lymphocytes. B lymphocytes show a comparatively modest proliferation after incubation with E. purpurea EPS. Thus, these compounds, which are at least in tissue culture completely nontoxic, may be suited to activate in vivo cells of the macrophage system to cytotoxicity. They may therefore be of relevance in tumor and infectious systems.

Tragni E Galli CL Tubaro A Del Negro P Della Loggia R
Anti-inflammatory activity of Echinacea angustifolia fractions separated on the basis of molecular weight.
Pharmacol Res Commun 1988 Dec;20 Suppl 5:87-90

Five fractions of an aqueous extract obtained from the roots of Echinacea angustifolia were separated on the basis of molecular weight. The topical anti-inflammatory activity of the fractions has been evaluated in mice using the Croton oil ear test. The fraction with a molecular weight between 30,000 and 100,000 was the most active in inhibiting the oedema; it also reduced the infiltration of inflammatory cells. The activity of this fraction was comparable with that of a raw polysaccharidic extract obtained from E. angustifolia roots by differential solubility. The high-molecular weight polysaccharides are therefore proposed as the anti-inflammatory principles of the plant.

Tubaro A Tragni E Del Negro P Galli CL Della Loggia R
Anti-inflammatory activity of a polysaccharidic fraction of Echinacea angustifolia.
J Pharm Pharmacol 1987 Jul;39(7):567-9

The anti-inflammatory activity of a polysaccharidic fraction (EPF) obtained from Echinacea angustifolia roots has been examined using the carrageenan paw oedema and the croton oil ear test. EPF (0.5 mg kg-1 i.v.) almost inhibited the carrageenan-induced oedema over 8 h and furthermore, EPF, topically applied, inhibited mouse ear oedema induced by croton oil. EPF also reduced the leukocytic infiltration of the croton oil dermatitis, evaluated both as peroxidase activity and histologically. After topical application EPF appears to be slightly inferior in potency to indomethacin. The results suggest that the anti-inflammatory activity of E. angustifolia resides in its polysaccharidic content.

Voaden D Jacobson M
Tumor inhibitors. 3. Identification and synthesis of an oncolytic hydrocarbon from American coneflower roots.
J Med Chem 15:619-23, 1972

Wacker A Hilbig W
[Virus-inhibition by echinacea purpurea (author's transl)]
Planta Med 1978 Feb;33(1):89-102 (Published in German)

Wagner V Proksch A Riess-Maurer et al
Immunostimulating polysaccharides (heteroglycanes) of higher plants—preliminary communications.
Arzneim Forsch 34:659-660, 1984

[Proceedings: Echinacea activates the properdin system]
Echinacea aktiviert das Properdinsystem
Med Monatsschr 1976 Jan;30(1):32-3 (Published in German)

Citations from the MEDLINE Database for the Genus *Eleutherococcus* (Siberian Ginseng)

Afanas'ev BG Zhestovskii VA Mazurov KV Maevskii KL
[Comparative evaluation of the effect of Eleutherococcus and an acid-saline beverage on the development of processes of adaptation to intermittent heat effects]
Vopr Pitan 1973 Jan-Feb;32(1):3-9 (Published in Russian)

Afanas'eva TN Lebkova NP
[Effect of Eleutherococcus on the subcellular structures of the heart in experimental myocardial infarct]
Biull Eksp Biol Med 1987 Feb;103(2):212-5 (Published in Russian)

Alekseeva LV Bykhovtsova TL Bezlepkin VG Motlokh NN Strizhov NI
[Effect of liquid extracts of ginseng and Eleutherococcus roots on cell carbohydrate-phosphorus metabolism in the rat liver]
Izv Akad Nauk SSSR [Biol] 1975 Jul-Aug(4):609-12 (Published in Russian)

Andreev IF
[Effect of Eleutherococcus extract on some functions of the digestive organs]
Vrach Delo 1976 Aug(8):40-1 (Published in Russian)

Anisimov MM Fronert EB Frolova GM Suprunov NI
[Effect of Eleutherococcus senticosus glycosides on early embryogenesis in the sea urchin]
Izv Akad Nauk SSSR [Biol] 1973 Jul-Aug;4:590-3 (Published in Russian)

Asano K Takahashi T Miyashita M Matsuzaka A Muramatsu S Kuboyama M Kugo H Imai J
Effect of Eleutherococcus senticosus extract on human physical working capacity.
Planta Med 1986 Jun(3):175-7

Barkan AI
Gaiduchenia LI Makarenko IuA
[Effect of Eleutherococcus on respiratory viral infectious morbidity in children in organized collectives]
Pediatriia 1980 Apr(4):65-6 (Published in Russian)

Batin VV Popov IuB Lifar VK
[Experience in using sugar and an Eleutherococcus extract with the workers of the hot shops and the night shifts of the Raichikhinsk Glass Plant]
Gig Tr Prof Zabol 1981 May(5):36-8 (Published in Russian)

Ben-Hur E Fulder S
Effect of Panax ginseng saponins and Eleutherococcus senticosus on survival of cultured mammalian cells after ionizing radiation.
Am J Chin Med 1981 Spring;9(1):48-56

Berdyshev VV
[Effect of the long-term intake of Eleutherococcus on the adaptation of sailors in the tropics]
Voen Med Zh 1981 May(5):57-8 (Published in Russian)

Berdyshev VV
[Effect of Eleutherococcus on body functions and the work capacity of sailors on a cruise]
Voen Med Zh 1981 Feb(2):48-51 (Published in Russian)

Bohn B Nebe CT Birr C
Flow-cytometric studies with eleutherococcus senticosus extract as an immunomodulatory agent.
Arzneimittelforschung 1987 Oct;37(10):1193-6

Boino-Iasenetskii AM
[Eleutherococcus extract in the treatment of acute pyelonephritis]
Urol Nefrol (Mosk) 1966 Nov-Dec;31(6):21-3 (Published in Russian)

Brekhman II Dardymov IV
Pharmacological investigation of glycosides from Ginseng and Eleutherococcus.
Lloydia 1969 Mar;32(1):46-51

Brekhman II Kirillov OI
Effect of eleutherococcus on alarm-phase of stress.
Life Sci 1969 Feb 1;8(3):113-21

Brekhman II Maianskii GM
[Eleutherococcus—a means of increasing the nonspecific resistance of the organism]
Izv Akad Nauk SSSR [Biol] 1965 Sep-Oct;5:762-5 (Published in Russian)

Bronnikov IuN
[Indications of the immunological effectiveness of the combined use of dysentery ultraviolet vaccines and Eleutherococcus under experimental conditions]
Zh Mikrobiol Epidemiol Immunobiol 1968 Nov;45(11):151

Buzlama VS Antipov VA Demchenko IuV Dolgopolou VN Retskiy MI
[Use of Eleutherococcus for preventing transportation stress in swine]
Veterinariia 1976 Apr(4) (Published in Russian)

Chenkov R
[Effectiveness of treating enuresis with Eleutherococcus (People's Republic of Bulgaria)]
Voen Med Zh 1984 Oct(10):60 (Published in Russian)

Chubarev VN Rubtsova ER Filatova IV Krendal' FP Davydova ON
[Immunotropic effect of a tincture of the tissue culture biomass of ginseng cells and of an Eleutherococcus extract in mice]
Farmakol Toksikol 1989 Mar-Apr;52(2):55-9 (Published in Russian)

Dzhioev FK
Effect of Eleutherococcus extract on adenomas induced by urethane in lungs of mice.
Fed Proc Transl Suppl 1966 Jul-Aug;25(4):651-3

Dzhioev FK
[Influence of extract of Eleutherococcus on urethane-induced lung adenomas in mice]
Vopr Onkol 1965;11(9):51-4 (Published in Russian)

Elizarov EN Khudoshin VA
[Effect of physical exercises and Eleutherococcus on lipid metabolic indices in submariners]
Voen Med Zh 1977 Apr(4):64-6 (Published in Russian)

Farnsworth NR Kinghorn AD Soejarto D Waller DP
Siberian Ginseng (Eleutherococcus senticosus): Current status as an adaptogen.
Economic Medicinal Plant Research 1:156-215, 1985

Gerling I Pribilla O
[Breath and blood alcohol concentration following intake of Eleutherococcus and Gallexier]
Blutalkohol 1986 Nov;23(6):400-6 (Published in German)

Golotin VG Gonenko VA Zimina VV Naumov VV Shevtsova SP
[Effect of ionol and eleutherococcus on changes of the hypophyseo-adrenal system in rats under extreme conditions]
Vopr Med Khim 1989 Jan-Feb;35(1):35-7 (Published in Russian)

Grigorian GS Manasian AV Manukian VA Petrosian SA
[Effect of an Eleutherococcus extract on the body of animals]
Veterinariia 1976 Apr(4):100-1 (Published in Russian)

Hikino H Takahashi M Otake K Konno C
Isolation and hypoglycemic activity of eleutherans A, B, C, D, E, F, and G: glycans of Eleutherococcus senticosus roots.
J Nat Prod 1986 Mar-Apr;49(2):293-7

Iaremenko KV Moskalik KG
[The combined effect of stress reactions and extracts of Eleutherococcus on the inoculation of tumor cells by intravenous administration]
Vopr Onkol 1967;13(9):65-9 (Published in Russian)

Kaloeva ZD
[Effect of the glycosides of Eleutherococcus senticosus on the hemodynamic indices of children with hypotensive states]
Farmakol Toksikol 1986 Sep-Oct;49(5):73 (Published in Russian)

Kupin VI Polevaia EB
[Stimulation of the immunological reactivity of cancer patients by Eleutherococcus extract]
Vopr Onkol 1986;32(7):21-6 (Published in Russian)

Liapustina TA
[The effect of Eleutherococcus extract on the sexual function of bulls]
Veterinariia 1967 Dec;44(12):83-5 (Published in Russian)

Maksimov IuL
[The use of eleutherococcus in animal husbandry]
Veterinariia 1966 Oct;43(10):52-3 (Published in Russian)

Martinez B Staba EJ
The physiological effects of Aralia, Panax and Eleutherococcus on exercised rats.
Jpn J Pharmacol 1984 Jun;35(2):79-85

Medon PJ Ferguson PW Watson CF
Effects of Eleutherococcus senticosus extracts on hexobarbital metabolism in vivo and in vitro.
J Ethnopharmacol 1984 Apr;10(2):235-41

Medon PJ Thompson EB Farnsworth NR
Hypoglycemic effect and toxicity of Eleutherococcus senticosus following acute & chronic administration in mice.
Chung Kuo Yao Li Hsueh Pao 1981 Dec;2(4):281-5

Minkova M Pantev T
Effect of Eleutherococcus extract on the radioprotective action of adeturone.
Acta Physiol Pharmacol Bulg 1987;13(4):66-70

Monakhov BV
[Reduction of the toxic effect of various antiblastic preparations by means of Eleutherococcus extract]
Vopr Onkol 1967;13(3):71-6 (Published in Russian)

Monakhov BV
[Extract of Eleutherococcus senticosus maxim and the therapeutic activity of cyclophosphane, ethymidine, and benzo-TEPA]
Vopr Onkol 1967;13(8):94-7 (Published in Russian)

Monokhov BV
[Influence of the liquid extract from the roots of Eleutherococcus senticosus on the toxicity and antitumor activity of cyclophosphan]
Vopr Onkol 1965;11(12):60-3 (Published in Russian)

Novozhilov GN Sil'chenko KK
[Mechanism of adaptogenic effect of Eleutherococcus on the human body during thermal stress]
Fiziol Cheloveka 1985 Mar-Apr;11(2):303-6 (Published in Russian)

Ronichevskaia GM
[The effect of large doses of extracts of ginseng and Eleutherococcus extracts on the occurrence of spontaneous tumors in hybrid mice]
Vopr Onkol 1967;13(3):67-71 (Published in Russian)

Sosnova TL
[The effect of Eleutherococcus spinosus on the color discrimination function of the visual analyzer in persons with normal trichromatic vision]
Vestn Oftalmol 1969;82(5):59-61 (Published in Russian)

Sosnova TL Bykova MI
[Experience in using Eleutherococcus for raising the level of the color discrimination function in railroad engineers]
Gig Sanit 1976 Jun(6):108-10 (Published in Russian)

Vereshchagin IA
[Treatment of dysentery in children with a combination of monomycin and Eleutherococcus]
Antibiotiki 1978 Jul;23(7):633-6 (Published in Russian)

Zaikova MV Verba AA Snegireva MP
[The use of Eleutherococcus in ophthalmology]
Vestn Oftalmol 1968 May-Jun;81(3):70-4 (Published in Russian)

Citations from the MEDLINE Database for the Genus *Eschscholzia* (California Poppy)

Rolland A Fleurentin J Lanhers MC Younos C Misslin R Mortier F Pelt JM
Behavioural effects of the American traditional plant Eschscholzia californica: sedative and anxiolytic properties.
Planta Med (1991 Jun) 57(3):212-6

Citations from the MEDLINE database for the Genus *Eucalyptus* (Eucalyptus)

Arustamov AS Udalov VA
[Treatment of rhinitis and rhinopharyngitis using a mixture of copper, Eucalyptus and tea]
Med Sestra 1980 Jul;37(7):38 (Published in Russian)

Bohlau V Schildwachter G
[Aerosol treatment of bronchitis]
ZFA (Stuttgart) 1977 Oct 31;53(30):1885-7 (Published in German)

Boyd EM
A review of studies on the pharmacology of the expectorants and inhalants.
Int Z Klin Pharmakol Ther Toxikol 1970 Jan;3(1):55-60

Burrow A Eccles R Jones AS
The effects of camphor, eucalyptus and menthol vapour on nasal resistance to airflow and nasal sensation.
Acta Otolaryngol (Stockh) 1983 Jul-Aug;96(1-2):157-61

Byers JF
To douche or not to douche.
Am Fam Physician 1974 Sep;10(3):135-9

Cohen BM Dressler WE
Acute aromatics inhalation modifies the airways. Effects of the common cold.
Respiration 1982;43(4):285-93

Demchenko P
[Aerosol therapy in the complex treatment of children with chronic pneumonia]
Pediatr Akush Ginekol 1966 Mar-Apr;2:11-4 (Published in Ukrainian)

Dzhanashiia NM Startsev VG
[Comparative evaluation of the effect of some species of Eucalyptus and of anti-biotics on peptic activity of gastric juice in monkeys]
Antibiotiki 1970 Jun;15(6):547-8 (Published in Russian)

Egawa H Tsutsui O Tatsuyama K Hatta T
Antifungal substances found in leaves of Eucalyptus species.
Experientia 1977 Jul 15;33(7):889-90

Goldstein E Cooper AD Tarkington B
Effect of inhaling medication vapors from a cold preparation on murine pulmonary bacterial defense systems.
J Toxicol Environ Health 1976 Nov;2(2):371-88

Jongkees LB
[Nose rinsing, gargling and steambaths]
Ned Tijdschr Geneeskd 1974 Aug 10;118(32):1227-9 (Published in Dutch)

Jori A Bianchetti A Prestini PE
Effect of essential oils on drug metabolism.
Biochem Pharmacol 1969 Sep;18(9):2081-5

Jori A Di Salle E Pescador R
On the inducing activity of eucalyptol.
J Pharm Pharmacol 1972 Jun;24(6):646-9

Kachnyi GG
[Use of chlorophyllypt 1 percent alcohol solution in chronic suppurative otitis media]
Zh Ushn Nos Gorl Bolezn 1977 Mar-Apr(3):85-6 (Published in Russian)

Koliadenko VG Levkovskii NM Golovchenko DIa
[Use of chlorophyllypt in the treatment of erosive-ulcerative skin diseases]
Vrach Delo 1976 Sep(9):121-2 (Published in Russian)

Kriazheva SS Khamaganova IV
[External use of eucalimine in pediatric practice]
Pediatriia 1989(8):97-8 (Published in Russian)

Lacroix R Merad MR Lacroix J Schoebel MF
[Broncho-pulmonary antiseptics in the traditional Algerian pharmacopoeia]
Tunis Med 1973 Sep;51(5):285-92 (Published in French)

Low D Rawal BD Griffin WJ
Antibacterial action of the essential oils of some Australian Myrtaceae with special references to the activity of chromatographic fractions of oil of Eucalyptus citriodora.
Planta Med 1974 Sep;26(2):184-5

Lysenko LV
[Anti-inflammatory effect of azulene of eucalyptus oil]
Farmakol Toksikol 1967 May-Jun;30(3):341-3 (Published in Russian)

Metaksa Glu Primachenko NB
[Use of chlorophyllypt for treating neurotoxoplasmosis]
Vrach Delo 1979 Jul(7):111-3 (Published in Russian)

Miao TJ Xiong RC
The use of Chinese herbs folium ilicis chinensis decoction plus eucalyptus distillate for preoperative preparation of intestinal tract.
J Tradit Chin Med 1984 Jun;4(2):149-52

Pochinok VIa
[Antibiotic substance, extracted from the leaves of the blue eucalyptus and its detoxication properties]
Farm Zh 1965;20(3):70-1 (Published in Ukrainian)

Pochinok VIa
[The effect of a detoxifying substance from eucalyptus leaves on the amino acid composition of diphtheria toxin]
Mikrobiol Zh 1972 Jan-Feb;34(1):7-8 (Published in Ukrainian)

Rodin VI Lozitskaia VI Foderman VM
[Use of chlorophilliptum in otorhinolaryngologic diseases of staphylococcal etiology]
Zh Ushn Nos Gorl Bolezn 1975 Nov-Dec(6):79-82 (Published in Russian)

Shramkevych AF Sol's'kyi IaP Rozumenko MB
[Antihypoxic effect of chlorophyllypt and the method for its clinical use in maternal and fetal tissue hypoxia]
Pediatr Akush Ginekol 1979 Sep-Oct(5):55 (Published in Ukrainian)

Tsvetkov VL Shevchenko NF
[The use of chlorophyllypt in eye practice]
Oftalmol Zh 1972;27(8):623-4 (Published in Russian)

Usenko GV
[Comparative evaluation of various methods for the overall treatment of inflammatory diseases of the internal female genitalia using chlorophyllypt]
Pediatr Akush Ginekol 1974 Sep-Oct(5):57-9 (Published in Ukrainian)

Vichkanova SA Dzhanashiia NM Goriunova LV
[The antiviral activity of the essential oil of E. viminalis and several other frost-hardy eucalypti]
Farmakol Toksikol 1973 May-Jun;36(3):339-41 (Published in Russian)

Zanker KS Tolle W Blumel G Probst J
Evaluation of surfactant-like effects of commonly used remedies for colds.
Respiration 1980;39(3):150-7

Citations from the MEDLINE Database for the Genus *Eupatorium* (Boneset, Gravel Root)

Cai DG
[Expectorant constituents of Eupatorium fortunei]
Chung Yao Tung Pao 1983 Nov;8(6):30-1 (Published in Chinese)

Gassinger CA Wunstel G Netter P
[A controlled clinical trial for testing the efficacy of the homeopathic drug eupatorium perfoliatum D2 in the treatment of common cold (author's transl)]
Klinische Prüfung zum Nachweis der therapeutischen Wirksamkeit des homoöpathischen Arzneimittels Eupatorium perfoliatum D 2 (Wasserhanf composite) bei der Diagnose "Grippaler Infekt 1."
Arzneimittelforschung 1981;31(4):732-6 (Published in German)

Hall TB Jr
Eupatorium perfoliatum. A plant with a history.
Mo Med 1974 Sep;71(9):527-8

Kupchan SM Sigel CW Hemingway RJ Knox JR Udayamurthy MS
Tumor inhibitors. 33. Cytotoxic flavones from eupatorium species.
Tetrahedron 1969 Apr;25(8):1603-15

Lexa A Fleurentin J Lehr PR Mortier F Pruvost M Pelt JM
Choleretic and hepatoprotective properties of Eupatorium cannabinum in the rat.
Planta Med 1989 Apr;55(2):127-32

Malingre TM
[Eupatorium cannabinum L., an old medicinal herb with new perspectives]
Eupatorium cannabinum L., een oud geneeskruid met nieuwe perspectieven.
Pharm Weekbl 1971 Sep 24;106(39):738-44 (Published in Dutch)

Rao KV Alvarez FM
Antibiotic principle of Eupatorium capillifolium.
J Nat Prod 1981 May-Jun;44(3):252-6

Triratana T Suwannuraks R Naengchomnong W
Effect of Eupatorium odoratum on blood coagulation.
J Med Assoc Thai 1991 May;74(5):283-7

Woerdenbag HJ
Eupatorium cannabinum L. A review emphasizing the sesquiterpene lactones and their biological activity.
Pharm Weekbl [Sci] 1986 Oct 17;8(5):245-51

Citations from the MEDLINE Database for Feverfew

Barsby R Salan U Knight DW Hoult JR
Irreversible inhibition of vascular reactivity by feverfew [letter]
Lancet 1991 Oct 19;338(8773):1015

Biggs MJ Johnson ES Persaud NP Ratcliffe DM
Platelet aggregation in patients using feverfew for migraine [letter]
Lancet 1982 Oct 2;2(8301):776

Collier HO Butt NM McDonald-Gibson WJ Saeed SA
Extract of feverfew inhibits prostaglandin biosynthesis [letter]
Lancet 1980 Oct 25;2(8200):922-3

Groenewegen WA Heptinstall S
Amounts of feverfew in commercial preparations of the herb [letter]
Lancet 1986 Jan 4;1(8471):44-5

Groenewegen WA Heptinstall S
A comparison of the effects of an extract of feverfew and parthenolide, a component of feverfew, on human platelet activity in-vitro.
J Pharm Pharmacol 1990 Aug;42(8):553-7

Groenewegen WA Knight DW Heptinstall S
Compounds extracted from feverfew that have anti-secretory activity contain an alpha-methylene butyrolactone unit.
J Pharm Pharmacol 1986 Sep;38(9):709-12

Hayes NA Foreman JC
The activity of compounds extracted from feverfew on histamine release from rat mast cells.
J Pharm Pharmacol 1987 Jun;39(6):466-70

Heptinstall S
Feverfew—an ancient remedy for modern times?
J R Soc Med 1988 Jul;81(7):373-4

Heptinstall S Groenewegen WA Spangenberg P Loesche W
Extracts of feverfew may inhibit platelet behaviour via neutralization of sulphydryl groups.
J Pharm Pharmacol 1987 Jun;39(6):459-65

Heptinstall S Groenewegen WA Spangenberg P Loesche W
Inhibition of platelet behaviour by feverfew: a mechanism of action involving sulphydryl groups.
Folia Haematol (Leipz) 1988;115(4):447-9

Heptinstall S White A Williamson L Mitchell JR
Extracts of feverfew inhibit granule secretion in blood platelets and polymorphonuclear leucocytes.
Lancet 1985 May 11;1(8437):1071-4

Johnson ES Kadam NP Anderson D Jenkinson PC Dewdney RS Blowers SD
Investigation of possible genotoxic effects of feverfew in migraine patients.
Hum Toxicol 1987 Nov;6(6):533-4

Johnson ES Kadam NP Hylands DM Hylands PJ
Efficacy of feverfew as prophylactic treatment of migraine.
Br Med J (Clin Res Ed) 1985 Aug 31;291(6495):569-73

Loesche W Groenewegen WA Krause S Spangenberg P Heptinstall S
Effects of an extract of feverfew (Tanacetum parthenium) on arachidonic acid metabolism in human blood platelets.
Biomed Biochim Acta 1988;47(10-11):S241-3

Loesche W Mazurov AV Voyno-Yasenetskaya TA Groenewegen WA Heptinstall S Repin VS
Feverfew—an antithrombotic drug?
Folia Haematol (Leipz) 1988;115(1-2):181-4

Loesche W Mazurov AV Heptinstall S Groenewegen WA Repin VS Till U
An extract of feverfew inhibits interactions of human platelets with collagen substrates.
Thromb Res 1987 Dec 1;48(5):511-8

Makheja AN Bailey JM
The active principle in feverfew [letter]
Lancet 1981 Nov 7;2(8254):1054

Makheja AN Bailey JM
A platelet phospholipase inhibitor from the medicinal herb feverfew (Tanacetum parthenium).
Prostaglandins Leukot Med 1982 Jun;8(6):653-60

Mervyn L
Standardised feverfew preparations [letter]
Lancet 1986 Jan 25;1(8474):209

Murphy JJ Heptinstall S Mitchell JR
Randomised double-blind placebo-controlled trial of feverfew in migraine prevention.
Lancet 1988 Jul 23;2(8604):189-92

O'Neill LA Barrett ML Lewis GP
Extracts of feverfew inhibit mitogen-induced human peripheral blood mononuclear cell proliferation and cytokine mediated responses: a cytotoxic effect.
Br J Clin Pharmacol 1987 Jan;23(1):81-3

Pattrick M Heptinstall S Doherty M
Feverfew in rheumatoid arthritis: a double-blind, placebo-controlled study.
Ann Rheum Dis 1989 Jul;48(7):547-9

Pugh WJ Sambo K
Prostaglandin synthetase inhibitors in feverfew.
J Pharm Pharmacol 1988 Oct;40(10):743-5

Sumner H Salan U Knight DW Hoult JR
Inhibition of 5-lipoxygenase and cyclo-oxygenase in leukocytes by feverfew. Involvement of sesquiterpene lactones and other components.
Biochem Pharmacol 1992 Jun 9;43(11):2313-20

Voyno-Yasenetskaya TA Loesche W Groenewegen WA Heptinstall S Repin VS Till U
Effects of an extract of feverfew on endothelial cell integrity and on cAMP in rabbit perfused aorta.
J Pharm Pharmacol 1988 Jul;40(7):501-2

Waller PC Ramsay LE
Efficacy of feverfew as prophylactic treatment of migraine [letter]
Br Med J (Clin Res Ed) 1985 Oct 19;291(6502):1128

Williamson LM Harvey DM Sheppard KJ Fletcher J
Effect of feverfew on phagocytosis and killing of Candida guilliermondii by neutrophils.
Inflammation 1988 Feb;12(1):11-6

Wind J Punt J
Efficacy of feverfew as prophylactic treatment of migraine [letter]
Br Med J (Clin Res Ed) 1985 Nov 23;291(6507):1508

Citations from the MEDLINE Database for the Genus *Filipendula* (Meadowsweet)

Barnaulov OD Denisenko PP
[Anti-ulcer action of a decoction of the flowers of the dropwort, Filipendula ulmaria (L.) Maxim]
Farmakol Toksikol (1980 Nov-Dec) 43(6):700-5

Kudriashov BA Liapina LA Azieva LD
[The content of a heparin-like anticoagulant in the flowers of the meadowsweet (Filipendula ulmaria)]
Farmakol Toksikol (1990 Jul-Aug) 53(4):39-41

Citations from the MEDLINE Database for the Genus *Foeniculum* (Fennel)

Abdul-Ghani AS Amin R
The vascular action of aqueous extracts of Foeniculum vulgare leaves.
J Ethnopharmacol 1988 Dec;24(2-3):213-8

Annusuya S Vanithakumari G Megala N Devi K Malini T Elango V
Effect of Foeniculum vulgare seed extracts on cervix and vagina of ovariectomised rats.
Indian J Med Res 1988 Apr;87:364-7

Chakurski I Matev M Koichev A Angelova I Stefanov G
[Treatment of chronic colitis with an herbal combination of Taraxacum officinale, Hypericum perforatum, Melissa officinalis, Calendula officinalis and Foeniculum vulgare]
Vutr Boles 1981;20(6):51-4 (Published in Bulgarian)

Malini T Vanithakumari G Megala N Anusya S Devi K Elango V
Effect of Foeniculum vulgare Mill. seed extract on the genital organs of male and female rats.
Indian J Physiol Pharmacol 1985 Jan-Mar;29(1):21-6

Citations from the MEDLINE Database for the Genus *Geranium* (Cranesbill)

Hodisan V Hintz IC
[The bacteriostatic activity of Geranium species]
Cercetari asupra actinunii bacteriostatics a speciei Geranium.
Rev Chir [Stomatol] 1984 Jul-Sep;31(3):173-6 (Published in Romanian)

Manolova N Gegova G Serkedzhieva Iu Maksimova-Todorova V Uzunov S
[Antiviral action of a polyphenol complex isolated from the medicinal plant Geranium sanguineum L. I. Its inhibiting action on the reproduction of the influenza virus]
Acta Microbiol Bulg 1986;18:73-7 (Published in Bulgarian)

Serkedzhieva Iu Manolova N
[The antiviral action of a polyphenol complex isolated from the medicinal plant Geranium sanguineum L. VI. Reproduction of the influenza virus pretreated with the polyphenol complex]
Acta Microbiol Bulg 1988;22:16-21 (Published in Bulgarian)

Serkedzhieva Iu Manolova N
[Antiviral effect of a polyphenolic complex isolated from the medicinal plant Geranium sanguineum L. V. Mechanism of the anti-influenzal effect in vitro]
Acta Microbiol Bulg 1987;21:66-71 (Published in Bulgarian)

Serkedzhieva Iu Manolova N Gegova G Maksimova-Todorova V Ivancheva S
[Antiviral action of a polyphenol complex isolated from the medicinal plant Geranium sanguineum L. II. Its inactivating action on the influenza virus]
Acta Microbiol Bulg 1986;18:78-82 (Published in Bulgarian)

Serkedzhieva Iu Manolova N Maksimova-Todorova V Gegova G
[Combined action of antiviral substances of natural and synthetic origin. I. The anti-influenza action of a combination of the polyphenol complex isolated from Geranium sanguineum L. and remantadine in vitro and in ovo]
Acta Microbiol Bulg 1986;19:18-22 (Published in Bulgarian)

Zgorniak-Nowosielska I Zawilinska B Manolova N Serkedjieva J
A study on the antiviral action of a polyphenolic complex isolated from the medicinal plant Geranium sanguineum L. VIII. Inhibitory effect on the reproduction of herpes simplex virus type 1.
Acta Microbiol Bulg 1989;24:3-8

Citations from the MEDLINE Database for the Genus Ginkgo (Ginkgo)

Agnoli A
Clinical and psychometric aspects of the therapeutic effects of GBE.
In: Effects of GBE and Organic Cerebral Impairment, Paris, London, John Lilley, 1985

Allard M
Treatment of the disorders of aging with Ginkgo biloba extract. From pharmacology to clinical medicine.
Presse Med 1986 Sep 25; 15(31):1540-5 (Published in French)

Auguet M DeFeudis FV Clostre F Deghenghi R
Effects of an extract of Ginkgo biloba on rabbit isolated aorta.
Gen. Pharmacol., 1982, 13, 225-230

Auguet M DeFeudis FV Clostre F
Effects of Ginkgo biloba on arterial smooth muscle responses to vasoactive stimuli.
Gen. Pharmacol., 1982, 13, 169-171

Auguet M Clostre F
Effects of an extract of Ginkgo biloba and diverse substances on the phasic and tonic components of the contraction of an isolated rabbit aorta.
Gen. Pharmacol., 1983, 14, 277-280

Auguet M Delaflotte S Hellegouarch A Clostre F
[Pharmacological bases of the vascular impact of Ginkgo biloba extract]
Bases pharmacologiques de l'impact vasculaire de l'extrait de Ginkgo biloba.
Presse Med (1986 Sep 25) 15(31):1524-8

Arrigo A Cattaneo S
Clinical and psychometric evaluation of Ginkgo biloba extract in chronical cerebrovascular diseases.
In: Effects of Ginkgo biloba on Organic Cerebral Impairment, Paris, London, John Lilley, 1985

Bauer U
Six months double-blind randomized clinical trial of Ginkgo biloba extract versus placebo in two parallel groups in patients suffering from peripheral arterial insufficiency.
Arzneim. Forsch./Drug Res., 1984, 34, 716-720

Boismare F
Étude de l'action hémodynamique de l'extrait concentré de Ginkgo biloba comparée a celle du gaz carbonique chez le sujet jeune et chez le sujet sénile.
Ouesl Medical, 1976, 29, 747-749

Bono Y Mouren P
L'insuffisance circulatoire cérébrale et son traitement par l'extrait de Ginkgo biloba.
Presse Med 1975,3,59-62

Boudouresques G Vigouroux R Boudouresques J
Intérêt et place de l'extrait de Ginkgo biloba en pathologie vasculaire cérébrale.
Médecine Practicienne, 1975,59, 75-78

Bourgain RH Maes L Andries R Braquet P
Thrombus induction by endogenic paf-acether and its inhibition by Ginkgo Biloba extracts in the guinea pig.
Prostaglandins (1986 Jul) 32(1):142-4

Chabrier PE Roubert P
[Effect of Ginkgo biloba extract on the hemato-encephalic barrier]
Effet de l'extrait de Ginkgo biloba sur la barrière hémo-encéphalique.
Presse Med (1986 Sep 25) 15(31):1498-501

Chaterjee G
Effects of Ginkgo biloba extract on cerebral metabolic processes.
In: Effects of GBE and Organic Cerebral Impairment, Paris, London, John Lilley, 1985

Gautherie M Bourjat P Grosshans E Quenneville Y
[Vasodilator effect of Gingko biloba extract determined by skin thermometry and thermography]
Therapie (Sep-Oct 72) 27(5):881-92

Clostre F
[From the body to the cell membrane: the different levels of pharmacological action of Ginkgo biloba extract]
Presse Med 1986 Sep 25; 15(31):1529-38 (Published in French)

Etienne A Hecquet F Clostre F
[Mechanism of action of Ginkgo biloba extract in experimental cerebral edema]
Mécanismes d'action de l'extrait de Ginkgo biloba sur l'oedème cérébral expérimental.
Presse Med (1986 Sep 25) 15(31):1506-10

Gessner B Voelp A Klasser M
Study of the long-term action of Ginkgo biloba extract on vigilance and mental performance as determined by means of quantitative pharmaco-EEG and psychometric measurements.
Arzneim. Forsch./Drug Res., 1985, 35, 1459-1465

Hofferberth B
The influence of Ginkgo Biloba Extract (GBE) on the Neurophysiological and Psychometrical Test results in patients suffering from organic cerebral Psychosyndrome: A Double-Blind Study Versus Placebo.
Conference at The Third Congress of the International Psychogeriatric Association, Chicago, August 1987.

Krauskopf R Guinot PH Peetz HG
Long term on line EEG analyses demonstrating the pharmaco-dynamic effect of a defined Ginkgo biloba extract.
Beaufour-Schwabe Internat. Report, 1983.

Otani M Chatterjee SS Gabard B Kreutzberg GW
Effect of an extract of Ginkgo biloba on triethyltin-induced cerebral edema.
Acta Neuropathol (Berl) (1986) 69(1-2):54-65

Pidoux B Bastien C Niddam S
Clinical and quantitative EEG double-blind study of GBE.
J Cerebral Blood Flow Metabolism, 1983, 3, 5556-5557

Pidoux B Bastien C Niddam S
Normalization of electroencephalographic activity in aging brain by an extract of Ginkgo biloba.
In: Bes. A. Braquet P., Paoletti R., Siesjo B.K. Eds., Cerebral Ischemia, Amsterdam, Excerpta Medica, 1984, 385-388

Pidoux B
[Effects of Ginkgo biloba extract on functional brain activity. An assessment of clinical and experimental studies]
Presse Med (1986 Sep 25) 15(31):1588-91

Racagni G Brunello N Paoletti R
[Neuromediator changes during cerebral aging. The effect of Ginkgo biloba extract]
Presse Med (1986 Sep 25) 15(31):1488-90

Stange G Benning CD Degenhardt M Ottinger E
[Adaptational behaviour of peripheral and central acoustic responses in guinea pigs under the influence of various fractions of an extract from *Gingko biloba* (author's transl)]
Arzneim Forsch (1976) 26(3):367-74

Subhan Z Hindmarch L
The psychopharmacological effects of Ginkgo biloba extract in normal healthy volunteers.
Internat. J. Clin. Pharmacol. Res., 1984, 4, 89-93

Taylor JE
The effects of chronic, oral Ginkgo biloba extract administration on neurotransmitter receptor binding in young and aged Fisher 344 rats.
In: Effects of Ginkgo biloba extract on organic cerebral impairment, Paris, London, John Lilley, 1985

Volkner JH
Inhalations of extracts from Gingko biloba in vasomotor rhinitis and in the bronchitic syndrome.
Dtsch Med J (5 Sep 67) 18(17):527-33

Warburton DM
Clinical psychopharmacology of *Ginkgo biloba* extract.
Presse Med 1986 Sep 25; 15(31):1595-604 (Published in French)

Citations from the MEDLINE Database for the Genus *Humulus* (Hops)

Bravo L Cabo J Fraile A Jimenez J Villar A
[Pharmacodynamic study of the lupulus' (Humulus lupulus L.) tranquilizing action]
Boll Chim Farm (1974 May) 113(5):310-5

Caujolle F Pham-Huu-Chanh Duch-Kan P Bravo-Diaz L
[Spasmolytic action of hop (Humulus lupulus, Cannabinacees)]
Agressologie (1969 Sep-Oct) 10(5):405-10

Hansel R Wagener HH
[Attempts to identify sedative-hypnotic active substances in hops]
Arzneimittelforschung (1967 Jan) 17(1):79-81

Hansel R Wohlfart R Coper H
[Sedative-hypnotic compounds in the exhalation of hops, II]
Z Naturforsch [C] (1980 Nov-Dec) 35(11-12):1096-7

Citations from the MEDLINE Database for the Genus *Hypericum* (St. John's Wort)

Aizenman Blu
[Antibiotic preparations from Hypericum perforatum L]
Mikrobiol Zh (1969 Mar-Apr) 31(2):128-33

Chaplinskaia MG Shteinberg MA Tribul'skaia ZF
[Study of the photodynamic action of Hypericum in its external use]
Farm Zh (1965) 20(2):47-53

Decosterd LA Hoffmann E Kyburz R Bray D Hostettmann K
A new phloroglucinol derivative from Hypericum calycinum with antifungal and in vitro antimalarial activity.
Planta Med (1991 Dec) 57(6):548-51

Derbentseva NA Mishenkova EL Garagulia OD
[Action of tannins from Hypericum perforatum L. on the influenza virus]
Mikrobiol Zh (1972) 34(6):768-72

Gurevich AI Dobrynin VN Kolosov MN Popravko SA Riabova ID
[Antibiotic hyperforin from Hypericum perforatum L]
Antibiotiki (1971 Jun) 16(6):510-3

Holzl J
[Is Hypericum perforatum phototoxic? (letter)]
Med Monatsschr Pharm (1991 Oct) 14(10):304-6

Ishiguro K Yamaki M Kashihara M Takagi S
Saroaspidin A, B, and C: additional antibiotic compounds from Hypericum japonicum.
Planta Med (1987 Oct) 53(5):415-7

Ishiguro K Yamaki M Kashihara M Takagi S Isoi K
Sarothralin G: a new antimicrobial compound from Hypericum japonicum.
Planta Med (1990 Jun) 56(3):274-6

Jayasuriya H Clark AM McChesney JD
New antimicrobial filicinic acid derivatives from Hypericum drummondii.
J Nat Prod (1991 Sep-Oct) 54(5):1314-20

Jayasuriya H McChesney JD Swanson SM Pezzuto JM
Antimicrobial and cytotoxic activity of rottlerin-type compounds from Hypericum drummondii.
J Nat Prod (1989 Mar-Apr) 52(2):325-31

Kosuge T Ishida H Satoh T
Studies on antihemorrhagic substances in herbs classified as hemostatics in Chinese medicine. IV. On antihemorrhagic principles in Hypericum erectum Thunb.
Chem Pharm Bull (Tokyo) (1985 Jan) 33(1):202-5

Matei I Gafitanu E Dorneanu V
[Value of Hypericum perforatum oil in dermatological preparations. I.]
Rev Med Chir Soc Med Nat Iasi (1977 Jan-Mar) 81(1):73-4

Melzer R Fricke U Holzl J
Vasoactive properties of procyanidins from Hypericum perforatum L. in isolated porcine coronary arteries.
Arzneimittelforschung (1991 May) 41(5):481-3

Meruelo D et al
Therapeutic agents with dramatic antiviral activity and little toxicity at effective doses: Aromatic polycyclicdiones hypericin and pseudohypericin.
Proceedings National Academy of Sciences 85:5230-34 1988

Muldner H Zoller M
[Antidepressive effect of a Hypericum extract standardized to an active hypericine complex. Biochemical and clinical studies]
Arzneimittelforschung (1984) 34(8):918-20

Okpanyi SN Weischer ML
[Animal experiments on the psychotropic action of a Hypericum extract]
Arzneimittelforschung (1987 Jan) 37(1):10-3

Suzuki O et al
Inhibition of monoamine oxidase by hypericin.
Planta Medica 50:272-4, 1984

Citations from the MEDLINE Database for the Genus *Hyssopus* (Hyssop)

Kreis W Kaplan MH Freeman J Sun DK Sarin PS
Inhibition of HIV replication by Hyssop officinalis extracts.
Antiviral Res (1990 Dec) 14(6):323-37

Crude extracts of dried leaves of Hyssop officinalis showed strong anti-HIV activity as measured by inhibition of syncytia formation, HIV reverse transcriptase (RT), and p17 and p24 antigen expression, but were non-toxic to the uninfected Molt-3 cells. Ether extracts from direct extraction (Procedure I), after removal of tannins (Procedure II), or from the residue after dialysis of the crude extract (Procedure III), showed good antiviral activity. Methanol extracts, subsequent to ether, chloroform and chloroform ethanol extractions, derived from procedure I or II, but not III, also showed very strong anti-HIV activity. In addition, the residual material after methanol extractions still showed strong activity. Caffeic acid was identified in the ether extract of procedure I by HPLC and UV spectroscopy. Commercial caffeic acid showed good antiviral activity in the RT assay and high to moderate activity in the syncytia assay and the p17 and p24 antigen expression. Tannic acid and gallic acid, common to other teas, could not be identified in our extracts. When commercial products of these two acids were tested in our assay systems, they showed high to moderate activity against HIV-1. Hyssop officinalis extracts contain caffeic acid, unidentified tannins, and possibly a third class of unidentified higher molecular weight compounds that exhibit strong anti-HIV activity, and may be useful in the treatment of patients with AIDS.

Citations from the MEDLINE Database for the Genus *Lavandula* (Lavender)

Atanassova-Shopova S Roussinov KS
On certain central neurotropic effects of lavender essential oil.
Izv Inst Fiziol (Sofiia) 1970;13:69-77

Buchbauer G Jirovetz L Jager W Dietrich H Plank C
Aromatherapy: evidence for sedative effects of the essential oil of lavender after inhalation.
Z Naturforsch [C] 1991 Nov-Dec;46(11-12):1067-72

Buckle J
Which lavender oil? Complementary therapies.
Nurs Times 1992 Aug 5-11;88(32):54-5

Delaveau P Guillemain J Narcisse G Rousseau A
[Neuro-depressive properties of essential oil of lavender]
C R Soc Sciences Soc Biol Fil 1989;183(4):342-8 (Published in French)

Frohlich E
[Lavender oil, review of clinical, pharmacological and bacteriologic studies. Contribution to clarification of the mechanism of action]
Wien Med Wochenschr 1968 Apr 13;118(15):345-50 (Published in German)

Gamez MJ Jimenez J Risco S Zarzuelo A
Hypoglycemic activity in various species of the genus Lavandula. Part 1: Lavandula stoechas L. and Lavandula multifida L.
Pharmazie 1987 Oct;42(10):706-7

Gamez MJ Zarzuelo A Risco S Utrilla P Jimenez J
Hypoglycemic activity in various species of the genus Lavandula. Part 2: Lavandula dentata and Lavandula latifolia.
Pharmazie 1988 Jun;43(6):441-2

Gruncharov V
[Clinico-experimental study on the choleretic and cholagogic action of Bulgarian lavender oil]
Vutr Boles 1973;12(3):90-6 (Published in Bulgarian)

Guillemain J Rousseau A Delaveau P
[Neurodepressive effects of the essential oil of Lavandula angustifolia Mill]
Ann Pharm Fr 1989;47(6):337-43 (Published in French)

Shimizu M Shogawa H Matsuzawa T Yonezawa S Hayashi T Arisawa M Suzuki S Yoshizaki M Morita N Ferro E et al
Anti-inflammatory constituents of topically applied crude drugs. IV. Constituents and anti-inflammatory effect of Paraguayan crude drug "alhucema" (Lavandula latifolia Vill.).
Chem Pharm Bull (Tokyo) 1990 Aug;38(8):2283-4

Tasev T Toleva P Balabanova V
[Neurophysical effect of Bulgarian essential oils from rose, lavender and geranium]
Folia Med (Plovdiv) 1969;11(5):307-17 (Published in French)

Citations from the MEDLINE Database for the Genus *Lycopus* (Bugleweed)

Wagner H Horhammer L Frank U
[Lithospermic acid, the antihormonally active principle of Lycopus europaeus L. and Symphytum officinale. 3. Ingredients of medicinal plants with hormonal and antihormonal-like effect]
Arzneimittelforschung (1970 May) 20(5):705-13

Winterhoff H Gumbinger HG Sourgens H
On the antigonadotropic activity of Lithospermum and Lycopus species and some of their phenolic constituents.
Planta Med (1988 Apr) 54(2):101-6

Citations from the MEDLINE Database for the Genus *Matricaria* (Chamomile)

Appelt GD
Pharmacological aspects of selected herbs employed in Hispanic folk medicine in the San Luis Valley of Colorado, USA: I. Ligusticum porteri (osha) and Matricaria chamomilla (manzanilla).
J Ethnopharmacol 1985 Mar; 13(1):51-5

Luppold E
[Matricaria chamomilla—an old and new medicinal plant]
Pharm Unserer Zeit (1984 May) 13(3):65-70 (Published in German)

Mariann S Gizella VP Ede F
[Antifungal effect of the biologically active components of Matricaria chamomilla L.]
Acta Pharm Hung (1976 Nov) 46(5-6):232-47 (Published in Hungarian)

Pasechnik IK
[Choleretic action of Matricaria officinalis]
Farmakol Toksikol (1966 Jul-Aug) 29(4):468-9 (Published in Russian)

Vilagines P Delaveau P Vilagines R
[Inhibition of poliovirus replication by an extract of Matricaria chamomilla (L)]
C R Acad Sci III (1985) 301(6):289-94 (Published in French)

Citations from the MEDLINE Database for the Genus *Melissa* (Lemon Balm)

Chakurski I Matev M Koichev A Angelova I Stefanov G
[Treatment of chronic colitis with an herbal combination of Taraxacum officinale, Hypericum perforatum, Melissa officinalis, Calendula officinalis and Foeniculum vulgare]
Vutr Boles 1981;20(6):51-4 (Published in Bulgarian)

Chlabicz J Galasinski W
The components of Melissa officinalis L. that influence protein biosynthesis in-vitro.
J Pharm Pharmacol 1986 Nov;38(11):791-4

Chlabicz J Rozanski A Galasinski W
Studies on substances of plant origin with anticipated cyto- and oncostatic activity. Part 1: The influence of water extracts from Melissa officinalis on the protein biosynthesis in vitro.
Pharmazie 1984 Nov;39(11):770

Glowatzki G
[Melissa, a drug for 2000 years]
Med Klin 1970 Apr 17;65(16):800-3 (Published in German)

Herrmann EC Jr Kucera LS
Antiviral substances in plants of the mint family (labiatae). II. Nontannin polyphenol of Melissa officinalis.
Proc Soc Exp Biol Med 1967 Mar;124(3):869-74

Kucera LS Herrmann EC Jr
Antiviral substances in plants of the mint family (labiatae). I. Tannin of Melissa officinalis.
Proc Soc Exp Biol Med 1967 Mar;124(3):865-9

Soulimani R Fleurentin J Mortier F Misslin R Derrieu G Pelt JM
Neurotropic action of the hydroalcoholic extract of Melissa officinalis in the mouse.
Planta Med 1991 Apr;57(2):105-9

Citations from the Medline Database for the Genus *Nepeta* (Catnip)

Harney JW Barofsky IM Leary JD
Behavioral and toxicological studies of cyclopentanoid monoterpenes from Nepeta cataria.
Lloydia (1978 Jul-Aug) 41(4):367-74

Hatch RC
Effect of drugs on catnip (Nepeta cataria)-induced pleasure behavior in cats.
Am J Vet Res (1972 Jan) 33(1):143-55

Sherry CJ Hunter PS
The effect of an ethanol extract of catnip (Nepeta cataria) on the behavior of the young chick.
Experientia (1979 Feb 15) 35(2):237-8

Citations from the MEDLINE Database for the Genus *Panax* (Ginseng—Korean, American, Chinese)

Avakia EV and Evonuk E
Effects of Panax ginseng extract on tissue glycogen and adrenal cholesterol depletion during prolonged exercise.
Planta Medica 36:43-8,1979

Banerjee U Izquierdo JA
Antistress and antifatigue properties of Panax ginseng: comparison with piracetum.
Acta Physiol Lat Am (1982) 32(4):277-85

Bombardelli E Cirstoni A and Lietti A
The effect of acute and chronic (Panax) ginseng saponins treatment on adrenal function; biochemical and pharmacological.
Proceedings 3rd International Ginseng Symposium, 1980, pp. 9-161

Brekhman II and Dardymov IV
New substances of plant origin which increase nonspecific resistance.
Ann Rev Pharmacol 9:419-30, 1969

Brekhman II and Dardymov IV
Pharmacological investigation of glycosides from ginseng and Eleutherococcus.
Lloydia 32:46-51, 1969

Chong SK Brown HA Rimmer E Oberholzer V Hindocha P Walker-Smith JA
In vitro effect of Panax ginseng on phytohaemagglutinin-induced lymphocyte transformation.
Int Arch Allergy Appl Immunol (1984) 73(3):216-20

D'Angelo L Grimaldi R Caravaggi M et al
A double-blind, placebo-controlled clinical study on the effect of a standardized ginseng extract on psychomotor performance in healthy volunteers.
J Ethnopharmacol 16:15-22, 1986

Fahim WS Harman JM Clevenger TE et al
Effect of Panax ginseng on testosterone level and prostate in male rats.
Arch Androl 8:261-3, 1982

Fels E
[Experiences with Panax, a new phenacetin-free analgesic drug]
Schweiz Rundsch Med Prax (1973 Aug 14) 62(33):1017-9

Feng LM Pan HZ Li WW
[Anti-oxidant action of Panax ginseng]
Chung Hsi I Chieh Ho Tsa Chih (1987 May) 7(5):288-90, 262

Fulder SJ
Ginseng and the hypothalamic-pituitary control of stress.
Am J Chin Med 9:112-8, 1981

Fulder SJ
The growth of cultured human fibroblasts treated with hydrocortisone and extracts of the medicinal plant Panax ginseng.
Exp Gerontol 12:125-31, 1977

Gupta S Agarwal LB Epstein G et al
Panax: a new mitogen and interferon producer.
Clin Res 28:504A, 1980

Hallstrom C Fulder S Carruthers M
Effect of ginseng on the performance of nurses on night duty.
Comp Med East & West 6:277-82, 1982

Hiai S Yokoyama H Oura H
Features of ginseng saponin-induced corticosterone secretion.
Endocrinol Japan 26:737-40, 1979

Hiai S Yokoyama H Oura H Kawashima Y
Evaluation of corticosterone secretion-inducing effects of ginsenosides and their prosapogenins and sapogenins.
Chem Pharm Bull 31:168-74, 1983

Hikino H Kiso Y Sanada S Shoji J
Antihepatotoxic actions of ginsenosides from Panax ginseng roots.
Planta Medica 52:62-4, 1985

Hong SA Park CW Kim JH et al
The effects of ginseng saponin on animal behavior.
Proceedings of the 1st International Ginseng Symposium, 1975, pp. 33-44

Hu GC Yang Q
[Effect of sapogenins from the leaves of Panax notoginseng on migraine]
Chung Hsi I Chieh Ho Tsa Chih (1988 Dec) 8(12):726-7, 709

Huo YS
[Anti-senility action of saponin in Panax ginseng fruit in 327 cases]
Chung Hsi I Chieh Ho Tsa Chih (1984 Oct) 4(10):593-6, 578

Jie YH Cammisuli S Baggiolini M
Immunomodulatory effects of Panax ginseng C.A. Meyer in the mouse.
Agents and actions 15:386-91, 1984

Joo CN
The preventative effect of Korean (P. ginseng) saponins on aortic atheroma formation in prolonged cholesterol-fed rabbits.
Proceeding 3rd International Ginseng Symposium, 1980, pp. 27-36

Kaku T Miyata T Uruno T Sako I Kinoshita A
Chemico-pharmacological studies on saponins of Panax ginseng C. A. Meyer. II. Pharmacological part.
Arzneimittelforschung (1975 Apr) 25(4):539-47

Katano M Matsunaga H Yamamoto H
[A tumor inhibitory substance from panax ginseng]
Nippon Geka Gakkai Zasshi (1988 Jun) 89(6):971

Katano M Yamamoto H Hisatsugu T
[Tumor growth inhibition by water-soluble substance from Panax ginseng]
Nippon Geka Gakkai Zasshi (1987 Dec) 88(12):1754

Katano M Yamamoto H Matsunaga H Mori M Takata K Nakamura M
[Cell growth inhibitory substance isolated from Panax ginseng root: panaxytriol]
Gan To Kagaku Ryoho (1990 May) 17(5):1045-9

Konno C Sugiyama K Kano M et al
Isolation and hypoglycaemic activity of panaxans A, B, C, D and E, glycans of Panax ginseng roots.
Planta Medica 51:434-6, 1984

Koriech OM
Ginseng and mastalgia (letter).
Br Med J i:1556, 1978

Lee FC Ko JH Park JK Lee JS
Effects of Panax ginseng on blood alcohol clearance in man.
Clin Exp Pharmacol Physiol (1987 Jun) 14(6):543-6

Lee KD Huemer RP
Antitumoral activity of Panax ginseng extracts.
Jap J Pharmacol 21:299-302, 1971

Ma EQ Luo CQ
[The effect of a compound panax-ginseng decoction in the treatment of adult acute respiratory insufficiency after burns]
Chung Hsi I Chieh Ho Tsa Chih (1982 Oct) 2(4):196, 224-5

Ng TB Yeung HW
Hypoglycemic constituents of Panax ginseng.
Gen Pharmacol 6:549-552, 1985-9

Oh JS Lim JK Park CW Han MH
The effect of ginseng on experimental hypertension.
Korean J Pharmacol 4:27-31, 1968

Oura H Hiai S Nabatini S Nakagawa H et al
Effect of ginseng on endoplasmic reticulum and ribosome.
Planta Medica 28:76-88, 1975

Oura H Nakashima S Tsukada K Ohta Y
Effect of radix ginseng on serum protein synthesis.
Chem Pharm Bull 20:980-6, 1972

Petkov W
Pharmacological studies of the drug P. ginseng C.A. Meyer.
Arzneim Forsch 9:305-11, 1959

Petkov W
The mechanism of action of P. ginseng.
Arzneim Forsch 11:288-95, 418-22, 1961

Punnonen R Lukola A
Oestrogen-like effect of ginseng.
Br Med J 281:1110, 1980

Scaglione F Ferrara F Dugnani S Falchi M Santoro G Fraschini F
Immunomodulatory effects of two extracts of Panax ginseng C.A. Meyer.
Drugs Exp Clin Res (1990) 16(10):537-42

Shibata S Tanaka O Shoji J Saito H
Chemistry and pharmacology of Panax.
Economic and Medicinal Plant Research 1:217-84, 1985

Siegel RK
Ginseng abuse syndrome.
JAMA 241:1614-5, 1979

Siegel RK
Ginseng and high blood pressure (letter).
JAMA 243:32, 1980

Singh VK Agarwal SS Gupta BM
Immunomodulatory activity of Panax ginseng extract.
Planta Medica 51:462-5, 1984

Tong LS Chao CY
Effects of ginsenoside Rg1 of Panax ginseng on mitosis in human blood lympho-cytes in vitro.
Am J Chin Med (1980 Autumn) 8(3):254-67

Xu CH
[Effect of Panax ginseng on 3H-thymidine incorporation into cultured liver cells in vitro]
Chung Yao Tung Pao (1985 May) 10(5):40-1, 16

Yamamoto M Uemura T Nakama S Uemiya M Kumagai A
Serum HDL-cholesterol-increasing and fatty liver-improving actions of Panax gin-seng in high cholesterol diet-fed rats with clinical effect on hyperlipidemia in man.
Am J Chin Med (1983) 11(1-4):96-101

Yamamoto M Kumagai A Yamamura Y
Stimulatory effect of P. ginseng principles on DNA and protein synthesis in rat testes.
Arzneim Forsch 27:1404-5, 1977

Yamamoto M Masaka K Yamada Y et al
Stimulatory effect of ginsenosides on DNA, protein and lipid synthesis in bone marrow.
Arzneim Forsch 28:2238-41, 1978

Yeung HW Cheung K Leung KN
Immunopharmacology of Chinese medicine. I. Ginseng induced immunosuppres-sion in virus infected mice.
Am J Chin Med 10:44-54, 1982

Yonezawa M
Restoration of radiation injury by intraperitoneal injection of ginseng extract in mice.
J Radiation Res 17:111-3, 1976

Yuan GC Chang RS
Testing of compounds for capacity to prolong postmitotic lifespan of cultured human amnion cells. Effect of steroids and Panax ginseng.
J Gerontol (1969 Jan) 24(1):82-5

Citations from the MEDLINE Database for the Genus *Peumus* (Boldo)

Lanhers MC Joyeux M Soulimani R Fleurentin J Sayag M Mortier F Younos C Pelt JM
Hepatoprotective and anti-inflammatory effects of a traditional medicinal plant of Chile, Peumus boldus.
Planta Med (1991 Apr) 57(2):110-5

Citations from the MEDLINE Database for the Genus *Populus* (Aspen, Balm of Gilead)

el-Ghazaly M Khayyal MT Okpanyi SN Arens-Corell M
Study of the anti-inflammatory activity of Populus tremula, Solidago virgaurea and Fraxinus excelsior.
Arzneimittelforschung 1992 Mar;42(3):333-6

Shen QL
[Antipyretic and analgesic constituents of the leaves of Populus tomentosa Carr]
Chung Yao Tung Pao 1988 Apr;13(4):36-7, 63 (Published in Chinese)

Van Hoof L Totte J Corthout J Pieters LA Mertens F Vanden Berghe DA Vlietinck AJ Dommisse R Esmans E
Plant antiviral agents, VI. Isolation of antiviral phenolic glucosides from Populus cultivar Beaupre by droplet counter-current chromatography.
J Nat Prod 1989 Jul-Aug;52(4):875-8

Whatley FR Greenaway W May J
Populus candicans and the Balm of Gilead.
Z Naturforsch [C] 1989 May-Jun;44(5-6):353-6

Citations from the MEDLINE Database for the Genus *Rheum* (Rhubarb)

Bi ZQ Zheng FL Kang ZQ
Treatment of chronic renal failure by retention-enema with rhizoma rhei compound decoction.
J Tradit Chin Med 1982 Sep;2(3):211-4

Chen HC Hsieh MT Tsai HY Chang HH Wang TF Shibuya T
Studies on the "San-Huang-Hsieh-Hsin-Tang" in the treatment of essential hypertension.
Taiwan I Hsueh Hui Tsa Chih 1984 Apr;83(4):340-6

Engelshowe R
[Rhubarb, an old drug—but still current]
Rhabarber, eine alte Droge—noch immer aktuell.
Pharm Unserer Zeit 1985 Mar;14(2):40-9 (Published in German)

Gao XS
[The effect of raw Chinese rhubarb on the activities of four digestive enzymes and the discussion on its medicine property (author's transl)]
Chung Yao Tung Pao 1981 May;6(3):25-9 (Published in Chinese)

Hu LH
[Experimental study of Rheum officinale Baill. in treating severe hepatitis and hepatic coma]
Chung Hsi I Chieh Ho Tsa Chih 1986 Jan;6(1):41-2, 5 (Published in Chinese)

Jiao DH
[Clinical research on the hemostatic effect of rhubarb on peptic ulcer with acute bleeding]
Chung Hsi I Chieh Ho Tsa Chih 1984 Oct;4(10):597-600, 579 (Published in Chinese)

Jiao DH
[Alcoholic extract tablet of rhubarb in treating acute upper gastrointestinal hemorrhage]
Chung Hsi I Chieh Ho Tsa Chih 1988 Jun;8(6):344-6, 324-5 (Published in Chinese)

Jiao DH Liu XC
[Resume of 1000 emergency cases of three kinds of digestive tract diseases treated with a single recipe rhubarb]
Chung Hsi I Chieh Ho Tsa Chih 1982 Apr;2(2):66-7, 85-7 (Published in Chinese)

Jiao DH Ma YH Chen SJ Liu CT Shu HN Chu CM
Resume of 400 cases of acute upper digestive tract bleeding treated by rhubarb alone.
Pharmacology 1980;20 Suppl 1:128-30

Jin YC
[Rheum and other individual medicinal herbs for the treatment of gastric hemorrhage]
Chung Hsi I Chieh Ho Tsa Chih 1983 Jul;3(4):251-2 (Published in Chinese)

Li T
[Rhubarb in the treatment of viral hepatitis and its mechanism of action]
Chung Hsi I Chieh Ho Tsa Chih 1985 Jun;5(6):383-4, 382 (Published in Chinese)

Liang ZJ
[Effect of Rheum palmatum L. on blood rheology in normal subjects]
Chung Hsi I Chieh Ho Tsa Chih 1984 Sep;4(9):560-2, 517 (Published in Chinese)

Mitsuma T Yokozawa T Oura H Terasawa K
[Rhubarb therapy in patients with chronic renal failure (Part 2)]
Nippon Jinzo Gakkai Shi 1987 Feb;29(2):195-207 (Published in Japanese)

Peigen X Liyi H Liwei W
Ethnopharmacologic study of Chinese rhubarb.
J Ethnopharmacol 1984 May;10(3):275-93

Ren S
[Role of a virus in hemorrhagic pancreatitis and the therapeutic effect of rhubarb]
Chung Hsi I Chieh Ho Tsa Chih 1990 Mar;10(3):162-3, 133 (Published in Chinese)

Sun DA
[Clinical evaluation of crude rhubarb powder and cimetidine in upper gastrointestinal bleeding]
Chung Hsi I Chieh Ho Tsa Chih 1986 Aug;6(8):458-9, 451 (Published in Chinese)

Wang GS
[Clinical and experimental study on the treatment of severe subacute hepatitis with traditional Chinese medicinal compounds]
Chung Hsi I Chieh Ho Tsa Chih 1985 Jun;5(6):329-31, 322 (Published in Chinese)

Wu CX
[A preliminary study on the effect of a single Rheum officinale in heavy doses in the treatment of acute icteric hepatitis]
Chung Hsi I Chieh Ho Tsa Chih 1984 Feb;4(2):88-9 (Published in Chinese)

Yuan ZD Di H Xu WZ
[Erythrocyte sodium pump activity in the human and the effect of Rheum palmatum on its activity]
Chung Hsi I Chieh Ho Tsa Chih 1988 Sep;8(9):536-7, 517 (Published in Chinese)

Yue R
[Experimental study and clinical uses of rhubarb]
Chung Hsi I Chieh Ho Tsa Chih 1990 May;10(5):310-3 (Published in Chinese)

Zhang WL
[Treatment of hemorrhage of the upper gastro-intestinal tract with the Chinese drug hai huang san. Analysis of 50 cases]
Chung Hsi I Chieh Ho Tsa Chih 1986 Nov;6(11):665-6, 644 (Published in Chinese)

Zhao SY
[Clinical studies on 2 acute diseases of the digestive tract treated with 2 kinds of radix et rhizoma Rhei]
Chung Yao Tung Pao 1986 Mar;11(3):58-60 (Published in Chinese)

Zhou H Jiao D
[312 cases of gastric and duodenal ulcer bleeding treated with 3 kinds of alcoholic extract rhubarb tablets]
Chung Hsi I Chieh Ho Tsa Chih 1990 Mar;10(3):150-1, 131-2 (Published in Chinese)

Zhou Z
[Application and mechanism of radix et rhizoma rhei in treating diseases of the digestive system]
Chung Kuo Chung Yao Tsa Chih 1989 Aug;14(8):501-3, 512 (Published in Chinese)

Citations from the MEDLINE Database for the Genus *Rosmarinus* (Rosemary)

Aruoma OI Halliwell B Aeschbach R Loligers J
Antioxidant and pro-oxidant properties of active rosemary constituents: carnosol and carnosic acid.
Xenobiotica 1992 Feb;22(2):257-68

Durakovic Z Durakovic S
The effect of rosemary oil on Candida albicans [letter]
J Indian Med Assoc 1979 Apr 1;72(7):175-6

Rulffs W
[Rosemary oil bath additive. Proof of effectiveness]
MMW Munch Med Wochenschr 1984 Feb 24;126(8):207-8 (Published in German)

Selmi G
[Therapeutic use of rosemary through the centuries]
Policlinico [Prat] 1967 Mar 27;74(13):439-41 (Published in Italian)

Steinmetz MD Vial M Millet Y
[Actions of essential oils of rosemary and certain of its constituents (eucalyptol and camphor) on the cerebral cortex of the rat in vitro]
J Toxicol Clin Exp 1987 Jul-Aug;7(4):259-71 (Published in French)

Zimmermann V
[Rosemary as a medicinal plant and wonder-drug. A report on the medieval drug monographs]
Sudhoffs Arch 1980;64(4):351-70 (Published in German)

Citations from the MEDLINE Database for the Genus *Ruta* (Rue)

al-Said MS Tariq M al-Yahya MA Rafatullah S Ginnawi OT Ageel AM
Studies on Ruta chalepensis, an ancient medicinal herb still used in traditional medicine.
J Ethnopharmacol 1990 Mar;28(3):305-12

Gandhi M Lal R Sankaranarayanan A Sharma PL
Post-coital antifertility action of Ruta graveolens in female rats and hamsters.
J Ethnopharmacol 1991 Aug;34(1):49-59

Kong YC Lau CP Wat KH Ng KH But PP Cheng KF Waterman PG
Antifertility principle of Ruta graveolens.
Planta Med 1989 Apr;55(2):176-8

Minker E Bartha C Koltai M Rozsa Z Szendrei K Reisch J
Effect of secondary substances isolated from the Ruta graveolens L. on the coronary smooth muscle.
Acta Pharm Hung 1980 Jan;50(1):7-11

Nieschulz O Schneider G
[Pharmacological findings on alkaloids from Ruta graveolens L]
Naturwissenschaften 1965 Jul;52(13):394-5 (Published in German)

Wehr K
[Criminal abortion using ruta roots (Ruta graveolens L.)]
Beitr Gerichtl Med 1974;32:126-31 (Published in German)

Citations from the MEDLINE Database for the Genus *Sanguinaria* (Bloodroot)

Frankos VH Brusick DJ Johnson EM Maibach HI Munro I Squire RA Weil CS
Safety of Sanguinaria extract as used in commercial toothpaste and oral rinse products.
J Can Dent Assoc (1990) 56(7 Suppl):41-7

Hannah JJ Johnson JD Kuftinec MM
Long-term clinical evaluation of toothpaste and oral rinse containing sanguinaria extract in controlling plaque, gingival inflammation, and sulcular bleeding during orthodontic treatment.
Am J Orthod Dentofacial Orthop (1989 Sep) 96(3):199-207

Harkrader RJ Reinhart PC Rogers JA Jones RR Wylie RE 2d Lowe BK McEvoy RM
The history, chemistry and pharmacokinetics of Sanguinaria extract.
J Can Dent Assoc (1990) 56(7 Suppl):7-12

Harper DS Mueller LJ Fine JB Gordon J Laster LL
**Effect of 6 months use of a dentifrice and oral rinse containing sanguinaria ex-
tract and zinc chloride upon the microflora of the dental plaque and oral soft
tissues.**
J Periodontol (1990 Jun) 61(6):359-63

Harper DS Mueller LJ Fine JB Gordon J Laster LL
**Clinical efficacy of a dentifrice and oral rinse containing sanguinaria extract and
zinc chloride during 6 months of use.**
J Periodontol (1990 Jun) 61(6):352-8

Karjalainen K Kaivosoja S Seppa S Knuuttila M
Effects of sanguinaria extract on leucocytes and fibroblasts.
Proc Finn Dent Soc (1988) 84(3):161-5

Kopczyk RA Abrams H Brown AT Matheny JL Kaplan AL
**Clinical and microbiological effects of a sanguinaria-containing mouthrinse and
dentifrice with and without fluoride during 6 months of use.**
J Periodontol (1991 Oct) 62(10):617-22

Kuftinec MM Mueller-Joseph LJ Kopczyk RA
**Sanguinaria toothpaste and oral rinse regimen clinical efficacy in short- and long-
term trials.**
J Can Dent Assoc (1990) 56(7 Suppl):31-3

Laster LL Lobene RR
**New perspectives on Sanguinaria clinicals: individual toothpaste and oral rinse
testing.**
J Can Dent Assoc (1990) 56(7 Suppl):19-30

Lobene RR Soparkar PM Newman MB
The effects of a sanguinaria dentifrice on plaque and gingivitis.
Compend Contin Educ Dent (1986) Suppl 7:S185-8

Mallatt ME Beiswanger BB Drook CA Stookey GK Jackson RD Bricker SL
Clinical effect of a sanguinaria dentifrice on plaque and gingivitis in adults.
J Periodontol (1989 Feb) 60(2):91-5

Miller RA McIver JE Gunsolley JC
Effects of sanguinaria extract on plaque retention and gingival health.
J Clin Orthod (1988 May) 22(5):304-7

Nikiforuk G
**The Sanguinaria story—an update and new perspectives (overview of the Toronto
symposium).**
J Can Dent Assoc (1990) 56(7 Suppl):5-6

Parsons LG Thomas LG Southard GL Woodall IR Jones BJ
**Effect of sanguinaria extract on established plaque and gingivitis when
supragingivally delivered as a manual rinse or under pressure in an oral irrigator.**
J Clin Periodontol (1987 Aug) 14(7):381-5

Schwartz HG
Safety profile of sanguinarine and sanguinaria extract.
Compend Contin Educ Dent (1986) Suppl 7:S212-7

Southard GL Harkrader RJ Greene JA
Efficacy and compatibility of a toothpaste containing sanguinaria extract and fluoride.
Compend Contin Educ Dent (1986) Suppl 7:S189-92

Southard GL Parsons LG Thomas LG Woodall IR Jones BJ
Effect of sanguinaria extract on development of plaque and gingivitis when supragingivally delivered as a manual rinse or under pressure in an oral irrigator [published erratum appears in J Clin Periodontol 1988 Jan;15(1):83]
J Clin Periodontol (1987 Aug) 14(7):377-80

Walker C
Effects of sanguinarine and Sanguinaria extract on the microbiota associated with the oral cavity.
J Can Dent Assoc (1990) 56(7 Suppl):13-30

Citations from the MEDLINE Database for the Genus *Serenoa, Sabal* (Saw Palmetto)

Boccafoschi Annoscia S
Comparison of Serenoa repens extract with placebo by controlled clinical trial in patients with prostatic adenomatosis.
Urologia 50:1257-68, 1983

Breu W Hagenlocher M Redl K Tittel G Stadler F Wagner H
[Anti-inflammatory activity of sabal fruit extracts prepared with supercritical carbon dioxide. In vitro antagonists of cyclooxygenase and 5-lipoxygenase metabolism]
Arzneimittelforschung (1992 Apr) 42(4):547-51

Champault G Bonnard AM Cauquil J Patel JC
Medical treatment of prostatic adenoma. Controlled trial: PA 109 vs. placebo in 110 patients.
Ann Urol 18:407-10, 1984

Champault G, Patel JC Bonnard AM
A double-blind trial of an extract of the plant Serenoa repens in benign prostatic hyperplasia.
Br J Clin Pharmacol 18:461-2, 1984

Cirillo-Marucco E Pagliarulo A Tritto G et al
Extract of Serenoa repens (Permixon) in the early treatment of prostatic hypertrophy.
Urologia 50:1269-77, 1983

Crimi A Russo A
Extract of Serenoa repens for the treatment of the functional disturbances of prostate hypertrophy.
Med Praxis 4:47-51, 1983

Duvia R Radice GP Galdini R
Advances in the phytotherapy of prostatic hypertrophy.
Med Praxis 4:143-8, 1983

Emili E Lo Cigno M Petrone U
Clinical trial of a new drug for treating hypertrophy of the prostate (Permixon).
Urologia 50:1042-8, 1983

Hiermann A
[The contents of sabal fruits and testing of their anti-inflammatory effect]
Arch Pharm (Weinheim) (1989 Feb) 322(2):111-4

Sultan C Terraza A Devillier C et al
Inhibition of androgen metabolism and binding by a liposterolic extract of "Serenoa repens B" in human foreskin fibroblasts.
J Steroid Biochem 20:515-9, 1984

Tarayre JP Delhon A Lauressergues H et al
Anti-edematous action of a hexane extract of the stone fruit of Serenoa repens Bartr.
Ann Pharm Franc 41:559-70, 1983

Tasca A Barulli M Cavazzana A et al
Treatment of obstructive symptomatology caused by prostatic adenoma with an extract of Serenoa repens. Double-blind clinical study vs. placebo.
Minerva Urol Nefrol 37:87-91, 1985

Timmermans LM Timmermans LG Jr
[Determination of the activity of extracts of Echinaceae and Sabal in the treatment of idiopathic megabladder in women]
Acta Urol Belg (1990) 58(2):43-59

Tripodi V Giancaspro M Pascarella M et al
Treatment of prostatic hypertrophy with Serenoa repens extract.
Med Praxis 4:41-6, 1983

Wagner H Flachsbarth H
[A new antiphlogistic principle from Sabal serrulata, I (author's transl)]
Planta Med (1981 Mar) 41(3):244-51

Citations from the MEDLINE Database for the Genus *Scutellaria* (Skullcap)

Konoshima T Kokumai M Kozuka M Iinuma M Mizuno M Tanaka T Tokuda H Nishino H Iwashima A
Studies on inhibitors of skin tumor promotion. XI. Inhibitory effects of flavonoids from Scutellaria baicalensis on Epstein-Barr virus activation and their anti-tumor-promoting activities.
Chem Pharm Bull (Tokyo) 1992 Feb;40(2):531-3

Li Z
[Progress in pharmacologic research on Scutellaria baicalensis]
Chung Hsi I Chieh Ho Tsa Chih 1989 Nov;9(11):698-700 (Published in Chinese)

Lin MT Liu GG Wu WL Chern YF
Effects of Chinese herb, Huang Chin (Scutellaria baicalensis George) on thermoregulation in rats.
Jpn J Pharmacol 1980 Feb;30(1):59-64

Nagai T Yamada H Otsuka Y
Inhibition of mouse liver sialidase by the root of Scutellaria baicalensis.

Citations from the MEDLINE Database for the Genus *Silybum* (Milk Thistle)

Antweiler, H.
Effects of silymarin on intoxication with ethionine and ethanol.
In: Symposium on the Pharmacodynamics of Silymarin, Cologne Nov. 1974. Braatz, R., Schneider, C.C. (eds.). Munchen-Berlin-Wien: Urban and Schwarzenberg, 1976, pp. 80-82

Bosisio E Benelli C Pirola O
Effect of the flavanolignans of Silybum marianum L. on lipid peroxidation in rat liver microsomes and freshly isolated hepatocytes.
Pharmacol Res 1992 Feb-Mar;25(2):147-54

Braatz R
Effects of silybin on phalloidine pretreated mice.
In: Symposium on the Pharmacodynamics of Silymarin, Cologne Nov. 1974. Braatz, R., Schneider, C.C. (eds.). Munchen-Berlin-Wien: Urban and Schwarzenberg, 1976, pp. 44-45

De Martiis M Fontana M Assogna G D'Ottavi R D'Ottavi O
[Milk thistle (Silybum marianum) derivatives in the therapy of chronic hepatopathies] Clin Ter 1980 Aug 15;94(3):283-315 (Published in Italian)

Desplaces A Choppin J Vogel G Trost W
Histochemical study on the treatment of the liver damage by phalloidine with silymarin, the active principle of the seed of *Silybum marianum* L. Gaertn.
Digestion 1 , 343-344 (1974)

Desplaces A Choppin J Vogel G Trost W
The effects of silymarin on experimental phalloidine poisoning.
Arzneim.-Forsch. 25, 89-96 (1975)

Desplaces A
The effect of silymarin on the histochemical picture in normal liver cells and in phalloidine-intoxicated liver cells.
In: Symposium on the Pharmacodynamics of Silymarin, Cologne Nov. 1974. Braatz, R., Schneider, C.C. (eds.). München-Berlin-Wien: Urban and Schwarzenberg, 1976, pp. 103-112

Fiebig M Wagner H
[New antihepatotoxic effects of flavonolignans of a white flowering variety of Silybum]
Planta Med 1984 Aug;50(4):310-3 (Published in German)

Floersheim GL
Antagonistic effects against single lethal doses of Amanita phalloides.
Naunyn-Schmiedebergs Arch. Pharmacol. 293, 171-174 (1976)

Floersheim GL
Treatment of experimental poisoning by extracts of Amanita phalloides.
Toxicol. Appl. Pharmacol. 34, 499-508 (1975)

Hahn G Lehmann HD Kurten M Uebel H Vogel G
[On the pharmacology and toxicology of silymarin, an antihepatotoxic active principle from Silybum marianum (L.) Gaertn.]
Arzneimittelforschung 1968 Jun;18(6):698-704 (Published in German)

Hikino H Kiso Y Wagner H Fiebig M
Antihepatotoxic actions of flavonolignans from Silybum marianum fruits.
Planta Med 1984 Jun;50(3):248-50

Morelli I
[Constituents of Silybum marianum and their therapeutic use]
Boll Chim Farm 1978 May;117(5):258-67 (Published in Italian)

Rumiantseva ZhN
[The pharmacodynamics of hepatic protectors from the lady's-thistle (Silybum marianum)]
Vrach Delo 1991 May(5):15-9 (Published in Russian)

Schriewer H Weinhold F
The influence of silybin from Silybum marianum (L.) Gaertn. on in vitro phosphatidyl choline biosynthesis in rat livers.
Arzneimittelforschung 1979;29(5):791-2

Sonnenbichler J Mattersberger J Rosen H
[Stimulation of RNA synthesis in rat liver and isolated hepatocytes by silybin, an antihepatotoxic agent from Silybum marianum L. Gaertn. (author's transl)]
Hoppe Seylers Z Physiol Chem 1976 Aug;357(8):1171-80 (Published in German)

Vogel G Trost W
Proceedings: Neutralization of the lethal effects of phalloidine and alpha-amanitine in animal experiments by substances from the seeds of Silybum marianum L. Gaertn.
Naunyn Schmiedebergs Arch Pharmacol 1974 Mar 22;282(0):suppl 282:R102

Vogel G Trost W Braatz R Odenthal KP Brusewitz G Antweiler H Seeger R
[Pharmacodynamics, site and mechanism of action of silymarin, the antihepatoxic principle from Silybum mar. (L.) Gaertn. 1. Acute toxicology or tolerance, general and specific (liver-) pharmacology]
Arzneimittelforschung 1975 Jan;25(1):82-9 (Published in German)

Wagner H Horhammer L Munster R
[On the chemistry of silymarin (silybin), the active principle of the fruits from Silybum marianum (L.) Gaertn. (Carduus marianus L.)]
Arzneimittelforschung 1968 Jun;18(6):688-96 (Published in German)

Wagner H Horhammer L Seitz M
[Chemical evaluation of a silymarin-containing flavonoid concentrate from Silybum marianum (L.) Gaertn.]
Arzneimittelforschung 1968 Jun;18(6):696-8 (Published in German)

Citations from the MEDLINE Database for the Genus *Smilax* (Sarsaparilla)

Giachetti D Taddei I Taddei E
Effects of Smilax macrophylla Vers. in normal or hyperuricemic and hyperuricosuric rats.
Pharmacol Res Commun (1988 Dec) 20 Suppl 5:59-62

Thurman FM
The treatment of psoriasis with Sarsaparilla compound.
NEJM 227:128-33, 1942

Wang WH
[Antagonistic effect of Smilax sp. on gossypol toxicity (author's transl)]
Chung Yao Tung Pao (1982 Jan) 7(1):32-4

Citations from the MEDLINE Database for the Genus *Solidago* (Goldenrod)

Bader G Binder K Hiller K Ziegler-Bohme H
[The antifungal action of triterpene saponins of Solidago virgaurea L.]
Pharmazie 1987 Feb;42(2):140 (Published in German)

Chodera et al
[Diuretic effect of the glycoside from a plant of the Solidago L. genus]
Acta Pol Pharm 1985;42(2):199-204 (Published in Polish)

Dittmann J
[Effect of extracts from Solidago virgaurea on the metabolism of rabbit brain slices (author's transl)]
Planta Med 1973 Dec;24(4):329-36 (Published in German)

el-Ghazaly M Khayyal MT Okpanyi SN Arens-Corell M
Study of the anti-inflammatory activity of Populus tremula, Solidago virgaurea and Fraxinus excelsior.
Arzneimittelforschung 1992 Mar;42(3):333-6

Matsunaga H Katano M Tasaki M Yamamoto H Mori M Takata K
Inhibitory effect of cis-dehydromatricaria ester isolated from Solidago altissima on the growth of mammalian cells.
Chem Pharm Bull (Tokyo) 1990 Dec;38(12):3483-4

Wagener HH
[On the pharmacology of a Solidago extract-containing venous drug]
Arzneimittelforschung 1966 Jul;16(7):859-66 (Published in German)

Citations from the MEDLINE Database for the Genus *Symphytum* (Comfrey)

Behninger C Abel G Roder E Neuberger V Goggelmann W
[Studies on the effect of an alkaloid extract of Symphytum officinale on human lymphocyte cultures]
Planta Med 1989 Dec;55(6):518-22 (Published in German)

Brauchli J Luthy J Zweifel U Schlatter C
Pyrrolizidine alkaloids from Symphytum officinale L. and their percutaneous absorption in rats.
Experientia 1982 Sep 15;38(9):1085-7

Culvenor CC Clarke M Edgar JA Frahn JL Jago MV Peterson JE Smith LW
Structure and toxicity of the alkaloids of Russian comfrey (symphytum x uplandicum Nyman), a medicinal herb and item of human diet.
Experientia 1980 Apr 15;36(4):377-9

Fell KR Peck JM
British medicinal species of the genus symphytum.
Planta Med 1968 May;16(2):208-16

Franz G
[Studies on the mucopolysaccharides of Tussilago farfara L., Symphytum officinalis L., Borago officinalis L. and Viola tricolor L.]
Planta Med 1969 Aug;17(3):217-20 (Published in German)

Gracza L Koch H Loffler E
[Biochemical-pharmacologic studies of medicinal plants. 1. Isolation of rosmarinic acid from Symphytum officinale L. and its anti-inflammatory activity in an in vitro model]
Arch Pharm (Weinheim) 1985 Dec;318(12):1090-5 (Published in German)

Hirono I Mori H Haga M
Carcinogenic activity of Symphytum officinale.
J Natl Cancer Inst 1978 Sep;61(3):865-9

Wagner H Horhammer L Frank U
[Lithospermic acid, the antihormonally active principle of Lycopus europaeus L. and Symphytum officinale. 3. Ingredients of medicinal plants with hormonal and antihormonal-like effect]
Arzneimittelforschung 1970 May;20(5):705-13 (Published in German)

Citations from the MEDLINE Database for the Genus *Taraxacum* (Dandelion)

Akhtar MS Khan QM Khaliq T
Effects of Portulaca oleracae (Kulfa) and Taraxacum officinale (Dhudhal) in normoglycaemic and alloxan-treated hyperglycaemic rabbits.
JPMA J Pak Med Assoc 1985 Jul;35(7):207-10

Baba K Abe S Mizuno D
[Antitumor activity of hot water extract of dandelion, Taraxacum officinale—correlation between antitumor activity and timing of administration (author's transl)]
Yakugaku Zasshi 1981 Jun;101(6):538-43 (Published in Japanese)

Chakurski I Matev M Koichev A Angelova I Stefanov G
[Treatment of chronic colitis with an herbal combination of Taraxacum officinale, Hipericum perforatum, Melissa officinalis, Calendula officinalis and Foeniculum vulgare]
Vutr Boles 1981;20(6):51-4 (Published in Bulgarian)

Racz-Kotilla E Racz G Solomon A
The action of Taraxacum officinale extracts on the body weight and diuresis of laboratory animals.
Planta Med 1974 Nov;26(3):212-7

Citations from the MEDLINE Database for the Genus *Trigonella* (Fenugreek)

Abdo MS al-Kafawi AA
Experimental studies on the effect of Trigonella foenum-graecum.
Planta Med 1969 Feb;17(1):14-8

Ahsan SK Tariq M Ageel AM al-Yahya MA Shah AH
Effect of Trigonella foenum-graecum and Ammi majus on calcium oxalate urolithiasis in rats.
J Ethnopharmacol 1989 Oct;26(3):249-54

Ajabnoor MA Tilmisany AK
Effect of Trigonella foenum-graecum on blood glucose levels in normal and alloxan-diabetic mice.
J Ethnopharmacol 1988 Jan;22(1):45-9

Elmadfa I Koken M
[Effect of vitamin E and protein quality on the hemolytic effect of Trigonella sapogenins in rats]
Z Ernahrungswiss 1980 Dec;19(4):280-9 (Published in German)

Ghafghazi T Sheriat HS Dastmalchi T Barnett RC
Antagonism of cadmium and alloxan-induced hyperglycemia in rats by Trigonella foenum-graecum.
Pahlavi Med J 1977 Jan;8(1):14-25

Mishkinsky JS Goldschmied A Joseph B Ahronson Z Sulman FG
Hypoglycaemic effect of Trigonella foenum-graecum and Lupinus termis (leguminosae) seeds and their major alkaloids in alloxan-diabetic and normal rats.
Arch Int Pharmacodyn Ther 1974 Jul;210(1):27-37

Citations from the MEDLINE Database for the Genus *Urtica* (Nettles)

Barsom S Bettermann AA
[Prostatic adenoma. The conservative therapy with urtica extract]
ZFA (Stuttgart) (1979 Nov 30) 55(33):1947-50

Czarnetzki BM Thiele T Rosenbach T
Immunoreactive leukotrienes in nettle plants (Urtica urens).
Int Arch Allergy Appl Immunol (1990) 91(1):43-6

Maitai CK Talalaj S Njoroge D Wamugunda R
Effect of extract of hairs from the herb Urtica massaica on smooth muscle.
Toxicon (1980) 18(2):225-9

Mittman P
Randomized, double-blind study of freeze-dried Urtica dioica in the treatment of allergic rhinitis.
Planta Med (1990 Feb) 56(1):44-7

Wagner H Willer F Kreher B
[Biologically active compounds from the aqueous extract of Urtica dioica]
Planta Med (1989 Oct) 55(5):452-4

Citations from the MEDLINE Database for the Genus *Valeriana* (Valerian)

Babichev VA
[Medicinal Valerian]
Feldsher Akush 1968 Oct;33(10):31-3 (Published in Russian)

Balderer G Borbely AA
Effect of valerian on human sleep.
Psychopharmacology (Berl) 1985;87(4):406-9

Boeters U
[Treatment of control disorders of the autonomic nervous system with valepotriate (Valmane)]
Munch Med Wochenschr 1969 Sep 12;111(37):1873-6 (Published in German)

Buchthala M
[Clinical observations on the use of a new tranquilizing agent]
Hippokrates 1968 Jun 30;39(12):466-8 (Published in German)

Buckova A Grznar K Haladova M Eisenreichova E
[Active substances in Valeriana officinalis L.]
Cesk Farm 1977 Sep;26(7):308-9 (Published in Slovak)

Cavazzuti GB
[Study of the clinical pharmacology of an association of gamma-amino-beta-hy-droxybutyric acid and plant extracts used in therapy of children with behavior disorders and sleep disorders]
Clin Ter 1969 Oct;51(1):15-29 (Published in Italian)

Chen SD Xie XL Du BN Su QH Wei QD Wang YQ Li HL Wang ZG Wang YH Cheng SJ et al
Infantile rotavirus enteritis treated with herbal Valeriana jatamansi (VJ).
J Tradit Chin Med 1984 Dec;4(4):297-300

Chirstl G
[Therapy with Cor-Vel liquid in pre-digitalization]
Z Allgemeinmed 1973 Jul 10;49(19):938-9 (Published in German)

de Romanis F Di Tondo U Renda F Sopranzi N
[Superficial and deep EEG recordings of valerian-related drugs]
Clin Ter 1988 Jul 31;126(2):101-8 (Published in Italian)

Della Loggia R Tubaro A Redaelli C
[Evaluation of the activity on the mouse CNS of several plant extracts and a combination of them]
Riv Neurol 1981 Sep-Oct;51(5):297-310 (Published in Italian)

Drozdov DD
[Use of aminazine with valerian in hypertensive disease]
Vrach Delo 1975 Jan(1):48-50 (Published in Russian)

Dymchenko EI
[Therapeutic dose of valerian tincture]
Vrach Delo 1969 Jul;7:141-2 (Published in Russian)

Eickstedt KW von
[Modification of the alcohol effect by valepotriate]
Arzneimittelforschung 1969 Jun;19(6):995-7 (Published in German)

Faust V Hole G
[Disturbed sleep II.: Therapy of sleep disorders]
ZFA (Stuttgart) 1980 Dec 20;56(35-36):2437-59 (Published in German)

Hartwell J
Plants used against cancer. A survey.
Lloydia 1971 Sep;34(3):310-61

Hazelhoff B Malingre TM Meijer DK
Antispasmodic effects of valeriana compounds: an in-vivo and in-vitro study on the guinea-pig ileum.
Arch Int Pharmacodyn Ther 1982 Jun;257(2):274-87

Houghton PJ
The biological activity of Valerian and related plants.
J Ethnopharmacol 1988 Feb-Mar;22(2):121-42

Klich R
[Behavior disorders in childhood and their therapy]
Med Welt 1975 Jun 20;26(25):1251-4 (Published in German)

Kohnen R Oswald WD
The effects of valerian, propranolol, and their combination on activation, performance, and mood of healthy volunteers under social stress conditions.
Pharmacopsychiatry 1988 Nov;21(6):447-8

Kornievskii Iul Rybal'chenko AS Stebliuk MV
[Antimicrobial properties of essential oils of Valeriana stolonifera Czern., Valeriana nitida Kreyer, Valeriana exaltata Mikan]
Zh Mikrobiol Epidemiol Immunobiol 1970 Nov;47(11):137-9

Kruse R
[Nervobaldon—a phytosedative with scopolamine. Clinical trial and EEG studies in children]
Med Klin 1966 Feb 4;61(5):190-3 (Published in German)

Last G
[On the treatment of insomnia]
Hippokrates 1969 Jan 15;40(1):28-33 (Published in German)

Leathwood PD Chauffard F
Quantifying the effects of mild sedatives.
J Psychiatr Res 1982-83;17(2):115-22

Leathwood PD Chauffard F
Aqueous extract of valerian reduces latency to fall asleep in man.
Planta Med 1985 Apr(2):144-8

Leathwood PD Chauffard F Heck E Munoz-Box R
Aqueous extract of valerian root (Valeriana officinalis L.) improves sleep quality in man.
Pharmacol Biochem Behav 1982 Jul;17(1):65-71

Lindahl O Lindwall L
Double-blind study of a valerian preparation.
Pharmacol Biochem Behav 1989 Apr;32(4):1065-6

Mayer B Springer E
[Psychoexperimental studies on the effect of a valepotriate combination as well as the combined effects of valtratum and alcohol]
Arzneimittelforschung 1974 Dec;24(12):2066-70 (Published in German)

Mirnov VN
[Change of the blood coagulation process under the action of valerian]
Farmakol Toksikol 1966 Mar-Apr;29(2):187-8 (Published in Russian)

Molodozhnikova LM
[Medicinal valerian]
Feldsher Akush 1988 Jan;53(1):44-6 (Published in Russian)

Muller-Limmroth W Ehrenstein W
[Experimental studies of the effects of Seda-Kneipp on the sleep of sleep disturbed subjects; implications for the treatment of different sleep disturbances (author's transl)]
Med Klin 1977 Jun 24;72(25):1119-25 (Published in German)

Pang QF Wan XB Chen SD Xie XL
Treatment of rotavirus infection in tree shrews (Tupaia belangeri yunalis) with herbal Valeriana jatamansi (VJ).
J Tradit Chin Med 1984 Dec;4(4):301-6

Petkov V
Plants and hypotensive, antiatheromatous and coronarodilating action.
Am J Chin Med 1979 Autumn;7(3):197-236

Sakamoto T Mitani Y Nakajima K
Psychotropic effects of Japanese valerian root extract.
Chem Pharm Bull (Tokyo) 1992 Mar;40(3):758-61

Schneider K
[Contribution to the treatment of the "nervous school child" in general practice]
Hippokrates 1967 Oct 31;38(20):820 (Published in German)

Sobocky L Cernacek J Wagnerova M
[Effect of Valman (complex of 3 alkaloids from Valeriana root) on the vegetative tonus and excitability in vegetative dysfunction of neurotic origin]
Cesk Neurol 1971 Sep;34(5):240-4 (Published in Slovak)

Straube G
[The importance of valerian roots in therapy]
Ther Ggw 1968 Apr;107(4):555-62 (Published in German)

Thierolf H
[Contribution on the treatment of nervous manifestations]
Landarzt 1964 Sep 10;40(25):1086-7 (Published in German)

Tresser E
[Psychopharmacologic agents in ENT practice. Experiences with a new phyto-ataxic agent]
Hippokrates 1969 Apr 30;40(8):314-6 (Published in German)

Tucakov J
[Comparative ethnomedical study of Valeriana officinalis L.]
Glas Srp Akad Nauka [Med] 1965(18):131-50 (Published in Serbo-Croatian, Cyrillic)

Veith J Schneider G Lemmer B Willems M
[The effect of degradation products of valepotriates on the motor activity of light-dark synchronized mice]
Planta Med 1986 Jun(3):179-83 (Published in German)

Verzarne PG Pethes D Marczal G Lemberkovics E
[Parameters of active ingredients of tinctures with special reference to Chamomilla and Valeriana]
Acta Pharm Hung 1977 Nov;47(6):273-82 (Published in Hungarian)

Wagner H Jurcic K
[On the spasmolytic activity of valeriana extracts (author's transl)]
Planta Med 1979 Sep;37(1):84-6 (Published in German)

Wohlfart R
[Radix valerianae. History of an old medical drug, its active substances and their importance in the modern therapy]
Z Allgemeinmed 1974 Jun 20;50(17):797-800 (Published in German)

Zhang BH Meng HP Wang T Dai YC Shen J Tao C Wen SR Qi Z Ma L Yuan SH
[Effects of Valeriana officinalis L. extract on cardiovascular system]
Yao Hsueh Hsueh Pao 1982 May;17(5):382-4 (Published in Chinese)

Citations from the MEDLINE Database for the Genus *Vitex* (Chasteberry)

Amann W
Improvement of acne vulgaris with Agnus castus (AgnolytTM)
Ther. d. Gegenw.(1967) 106: 124-6

Attelmann H et al
Investigation of the treatment of female imbalances with Agnolyt.
Geriatrie (1972) 2: 239

Bhargava SK
Antiandrogenic effects of a flavonoid-rich fraction of Vitex negundo seeds: a histological and biochemical study in dogs.
J Ethnopharmacol (1989 Dec) 27(3):327-39

Brantner F
Sexual hormones from plants in female medicine.
Ehk. (1979) 28:413

Hahn G et al
Monk's pepper.
Notabene medici (1986) 16: 233-6, 297-301

Kayser HW Istanbulluoglu S
Treatment of PMS without hormones.
Hippokrates 25:717

Citations from the MEDLINE Database for the Genus *Zingiber* (Ginger)

Backon J
Ginger as an antiemetic: possible side effects due to its thromboxane synthetase activity.
Anaesthesia 1991 Aug;46(8):705-6

Backon J
Ginger in preventing nausea and vomiting of pregnancy; a caveat due to its thromboxane synthetase activity and effect on testosterone binding [letter; comment]
Eur J Obstet Gynecol Reprod Biol 1991 Nov 26;42(2):163-4

Backon J
Ginger: inhibition of thromboxane synthetase and stimulation of prostacyclin: relevance for medicine and psychiatry.
Med Hypotheses 1986 Jul;20(3):271-8

Bone ME Wilkinson DJ Young JR McNeil J Charlton S
Ginger root—a new antiemetic. The effect of ginger root on postoperative nausea and vomiting after major gynaecological surgery [see comments]
Anaesthesia 1990 Aug;45(8):669-71

Cai R Zhou A Gao H
[Study on correction of abnormal fetal position by applying ginger paste at zhihying acupoint A. Report of 133 cases]
Chen Tzu Yen Chiu 1990;15(2):89-91 (Published in Chinese)

Datta A Sukul NC
Antifilarial effect of Zingiber officinale on Dirofilaria immitis.
J Helminthol 1987 Sep;61(3):268-70

Fischer-Rasmussen W Kjaer SK Dahl C Asping U
Ginger treatment of hyperemesis gravidarum [see comments]
Eur J Obstet Gynecol Reprod Biol 1991 Jan 4;38(1):19-24

Gomita Y Uchikado A Moriyama M Ichimaru Y Kawasaki H Nonaka G Nishioka I
[Pharmacological study of Zingiber mioga Roscoe: effects on thiopental sleeping time and intracranial self-stimulation behavior (author's transl)]
Yakugaku Zasshi 1980 Apr;100(4):452-6 (Published in Japanese)

Grontved A Brask T Kambskard J Hentzer E
Ginger root against seasickness. A controlled trial on the open sea.
Acta Otolaryngol (Stockh) 1988 Jan-Feb;105(1-2):45-9

Grontved A Hentzer E
Vertigo-reducing effect of ginger root. A controlled clinical study.
ORL J Otorhinolaryngol Relat Spec 1986;48(5):282-6

Gugnani HC Ezenwanze EC
Antibacterial activity of extracts of ginger and African oil bean seed.
J Commun Dis 1985 Sep;17(3):233-6

Henry CJ Piggott SM
Effect of ginger on metabolic rate.
Hum Nutr Clin Nutr 1987 Jan;41(1):89-92

Holtmann S Clarke AH Scherer H Hohn M
The anti-motion sickness mechanism of ginger. A comparative study with placebo and dimenhydrinate.
Acta Otolaryngol (Stockh) 1989 Sep-Oct;108(3-4):168-74

Huang Q Matsuda H Sakai K Yamahara J Tamai Y
[The effect of ginger on serotonin induced hypothermia and diarrhea]
Yakugaku Zasshi 1990 Dec;110(12):936-42 (Published in Japanese)

Kanjanapothi D Soparat P Panthong A Tuntiwachwuttikul P Reutrakul V
A uterine relaxant compound from Zingiber cassumunar.
Planta Med 1987 Aug;53(4):329-32

Kawasaki H Gomita Y Fukamachi K Moriyama M Ichimaru Y Uchikado A Nonaka G Nishioka I
[Behavioral and EEG effects of Zingiber mioga Roscoe (water soluble fraction) (author's transl)]
Nippon Yakurigaku Zasshi 1979 Sep;75(6):601-15 (Published in Japanese)

Kiuchi F Shibuya M Sankawa U
Inhibitors of prostaglandin biosynthesis from ginger.
Chem Pharm Bull (Tokyo) 1982 Feb;30(2):754-7

Liu WH
Ginger root, a new antiemetic [letter; comment]
Anaesthesia 1990 Dec;45(12):1085

Mascolo N Jain R Jain SC Capasso F
Ethnopharmacologic investigation of ginger (Zingiber officinale).
J Ethnopharmacol 1989 Nov;27(1-2):129-40

Meng HQ
[Pharmacological effects of fresh ginger and dried ginger]
Chung Hsi I Chieh Ho Tsa Chih 1990 Oct;10(10):638-40 (Published in Chinese)

Mowrey DB Clayson DE
Motion sickness, ginger, and psychophysics.
Lancet 1982 Mar 20;1(8273):655-7

Mustafa T Srivastava KC
Ginger (Zingiber officinale) in migraine headache.
J Ethnopharmacol 1990 Jul;29(3):267-73

Nakamura H Yamamoto
T Mutagen and anti-mutagen in ginger, Zingiber officinale.
Mutat Res 1982 Feb;103(2):119-26

Ozaki Y Kawahara N Harada M
Anti-inflammatory effect of Zingiber cassumunar Roxb. and its active principles.
Chem Pharm Bull (Tokyo) 1991 Sep;39(9):2353-6

Qian DS Liu ZS
[Pharmacologic studies of antimotion sickness actions of ginger]
Chung Kuo Chung Hsi I Chieh Ho Tsa Chih 1992 Feb;12(2):95-8, 70 (Published in Chinese)

Shoji N Iwasa A Takemoto T Ishida Y Ohizumi Y
Cardiotonic principles of ginger (Zingiber officinale Roscoe).
J Pharm Sci 1982 Oct;71(10):1174-5

Srivastava KC
Effects of aqueous extracts of onion, garlic and ginger on platelet aggregation and metabolism of arachidonic acid in the blood vascular system: in vitro study.
Prostaglandins Leukot Med 1984 Feb;13(2):227-35

Srivastava KC
Aqueous extracts of onion, garlic & ginger inhibit platelet aggregation and alter arachidonic acid metabolism.
Biomed Biochim Acta 1984;43(8-9):S335-46

Srivastava KC
Effect of onion and ginger consumption on platelet thromboxane production in humans.
Prostaglandins Leukot Essent Fatty Acids 1989 Mar;35(3):183-5

Srivastava KC Mustafa T
Ginger (Zingiber officinale) and rheumatic disorders.
Med Hypotheses 1989 May;29(1):25-8

Stewart JJ Wood MJ Wood CD Mims ME
Effects of ginger on motion sickness susceptibility and gastric function.
Pharmacology 1991;42(2):111-20

Xiong HX
[Changes in multihormones in treating male sterility with acupuncture and indirect moxibustion using ginger slices on the skin]
Chung Hsi I Chieh Ho Tsa Chih 1986 Dec;6(12):726-7, 708 (Published in Chinese)

Yamahara J Huang QR Li YH Xu L Fujimura H
Gastrointestinal motility enhancing effect of ginger and its active constituents.
Chem Pharm Bull (Tokyo) 1990 Feb;38(2):430-1

Yamahara J Miki K Chisaka T Sawada T Fujimura H Tomimatsu T Nakano K Nohara T
Cholagogic effect of ginger and its active constituents.
J Ethnopharmacol 1985 May;13(2):217-25

The Crossing Press

publishes a full selection
of Health titles.
To receive our current catalog,
please call, toll-free,
800/777-1048.